GIS and Spatial Analysis in Veterinary Science

GIS and Spatial Analysis in Veterinary Science

Edited by

P.A. Durr
Veterinary Laboratories Agency
UK

and

A.C. Gatrell
Lancaster University
UK

CABI Publishing

CABI Publishing is a division of CAB International

CABI Publishing
CAB International
Wallingford
Oxfordshire OX10 8DE
UK

Tel: +44 (0)1491 832111
Fax: +44 (0)1491 833508
E-mail: cabi@cabi.org
Website: www.cabi-publishing.org

CABI Publishing
875 Massachusetts Avenue
7th Floor
Cambridge, MA 02139
USA

Tel: +1 617 395 4056
Fax: +1 617 354 6875
E-mail: cabi-nao@cabi.org

A catalogue record for this book is available from the British Library, London, UK.

Library of Congress Cataloging-in-Publication Data

GIS and spatial analysis in veterinary science / edited by P.A. Durr and A.C. Gatrell.
p. cm.
Includes bibliographical references (p.).
ISBN 0-85199-634-5 (alk. paper)
1. Veterinary epidemiology--Data processing. 2. Geographic information systems. 3. Spatial analysis (Statistics) I. Durr, P. A. (Peter A.) II. Gatrell, A. C. (Anthony C.)

SF780.9.G56 2004
636.089'44--dc22 2003017938

ISBN 0 85199 634 5

Typeset by Servis Filmsetting Ltd, Manchester
Printed and bound in the UK by Cromwell Press, Trowbridge

Contents

The colour plate section can be found following p. 118.

List of Contributors

Jan Biesemans, Avia-GIS, Risschotlei 33, 2980 Zoersel, Belgium (jan.biesemans@skynet.be)

Reginald de Deken, Institute for Tropical Medicine, Nationalestraat 101, B-2000 Antwerp, Belgium

Peter J. Diggle, Medical Statistics Unit, Department of Mathematics and Statistics, Lancaster University, Lancaster LA1 4YT, UK (p.diggle@lancaster.ac.uk)

Peter A. Durr, Department of Epidemiology, Veterinary Laboratories Agency, New Haw, Addlestone, Surrey KT14 3NB, UK (p.durr@vla.defra.gsi.gov.uk)

Nigel P. French, Division of Farm Animal Studies, University of Liverpool Veterinary Teaching Hospitals, Leahurst, Neston, South Wirral CH64 7TE, UK (n.p.french@liverpool.ac.uk)

Anthony C. Gatrell, Institute for Health Research, Lancaster University, Lancaster LA1 4YT, UK (a.gatrell@lancaster.ac.uk)

Guy Hendrickx, Avia-GIS, Risschotlei 33, 2980 Zoersel, Belgium (ghendrickx@pandora.be)

Giles Innocent, Comparative Epidemiology and Informatics, Department of Veterinary Clinical Studies, University of Glasgow

Veterinary School, Bearsden Road, Glasgow G61 1QH, UK (g.innocent@ vet.gla.ac.uk)

Joanna S. McKenzie, EpiCentre, Institute of Veterinary, Animal and Biomedical Sciences, Massey University, Palmerston North, New Zealand (j.s.mckenzie@massey.ac.nz)

Dominic Mellor, Department of Veterinary Clinical Studies, University of Glasgow Veterinary School, Bearsden Road, Glasgow G61 1QH, UK (d.mellor@vet.gla.ac.uk)

Dirk U. Pfeiffer, The Royal Veterinary College, University of London, Hawkshead Lane, North Mimms, Hatfield AL9 7TA, UK (pfeiffer@ rvc.ac.uk)

Stuart Reid, Comparative Epidemiology and Informatics, Universities of Glasgow and Strathclyde, Bearsden Road, Glasgow G61 1QH, UK (s.reid@vet.gla.ac.uk)

Robert L. Sanson, AgriQuality New Zealand, PO Box 585, Palmerston North, New Zealand (sansonr@agriquality.co.nz)

Christoph Staubach, Bundesforchunganstalt für Viruskrankheiten der Tiere, Seestrasse 55, 16868 Wusterhausen, Germany (Christoph.Staubach@Wus.BFAV.DE)

Nigel Tait, Department of Epidemiology, Veterinary Laboratories Agency, New Haw, Addlestone, Surrey KT14 3NB, UK (n.tait@vla.defra.gsi.gov.uk)

Piran C.L. White, The Environment Department, University of York, Heslington, York YO10 5DD, UK (pclw1@york.ac.uk)

Preface

This volume has its origins in a visit made by Peter Durr (Veterinary Laboratories Agency) to Tony Gatrell (Lancaster University) in 1999. Peter was aware of Tony's interests in applied spatial analysis, in particular the book he had co-authored with Trevor Bailey in 1995. He was interested in using some of the methods discussed in that book in a veterinary epidemiological context. Tony, in turn, had long-standing interests in the application of spatial analysis to epidemiological problems, though he had worked exclusively on human rather than on animal health. From these early discussions emerged the idea for a scientific meeting that would bring together the relatively small group of veterinary scientists interested in making use of spatial statistical ideas in their work, and others who recognized the value of spatial analysis and geographical information systems (GIS) in a veterinary context.

We therefore brought together a group of 75 people for a conference at Lancaster University in September 2001. This was the first of what we hope will be a series of 'GisVet' scientific meetings, designed to explore the applications of GIS and spatial analysis in veterinary science. Along with a special issue of *Preventive Veterinary Medicine* (2002, volume 56, issue 1), the edited collection that follows is one of the outputs from this scientific meeting. It includes revised and expanded versions of several of the papers delivered there, together with one additional invited contribution.

The book is divided into three parts. Part 1 sets the scene with two chapters that introduce basic concepts and principles and offer some illustrative examples of the relevance of GIS and spatial analysis in a veterinary context. The second part consists of two further chapters that set this work in a broader context, with reference to biomedical applications and those in a human public health context. The chapters in the final part of the book deal with applications in various domains, ranging from parasitic disease through to companion animals, wildlife disease, epidemic disease response and disease spread.

We have created a website that contains further information and resources relating to GIS and spatial analysis in animal health: www.gisvet.org. Readers are invited to explore this site.

We are grateful to a number of individuals for their help in promoting and organizing the first GisVet conference and for subsequent assistance in delivering this edited collection. First, generous financial support from the Chief Veterinary Officer for Great Britain and the Veterinary Laboratories Agency ensured the viability of the scientific meeting. Much hard work before and during the conference was undertaken by Alice Froggatt (formerly of the Veterinary Laboratories Agency), and we thank her for this. Duncan Whyatt (Department of Geography, Lancaster University) convened an introductory workshop on GIS as part of the conference, and is thanked for devising a very useful programme. Administration of the conference was undertaken with great efficiency and good humour by Teresa Wisniewska. We appreciate greatly the support and interest shown in an edited collection by Tim Hardwick of CABI Publishing. Lastly, we offer our sincere thanks to our authors, who kept to our deadlines for their contributions to the volume.

Although the conference was a successful venture, it was overshadowed by news of the terrorist attacks in the USA that filtered in on the morning of 11 September 2001. The true impact of these events became clear only after the conference had ended, but all who attended were deeply affected by the news.

Peter Durr
Tony Gatrell

The Tools of Spatial Epidemiology: GIS, Spatial Analysis and Remote Sensing

1

Peter A. Durr and Anthony C. Gatrell

1.1 Starting out: what is GIS?

Everyone encountering for the first time the term 'GIS' or 'geographical information system', whether at a presentation, in a book title or as a mention in a scientific article, will ask themselves: 'Exactly what *is* a GIS?' A superficial answer is that it has something to do with using computer software to produce maps; it seems to be an information system that turns spatial data into meaningful mapped output. Accordingly, it is comparable to any other data-handling tool, be it a spreadsheet, a database or a statistics package (Fig. 1.1). Nevertheless, while this definition of GIS as just another database may satisfy some, for many it does not quite convince. GIS seems somehow different: to promise more, to be about something bigger.

Why, then, should GIS be different? To a large part this is to do with the power of maps. In many countries, maps are things to be taken for granted, be they in the form of atlases, fold-up sheets or bound street guides. However, one only needs the experience of arriving in a strange city or country without a map to realize what an essential and powerful tool they are. Finding a stranger to point you in the right direction may help, but buying a map and sitting down to understand it can transform the situation. One goes from being lost and frustrated one minute to being able to make sense of one's surroundings the next. In this sense, maps are one of the key tools – like pens and paper and books – that underlie and make possible our civilization. It is little wonder that in preindustrial times mapmakers (cartographers) were highly valued professionals, and governments embarking on nation-building and/or

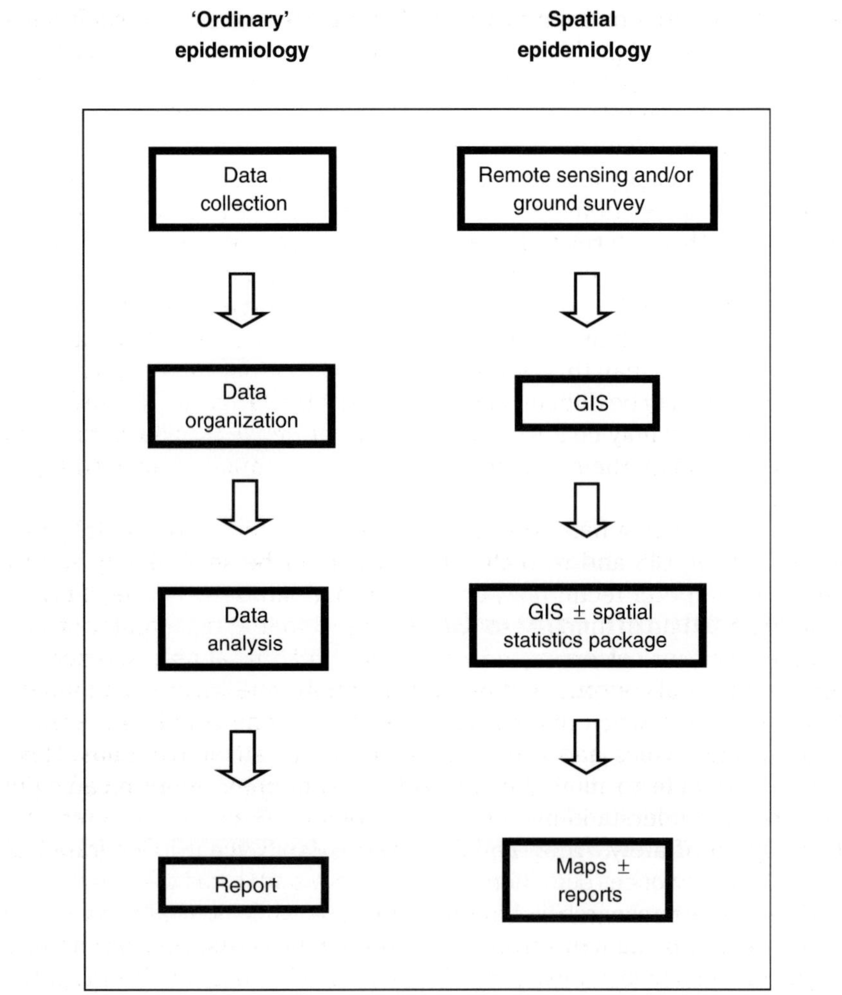

Fig. 1.1. GIS in relation to the usual epidemiological activities of data collation, data management, analysis and reporting.

imperialistic ventures saw the founding of a national mapping institute as an essential investment. One sees the relics of this in the naming of national mapping agencies, such as the Ordnance Survey of Great Britain.

With a GIS, therefore, we seem to be presented with the key to the magic of maps. Suddenly we are no longer dependent upon maps already published but can create our own. Even better, GIS software has now become so user-friendly that, once one has the data, producing a map can be undertaken literally in a matter of minutes. But therein lies one of the problems with GIS – one needs the spatial data, and collecting this may take months or even years. And there are many more such data-related issues and problems. For example, what exactly do we mean by 'location' for people and animals, which are constantly on the move? Should we define this simply as the place where they spend more time than anywhere else (for instance, the place or farm of residence), or should we be asking for more detail – where they were born, where they work, what proportion of the day they spend travelling? The more one delves into this and related questions, the more one realizes that 'location' and 'space' are complex and subtle concepts, and this leaves one wondering how a GIS can deliver anything meaningful. There are further issues that arise when one actually starts producing maps. For example, do we produce a map that purports to show farms as discrete point locations (which may be difficult at some scales if the farms are located close together – they may coalesce on the map), or do we transform the data so that we map their density (i.e. count the number of farms per hectare)?

We are starting here to understand some of the fundamental problems of using GIS and to realize that it cannot be seen simply as just another computer technology or just another database. Rather, it is intimately bound up in fundamental questions of spatial representation and spatial relations, of error and uncertainty, of the appropriateness of forms of (visual) output, and of interpretation. The nature of a modern GIS means that, when one starts out as a user, one could ignore these fundamental issues and produce colourful and attractive maps. However, to be able to move beyond this to something more meaningful requires an understanding of the bigger picture. This has been termed, quite appropriately, 'geographical information *science*'. Geographical information science (see Chapter 3) is a large and expanding discipline, with an active research community and specialist journals. As whole texts are now being written about its component parts, such as computing algorithms (see, for example, Worboys, 1995; Jones, 1997) and spatial uncertainty and indeterminacy (Burrough and Frank, 1996; Foody and Atkinson, 2002), not to mention public health applications (Gatrell and Löytönen, 1998; Cromley and McLafferty, 2002), it is increasingly difficult to summarize all aspects in a single chapter. This is especially so because GIS is only one of the software tools available to the epidemiologist interested in spatial issues, the other two being software environments that allow spatial statistical analyses (Robinson, 2000) and the processing of remote sensing imagery (Hay *et al.*, 2000; Messina and Crews-Meyer, 2000a,b).

Accordingly, what follows is an attempt to introduce some of the basic ideas of GIS, spatial analysis and remote sensing, using worked examples of real problems and real spatial data. To make things even more practical, we have chosen as examples material already published in the veterinary literature, which can be referred to for background concerning the actual scientific problem. Three examples will be discussed, which focus in turn on the component technologies of geographical information science: GIS proper, spatial data analysis and remote sensing. Before we introduce these examples, however, we give a brief historical overview of developments in GIS.

1.2 Historical overview

Many of the key texts and edited collections on GIS (see Chapter 11) describe the evolution of the systems or technology and (to a lesser extent) the science (for a recent overview see Longley *et al.*, 1999). At the risk of oversimplification (for a good overview see http://www.casa.ucl.ac.uk/gistimeline), we point to the key developments in automated cartography both in the UK and USA (notably at the Harvard Laboratory for Computer Graphics). Here, early line-printer-based systems (such as SYMAP) gave way to more sophisticated vector-based mapping packages, which in turn evolved into early GISystems (such as ODYSSEY, the forerunner of ARCINFO – perhaps the most well-known and widely used software product in this field). Other researchers, both in Britain and North America, had recognized the importance of early-generation computers in handling spatial data (from agricultural censuses and land-use inventories, for example) and had sown the seeds of early GISystems. Here, due prominence is given to the Canada Geographic Information System, 'widely acknowledged to be the first real GIS' (Longley *et al.*, 1999, p. 2). In all these early developments the importance of hardware developments (digitizers, plotters, graphics terminals and scanners) needs due recognition.

Paralleling these developments in both software and hardware were other concerns, such as the need for more sensitive environmental planning. Correspondingly, McHarg's (1969) notion of *map overlay*, whereby the world was conceived as a series of environmental 'layers' (each comprising one feature of the environment, such as natural vegetation, soil cover, and so on), provided some impetus for other developments. The digital representation of these data layers (as a series of cell-based coverages) led directly to raster-based systems (see below).

In the 1980s there emerged a number of proprietary systems running on workstations and minicomputers. Companies such as ESRI, Intergraph and LaserScan emerged as prominent vendors of such software systems. While the vendor scene continues to evolve, the contemporary software and hardware scene looks very different from how it appeared only 5 or 10 years ago. Here, the following developments are of note. First, desktop systems are in wide use on increasingly powerful PCs (many of which are portable and used in the field for both data collection and processing). Secondly, distributed systems have emerged, with greater interoperability of services; the Open GIS Consortium (http://www.opengis.org) plays a key role here. Thirdly, the availability of powerful software has spawned applications in all areas of the social and environmental sciences. Fourthly, and most significantly, the use of the World Wide Web (Thrall and Thrall, 1999) has transformed the use of GIS. Forer and Unwin (1999) trace this rapid change, emphasizing in particular the shift from a narrow technical focus towards GIS as an enabling technology. From an academic perspective, the transition to a concern with the basic science has been hugely significant (epitomized in the change of name of the premier journal from the *International Journal of Geographical Information Systems* to the *International Journal of Geographical Information Science*).

All these changes have seen the emergence of numerous texts and specialist journals to cater for both conceptual developments and areas of application. The number of courses, at both undergraduate and postgraduate level, has grown rapidly and has taken different forms. For example, the US National Center for Geographic Information and Analysis (NCGIA) devised a core curriculum that saw widespread take-up (http://www.ncgia.ucsb.edu/giscc), while both in North America and Europe several institutions have collaborated on courses offered as distance learning.

1.3 The gis(t) of GIS: an example from veterinary epidemiology

In 1970, Reif and Cohen published one of the first environmental epidemiological studies for companion animals. They were interested in the effect of living in cities on chronic pulmonary disease (CPD) in dogs, and were looking indirectly to test the hypothesis that urban air pollution may be a risk factor for the disease (Reif and Cohen, 1970). Their method was to select a sample of dogs from both urban and rural areas and to X-ray their lungs for evidence of the disease. They also constructed a simple map of atmospheric dust concentrations, which were ranked into four classes (Fig. 1.2).

Imagine a postgraduate student interested in the same question 30–35 years later. Her supervisor suggests that she should contact a random sample of veterinary practices in Philadelphia County and request they let her visit and examine some of their case X-rays of dogs with CPD. Having obtained such data, she might then hope to associate the incidence of CPD with appropriate measures of air pollution or, more simply, to test the hypothesis that the incidence of CPD is higher in the urban areas. Obtaining a list of practices is easily done by visiting online yellow pages (http://www.yellow.com), during which she notices that each listing links her to a small map (http://www.mapquest.com) showing the location of the practice within the city. She thinks that it

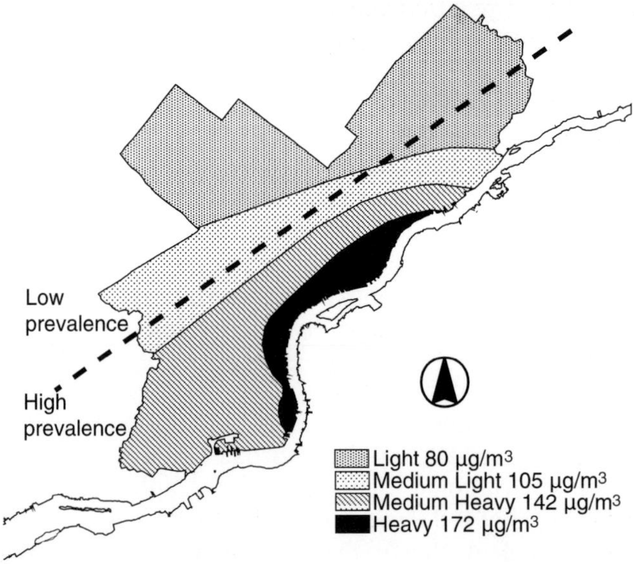

Fig. 1.2. Levels of atmospheric dust concentration in Philadelphia cited in the study by Reif and Cohen (1970) and the relative prevalence (high versus low) of chronic pulmonary disease in dogs aged 7–12 years. The dividing line between areas of high and low prevalence was equated with urban and rural land use. Redrawn from Reif and Cohen (1970).

would be good to combine these individual maps into a single one, to let her see at a glance how the veterinary practices are distributed in the city. Having produced the maps of the practices over the web in seconds, she imagines this will be a trivial task.

As the student will shortly find out, this is going to prove quite a difficult task, since what she has been accessing to obtain her location maps is in fact a sophisticated and functional GIS. This online GIS has been customized to produce, very efficiently, a base map of the streets, with a symbol locating the veterinary practice and a facility to zoom in and out and thereby show different levels of detail or scale. While it would have been very simple for the developers of the online street-map to provide a facility that maps a group of specially selected addresses, this would have been a specialist use, probably of limited interest to the vast majority of visitors to their site.

Feeling a bit frustrated, our researcher visits a student friend in the Geography Department and asks for some assistance. This friend has just completed an introductory course in GIS and is quite willing to help. He gives a demonstration of the software package he has on his PC, pointing out the essential components, such as the spreadsheet where the map's data are stored, and how this relates to features being dis-

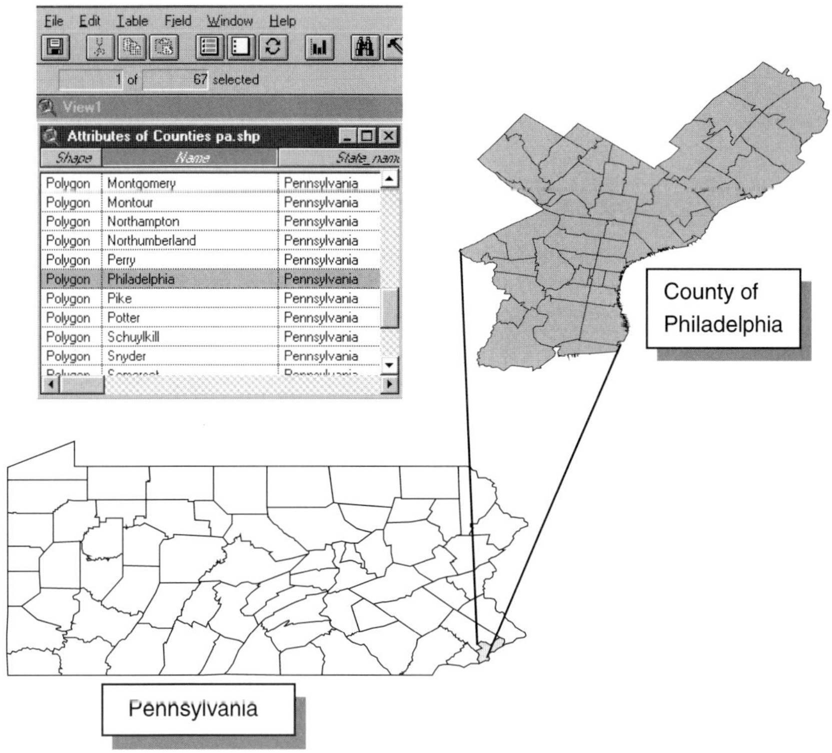

Fig. 1.3. The relationship between spatial (mapped) and attribute (spreadsheet) data in a GIS package, used in this example to extract the county of Philadelphia from the state of Pennsylvania.

played on the screen. The package he uses comes with digital maps of the larger cities of the USA, and although hc nccds to do some work to extract the county of Philadelphia from the rest of Pennsylvania, an attractive base-map is produced (Fig. 1.3). Here, there is a relationship between the spreadsheet, which stores the attribute data in a GIS, and a map based upon it. The spreadsheet consists of a row for each map feature (e.g. the counties of Pennsylvania) and a column for each attribute (e.g. the county's name or area). A true GIS, however, needs to contain additional files, i.e. those that store information about the spatial relations between the map features.

Our student's friend points out that there are, in essence, two different ways of producing a digital base-map, the simplest being to use a scanner to take an image of an existing paper map. While such raster or pixellated base-maps are quick and efficient to produce, they are not ideal, as each pixel in the map is autonomous with respect to its neighbours (Fig. 1.4b). Thus, a road will be displayed as a series of dark pixels on a light background, which, except at all but the highest resolution (i.e. with a very small pixel area), will generally display with a fuzzy edge. The alternative is a vector base-map in which the map features themselves (roads, buildings, lakes etc.) are treated as the fundamental units (Fig. 1.4a). In order to produce vector base-maps, the features had, at some stage, to be electronically traced (i.e. digitized) from a paper map, an activity that requires training and considerable skill, particularly for complex features. Accordingly, vector base-maps are costly to produce and, depending upon the size of the GIS market, can be very expensive to purchase.

Having extracted a vector street-map of Philadelphia, our student's next task is to add the veterinary practices, a task she thinks should be easy. However, her friend explains that this is a bit harder, as what will be needed to map them is their locational co-ordinates – their latitude and longitude. He explains that what the Internet street mapping sites do is to search a database that links street addresses to approximate latitudes and longitudes, and this requires an expensive 'geocoding' extension to his GIS package. He shows how geocoding works using the postal codes (zip codes) of the veterinary practices obtained from the online yellow pages, but these only put each practice in its approximately correct location, and quite a few end up on the same point, the zip-code 'centroid'. To overcome this, he initially suggests a visit to each practice to determine the exact co-ordinates by the use of a hand-held global positioning system device (GPS). However, the student is understandably reluctant to do this, as there are over 60 practices, so her friend comes up with a more practical solution using the Zip+4 codes, which can de downloaded over the Internet. These cover a smaller area than the normal zip codes and, accordingly, their centroids will be a lot closer to their true locations.

As we suggested earlier, locating features of interest (georeferencing) is a key data requirement for effective GIS, but is always bound up with various degrees of approximation and error. Of course, in reality veterinary practices are buildings that occupy an area on the ground; however, they are sufficiently small in relation to the city for us sensibly to approximate them to a single point. Indeed, at this scale of resolution, producing vector outlines of the buildings (which in theory could be easily done using areal photographs) would be a waste of time and effort. However, in this example we are using Zip+4 codes, which do have locational error, and this results in some practices not being located exactly on the correct roads. Is this important and should an effort be made to get the locations more geographically correct? The answer depends on the question being asked, or the hypothesis one wishes to test. If one were doing a study examining the association between the incidence of canine pulmonary disease and whether the dog lived in a home located directly on a main road, such locational error

(a)

(b)

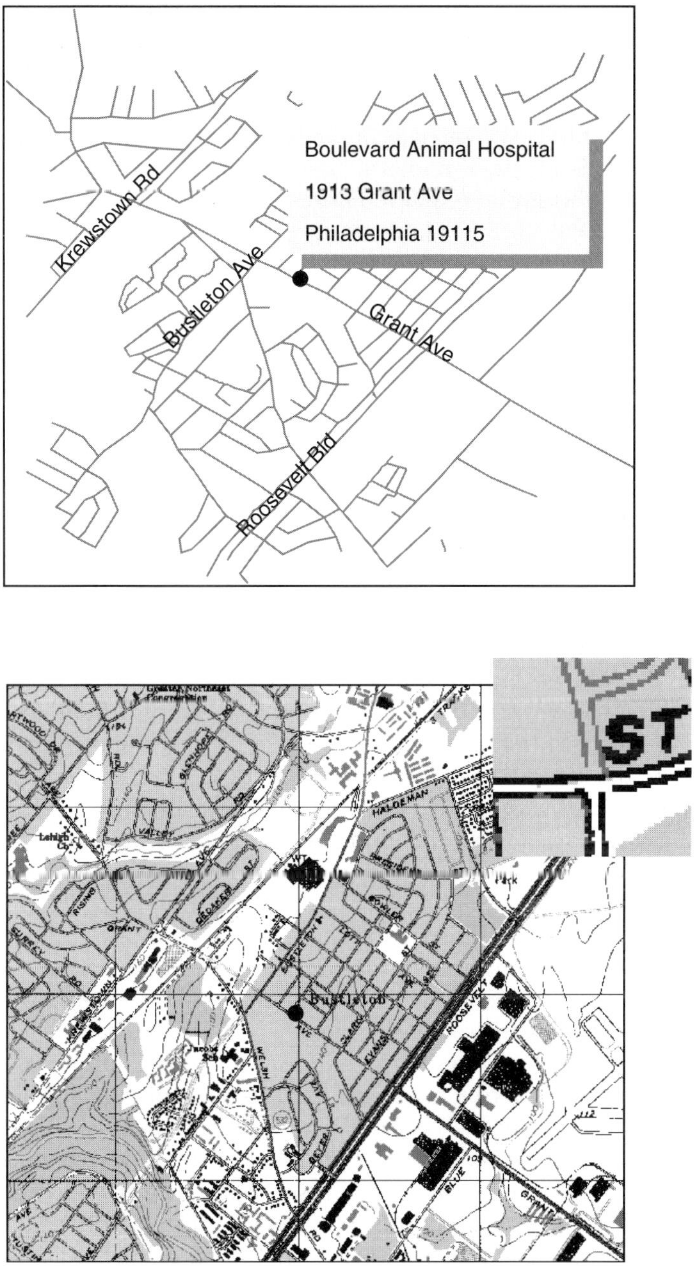

Fig. 1.4. Comparison between a vector map (a) and a raster map (b) of an approximately similar area within Philadelphia, showing the location of a single veterinary practice. The vector map is better for visualizing the veterinary practices as it lacks the clutter of the raster map. Raster map data obtained from the US Geological Survey, EROS Data Center, Sioux Falls, South Dakota.

may well be unacceptable. This demonstrates an important principle of GIS data collection: that issues of error and uncertainty are closely bound up with both the geographical scale of the study and the nature of the intended analysis.

In our example, the same person is undertaking both the spatial data collection and the data analysis, so she can make her own decisions about what is acceptable error. However, she or her supervisor might make her spatial data available to a geographer who is examining the spatial distribution of veterinary practices in Philadelphia in relation to the time taken by clients to travel to the practices. Not unreasonably, he may assume that the locational coordinates of the practices are very accurate, and may thus proceed to undertake a network analysis without first checking the data. This may lead to a flawed analysis.

Returning to the hypothetical example in Philadelphia, our student discusses with her supervisor the best way to select a set of practices in order to test a hypothesis concerning the relationship between disease and pollution. A simple method would be to take a random sample of, say, between 10 and 15 practices, but since the study aims to test the hypothesis of differences between urban and rural dogs suffering from chronic pulmonary disease, this is not entirely satisfactory. They therefore agree that it might be better to obtain an equal number of practices in both groups. They reason that, because a majority of clients visit nearby practices, a rural practice is more likely to have dogs that live in rural areas, and vice versa. They appreciate that some practices will have a mix of urban and rural clients, but agree that, for the purposes of their study, this will be acceptable error.

The problem now is how to classify each veterinary practice as predominately rural or urban. By now the student has obtained a copy of a GIS package and notices that it includes a CD containing demographic data from the 1999 US Census. These data are at quite a high spatial resolution, the average 'census tract' having an area of 0.39 square miles. After some searching on the US Census website (http://www.census.gov), she finds that the standard definition used for 'rural' is a population density of fewer than 1000 people per square mile. She uses this classification to produce a shaded map of the county of Philadelphia, with each tract classified as 'rural' or 'urban' (Fig. 1.5a). However, she notices that it does not correspond to her own intuitive sense of the county, especially as the map does not show an important feature – the substantial suburban areas. As the division between rural and urban is so important for the intended work, she decides to visit the library to find out more about classifying land use. She quickly discovers that this is a very contentious subject, and that most of the books and articles on the subject disagree about where the class divisions should be drawn. She notes down several of these schemes and plots these using the GIS. Figure 1.5b is just one example that incorporates a 'suburban' class of

(a)

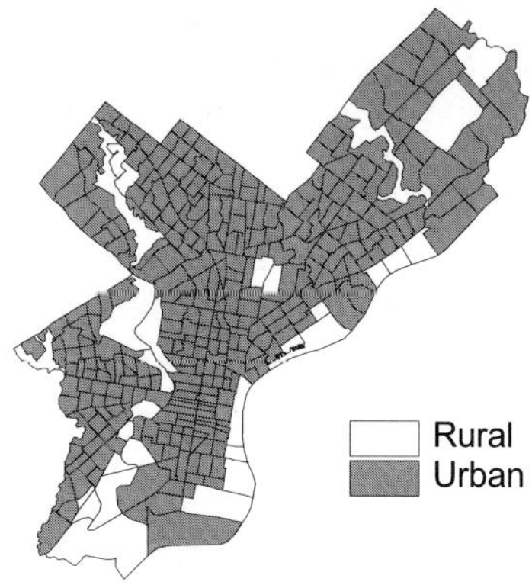

(b)

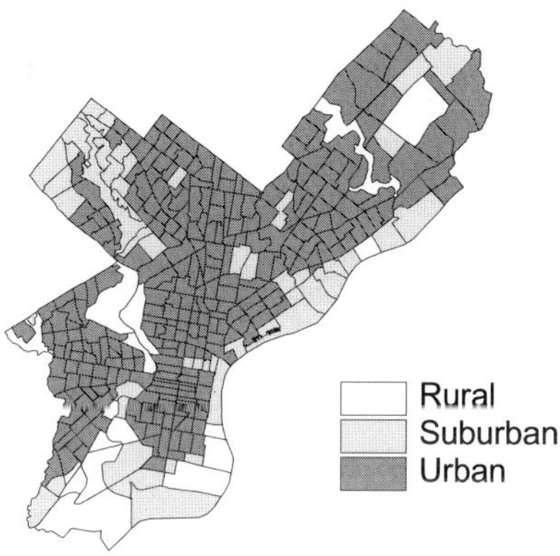

(c)

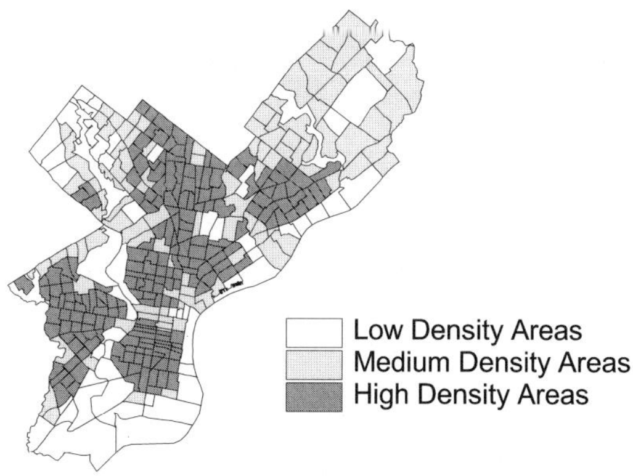

Fig. 1.5. Alternative ways to classify Philadelphia's 1999 census tracts according to their population density using (a) the US Bureau of Census' threshold of 1000 persons per square mile, (b) incorporating a suburban class defined as low-to-medium density residential with a population density of between 130 and 5180 persons per square mile and (c) a simple GIS-calculated classification into three areas of equal population density.

low to medium residential density. However, she now starts to feel uneasy because, while all the maps have some features in common, they all look rather different. After further thought and discussion, she decides that the best thing to do is simply to divide the county into three equal-area classes of high, medium and low population density (Fig. 1.5c). After all, she reasons, this classification is a true description of the data and has none of the connotations of the terms ‘urban’, ‘suburban’ and ‘rural’.

The problem encountered in classifying spatial data attributes and their visual display is one commonly encountered by all GIS users. The essence of the power of maps to convey complex information is the human brain’s highly developed capacity for pattern recognition and for imposing meaning on these patterns on the basis of previous experience. For example, anyone viewing the first map of the county would have their eye drawn to the two irregular belts of ‘rural’ low population density in the west and east of the county. A reasonable hypothesis, based upon experience of viewing maps of urbanized areas in other locations of the world, is that these correspond to rivers, where the low density of housing reflects a combination of conservation and avoidance of flooding. However, the western river area is not as obvious in the second map when the suburban class is added. If this map alone had been drawn, we would probably have missed learning something about the county. In our example, this does not matter as we are not fundamentally interested in the geography of Philadelphia. But by extension one can see that if this were a disease map, failure to recognize higher incidence of disease alongside a river might lead to something important being missed. In the days before computerized cartography and GIS, a large part of the art of map design was given over to how best to display the data to enable the user to see patterns and relationships. This is a tacit skill that very few GIS users learn, or even appreciate, and so many GIS-generated maps that find their way into the literature often do more to deceive their users than to help them understand the data (MacEachren, 1995; Monmonier, 1996).

Our student finally now has all the data necessary to complete her task, and randomly selects two or three veterinary practices in each of the three population densities of the county (Fig. 1.6). In arriving at this map, she has learnt quite a lot about GIS and spatial data. In particular, she has been impressed by the power of a GIS to undertake a meaningful display of spatial data, once these are assembled. But, as she discovered in trying to locate the veterinary practices on a map, collating the data can be a tedious and time-consuming process. In addition, she has learnt that even when spatial data are available, as with census tract population density, there is frequently no unambiguous way to classify and/or interpret it. Probably most importantly, she has learnt quite a bit about her research subject. For example, she suspects that Reif and

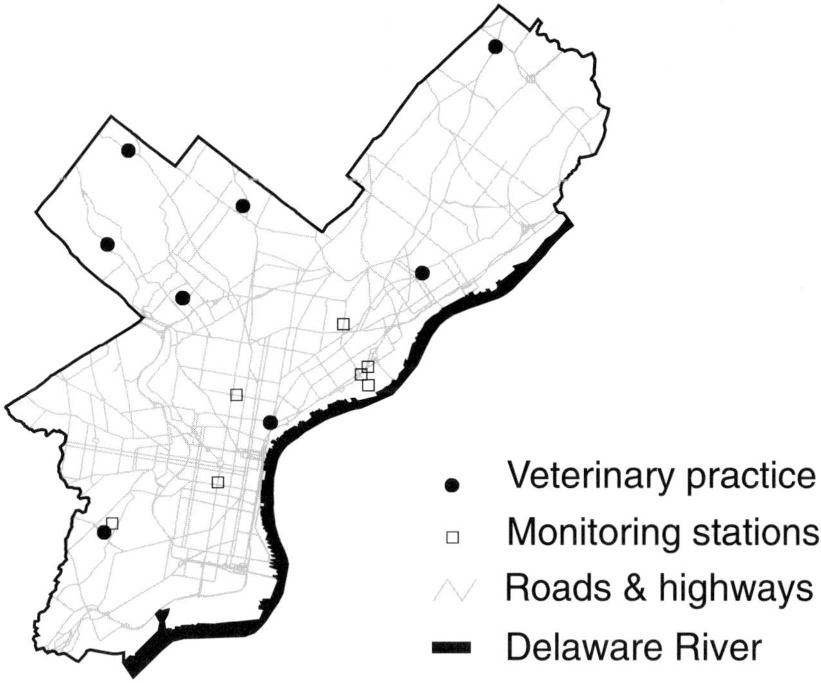

Fig. 1.6. A subset of veterinary practices in the county of Philadelphia, selected by their location within the areas of the population density classes of Fig. 1.5c. Locations where air pollution levels are currently measured in the city are also shown.

Cohen greatly simplified their dividing lines between 'urban' and 'suburban' in their publication (Fig. 1.2). In addition, she thinks that dividing the county by population density may not be the best way to test the hypothesis, since if cars are the major cause of particulate pollution, traffic loads or even street density might be a better measure of risk. However, she appreciates that she must complete her thesis, and now is the time to go and examine the X-rays in the veterinary practices. She will examine a random sample of X-rays from veterinary records and, using appropriate statistical techniques, will compare the proportions of dogs with and without CPD in each of the three groups, after adjustment for possible confounding factors.

1.4 Spatial analysis: autocorrelation, interpolation and spatial regression

In the last section we showed how a GIS could help develop an appropriate sampling strategy for a relatively simple epidemiological study relating chronic pulmonary disease in dogs to possible levels of air pollution in Philadelphia. However, air pollution was not considered in a direct way. What data and methods might be available to allow us to characterize this better?

Suppose air quality data are collected at only a small number of monitoring stations throughout the city (Fig. 1.6). Immediately, we see that there will be a problem in assigning levels of pollutants to the veterinary practices in our sample. For example, while it is reasonable to assign the measured value of a pollutant to a practice when it is located close to a recording station, what value should be assigned when the practice is located between two stations that have recorded widely different values? Intuitively, the practice should be assigned a value that is intermediate between those of the two sampling stations. This problem of interpolating values between sampling points is a common one in spatial statistics – that branch of statistics concerned with spatial data such as these. Before we consider a possible solution to the interpolation problem we need to consider some other issues concerned with spatial statistical analysis.

In order to do so, consider another veterinary epidemiology example, taken from the state of Victoria, Australia. In this state, fasciolosis (caused by the liver fluke *Fasciola hepatica*) is an important disease in both cattle and sheep. In 1977 a detailed abattoir study was undertaken in Melbourne in which the *Fasciola* status of over 25,000 cattle was recorded (G.E.L. Watt (1977) An abattoir survey of the prevalence of *Fasciola hepatica* affected livers in cattle in Victoria. Unpublished MSc thesis, University of Melbourne, Melbourne, Australia; Watt, 1980). Evidence of fasciolosis severe enough to entail condemnation of the liver for human consumption was found in 42% of animals. An important feature of this study was that the investigator was able to identify, by a system of tail tags, the local administrative division (shire) from which about 85% of animals originated. Accordingly, he could produce a shaded choropleth map showing where in Victoria serious liver fluke in cattle was most prevalent (Fig. 1.7). The author went on to explain the distribution of the high-prevalence areas, especially in the north-east part of the state, in terms of environmental risk factors, such as rainfall and irrigation.

Looking at his map, there are two obvious patterns. First, over the whole state there is a distinct trend, with all the high prevalence areas in the north and east of the state, while to the west and the south the prevalence is much lower. Secondly, within both the high and low prev-

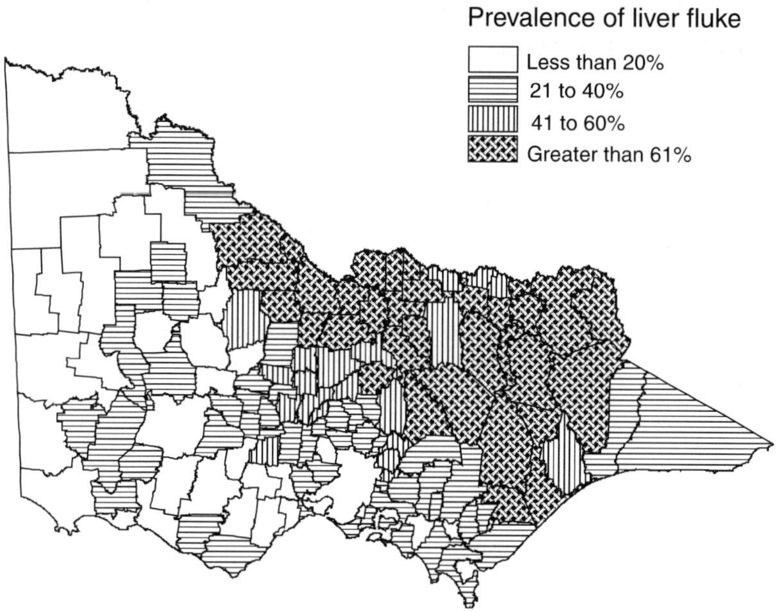

Fig. 1.7. Percentage of bovine livers seriously affected by fluke (*Fasciola hepatica*) by shire of origin, as determined by a survey at a Melbourne abattoir in 1977. Redrawn from Watt (1977).

alence areas, the recorded value for each shire tends to be similar to those of its immediate neighbours. The tendency for nearby spatial units to record similar values is very common, and is termed *spatial autocorrelation*.

The fact that spatial autocorrelation is so common has led to a number of statistical techniques to measure it. For the liver fluke data set, where the spatial unit is an area or polygon, an appropriate measure is Moran's *I* coefficient, which is essentially a modification of the ordinary (Pearson) correlation coefficient but with an added term which measures spatial proximity between areas (Bailey and Gatrell, 1995). However, we need to define what is meant by 'proximity'. One common definition is that the areal units must have a common boundary (i.e. they are contiguous). Alternatively, if the distance between the centres (centroids) of pairs of zones is measured, proximity can be defined in terms of a threshold distance. Neighbourhood relationships can be visualized by forming a network in which the centroid of the area is identified as a point and a line indicates neighbours (Cliff and Haggett, 1988). In the case of the shires of Victoria, these two definitions result in different networks of connectedness. An advantage of the distance-based measure is that there are no 'islands', but a disadvantage is that in some regions, such as that around the city of Melbourne, with its many small suburban

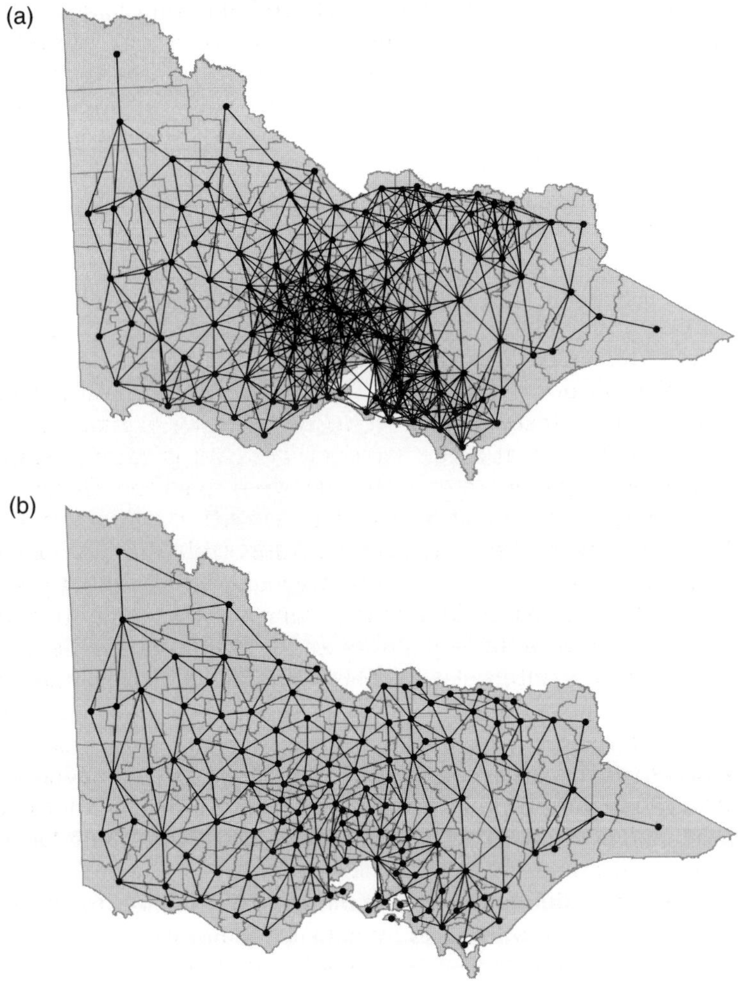

Fig. 1.8. Neighbourhood lattices of the shires of Victoria as defined by (a) a common border and (b) having a centroid within 43.2 km, the mean intercentroid distance over the whole state.

shires, there is a complex matrix (Fig. 1.8a and b). Regardless of which definition of proximity is used, the result is that there is a significant level of positive spatial autocorrelation, as measured by the Moran statistic.

Although testing for autocorrelation is an important exploratory step in spatial analysis, there are some important caveats to consider in the interpretation of significant and non-significant results. First, autocorrelation tends to be overestimated in the presence of a strong spatial trend. This is a common problem in spatial analysis, in that many statistics measuring spatial association rest on the assumption that there is an absence of a trend, an assumption referred to in the statistical literature as 'stationarity'. One of the simplest ways to overcome this is to 'detrend' the variable by undertaking multiple regression analysis with latitude and longitude (and various polynomial transformations of them) as the independent variables, and then testing for autocorrelation among the residuals. In the case of our data set, the spatial autocorrelation is reduced but is still highly significant after the data have been detrended in this way. The second caveat about the use of statistics such as Moran's *I* is that they are global, in that they test for spatial structure over the entire data set. The situation can arise in which there are pockets of autocorrelation ('hotspots') that are masked by an overall absence, as shown by the whole-map Moran statistic. This is obviously not a problem in our data set, but, should autocorrelation not occur when it is expected, tests for local autocorrelation are recommended. An example of such a local autocorrelation statistic is the G_I^* statistic, which can be implemented in the SPACESTAT package (http://www.spacestat.com). Autocorrelation is discussed further in Chapter 3.

Although, as we will see later, spatial autocorrelation is problematic for statistical modelling, it is also advantageous as it makes it possible to estimate data values for locations (either areas or point locations), provided the values of its neighbours are known. This can be demonstrated by using it to interpolate climate values from weather stations to provide us with mean estimates for each shire. In this instance, we are not simply interested in working out if there is significant spatial autocorrelation over the whole data set but in defining how it operates at a local level. For example, does the degree of spatial dependence extend to a large distance beyond the recording stations, or does it fall away quickly beyond a few kilometres? An important tool for defining local spatial autocorrelation is the *variogram*, in which the 'semivariance' in the values between measuring points is computed. Semivariance ('gamma') is the converse of autocorrelation, in that it is low in the presence of local spatial effects and increases to a maximum where there is no longer any spatial dependence.

Victoria has an extensive network of weather stations, over 100 of which record both temperature and precipitation. Variogram plots of the mean annual temperature and the total annual rainfall from these stations over the period 1972–1977 show strong spatial autocorrelation, in both cases gradually reducing to insignificance at a distance of about 200–300 km (Fig. 1.9a). Rainfall has a much higher variability than temperature, even allowing for the difference in units, and this justifies the fact that most countries have a much more extensive network for recording rainfall than for other climate variables. In order to make use of the variogram for spatial interpolation, the common practice is to model it using a mathematical function and thereby derive parameters that can be used in the interpolation. These parameters are referred to in the

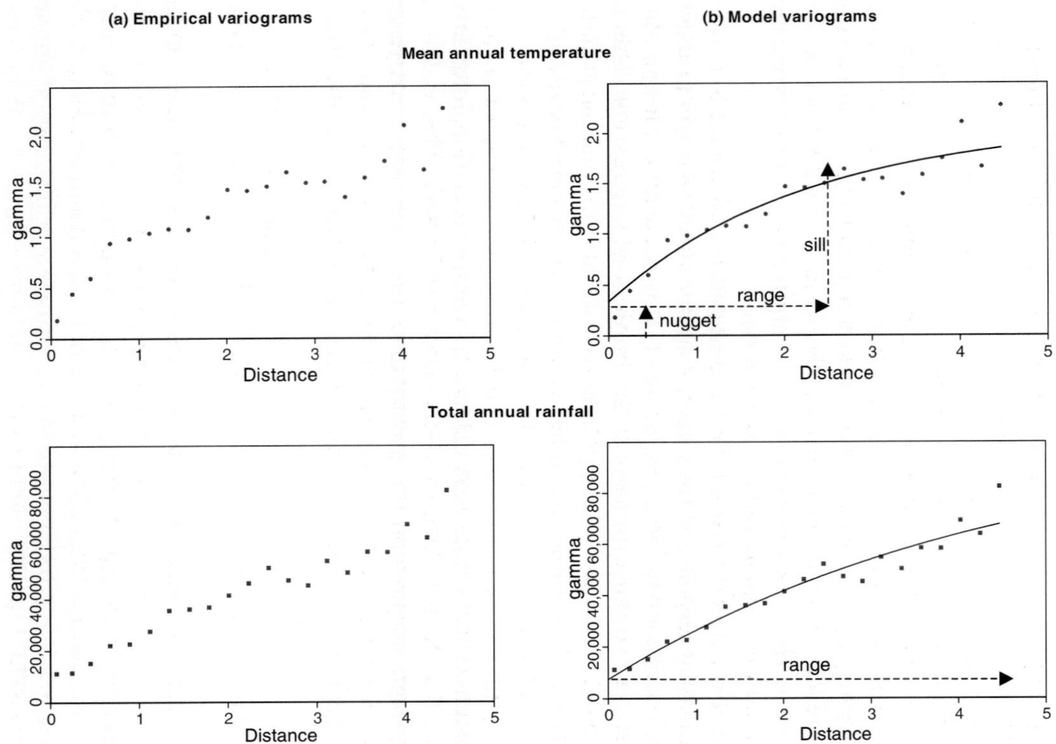

Fig. 1.9. Empirical (a) and exponential model (b) variograms for mean annual temperature and total annual rainfall for 124 recording stations in Victoria, Australia 1974–1977. Note that distance units are in degrees of latitude and longitude, which equate to 89 km over the study area. Data supplied by the Australian Bureau of Meteorology.

geostatistical literature as the 'range' (the distance over which spatial dependence operates), the 'nugget' (the semivariance at zero distance and a measure of small-scale variability and sampling errors) and the 'sill' (the maximum semivariance minus any nugget effect). In the case of our data set, an exponential function is effective in modelling the empirical variogram (Fig. 1.9b).

Variograms are generally associated with a geostatistical interpolation technique known as *kriging* (see Chapter 4 in Bailey and Gatrell, 1995). This can be viewed as a modification of inverse distance weighting, one of the simplest interpolation techniques, in which the weighting given to the value of a neighbouring measured point is determined by the inverse of the distance separating it from the point to be estimated. In ordinary kriging, the weightings of these neighbouring measurements are, in essence, derived from the modelled values of semivariance. If a trend exists in the data, the calculations are adjusted using an extension of the technique, termed 'universal kriging'.

While it is perfectly feasible for us to use universal kriging to undertake a climate interpolation for Victoria for our study years, in practice this would not be advisable. First, we do not have data for the neighbouring states, and so our estimates at the borders will be too low. This is because most packages for interpolation will misinterpret missing values at the edges as being zero. Secondly, climate variables are heavily influenced not just by neighbouring values but also by altitude, and so we will require digital elevation data and considerably more complex calculations. Fortunately, there already exists a moderate-resolution, long-term interpolated data set (http://www.bom.gov.au/climate). This is based upon a period longer than the study (1961–1990) and uses a different method of interpolation (thin-plate smoothing splines; Hutchinson, 1995) but it is unlikely to differ from one estimated specifically for the study years (Colour Plate 1).

Now that we have interpolated values of total annual rainfall, we are in a position to test the hypothesis of an association between precipitation and the proportion of livers found to be seriously affected with fasciolosis. This is an example of spatial correlation, which differs from spatial autocorrelation in that it involves two variables. When one of these variables is thought to be causative, it is more correct to refer to the procedure as spatial regression. Spatial regression can be considered in essence as akin to normal linear regression with added terms to allow for possible spatial autocorrelation.

The scatterplot of the percentage of condemned livers for each shire against total annual rainfall shows a poor overall relationship (Fig. 1.10). However, when we examine the scatterplot carefully we notice a cluster of shires having a much higher than expected prevalence, given their low rainfall. To understand more fully why this might be the case, we need a modern GIS package that enables us to select points of interest

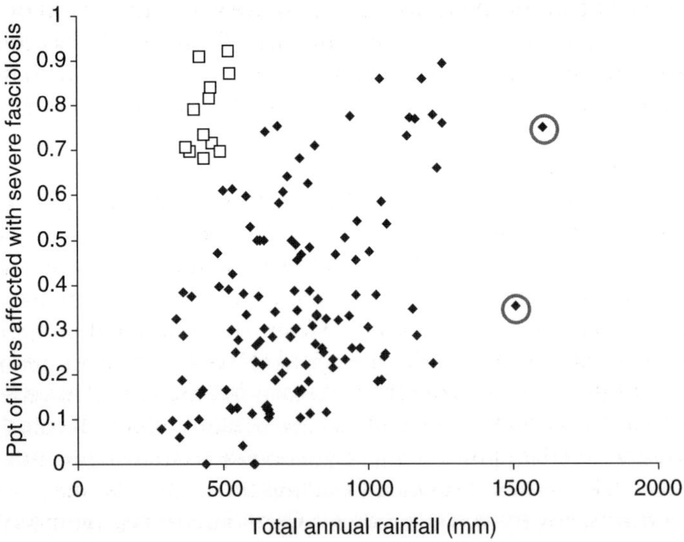

Fig. 1.10. Scatterplot of total annual rainfall versus percentage of livers found to be seriously affected with liver fluke in the abattoir survey of Watt (1977). The cluster of values to the top left corresponds to the irrigated areas marked on Colour Plate 1. The two outliers (circled) did not have any obvious explanation and may be a result of data errors.

on a graph (here, a scatterplot) and to visualize them simultaneously on a map. This way it becomes easier to give spatial meaning to clusters and outliers. In the case of the scatterplot of the condemned livers, when we mark on the screen the cluster at the top left corner of the plot (Fig. 1.10), we notice on the map that these shires are spatially clustered, along the Murray River in the north of the state (highlighted in Colour Plate 1). Finding such a marked spatial cluster is generally indicative of an additional variable needed to understand the disease distribution. This turns out to be the case, since all these shires use supplementary irrigation, something which would be likely to increase the population of the snail intermediate host (Colour Plate 1). In our interactive software environment (where we scan the scatterplot and map together) we also notice some outliers, but in this case there is no corresponding spatial clustering, and the outliers probably represent random variability or possibly measurement or recording error.

Following on from this exploratory analysis of the data, we are now ready to try to build a parsimonious model, one that explains variation in disease incidence using a minimum number of variables. In this case we have decided upon two possible explanatory variables – total annual rainfall and the presence or absence of irrigation. We might also like to consider temperature, as an extensive series of field studies in south-eastern Australia in the 1960s found that there was a threshold of development at 10°C for the snail intermediate host (Boray, 1969). Accordingly, we may hypothesize that the mountainous areas of Victoria, with its high precipitation, might not necessarily be fluke country on account of the extended period when the mean temperature is less than the threshold.

Proceeding with the model-building in an interactive way in which terms are added and removed, and their effect on the fit tested at each step, we arrive at a final model in which only total annual precipitation and the irrigation terms are statistically significant. This fully satisfies our requirement for a parsimonious model and, as judged by the R^2 value, accounts for 37% of the variance. The indication that temperature had little effect is of some epidemiological interest. However, before we conclude that the disease is determined only by humidity it is necessary to stress that this is really only true for the scale at which the study was done. If we reduce the spatial scale, for example to that of the individual farm, other risk factors, especially management factors, may become more important. For example, cattle on dairy farms may be more likely to receive preventative treatment compared with beef animals.

Having established a useful model, we would next like to use it for prediction. However, there is a problem with the parameters we have derived from it in that they have ignored the spatial autocorrelation we detected earlier through the use of Moran's *I* statistic. This is particularly problematic because the validity of regression modelling is critically dependent upon a number of assumptions, one of which is the independence of the sampling units. To adjust for the lack of independence in our data, we therefore rerun the modelling exercise, but this time we include a spatial autoregressive term; this means that we allow for the fact that values of the dependent variable in nearby zones can influence that of the zone whose value is being predicted. The result of doing this does not change the two variables that we have selected for our parsimonious model, but does alter the parameter estimates and their standard errors.

The statistically astute may have detected a fundamental problem with the approach we have adopted, in that we have applied models formulated for continuous response variables to data that are essentially proportions. This is a valid criticism, and thus our model is misspecified. Nevertheless, there is a good reason for adopting a simple approach, since attempts to model spatial structure for presence/absence, count or proportional data become very complex. In fact, only recently have software routines become available for such analysis, and these are only just entering mainstream spatial statistical analysis (Lawson *et al.*, 2003).

1.5 Setting the scene: remote sensing and image analysis

In the previous section we showed that there was a broad association between severe liver fluke in cattle and total annual rainfall. While it was not possible to explain the inconsistencies for the entirety of the study area (for one part, along the Murray River in the north), the higher than expected prevalence of disease was identified as possibly resulting from irrigation. This area was sketched in a hand-drawn map in Watt's thesis (G.E.L. Watt (1977) An abattoir survey of the prevalence of *Fasciola hepatica* affected livers in cattle in Victoria. Unpublished MSc thesis, University of Melbourne), but to help us delineate it more exactly we might have attempted to obtain a data set on water use in the state. Nevertheless, this is not a data set in the public domain, and would probably take considerable effort to obtain. An alternative representation would be an indirect measure of where irrigation is used. For example, one might suspect that since irrigation is used in areas of low rainfall such zones would be greener than the surrounding ones. If greenness could be detected over the whole state, all we would need to do would be to separate greenness resulting from rainfall from that resulting from irrigation. This might be achievable by measuring greenness in the dry season (Colour Plate 2) and comparing it with greenness in the wet season. The need to obtain information about the earth's surface systematically over areas and to be able to compare results between points in time is essentially the motivation for the use of remote sensing in a host of environmental and epidemiological studies (for reviews, see Hay *et al.*, 2000; Messina and Crews-Meyer, 2000a,b).

Although remote sensing is now firmly associated with satellites, all the concepts and the technology were largely refined a long time before satellites came into use for this purpose, through the use of radiation sensors (or radiometers) carried upon aircraft. When satellite technology was developed in the 1960s, radiometers of a similar type were mounted on the satellites. Some of the greatest technical hurdles in the early years of remote sensing were not in the design of the radiometers, but rather in developing systems for processing the immense amounts of data generated by the sensing, both for storage on board and for transmission back to the earth.

While there are now a large number of earth observation satellites, very few have found any application in epidemiology. By far the most important have been the Landsat and the NOAA (National Oceanic and Atmospheric Administration, USA) series, both of which orbit the earth between 700 and 900 km above its surface and circumnavigate the poles (Colour Plate 3). A comparison of these two satellites demonstrates the trade-offs that occur with satellite imagery in terms of spatial and temporal resolution (Fig. 1.11). The radiometers on board the Landsat

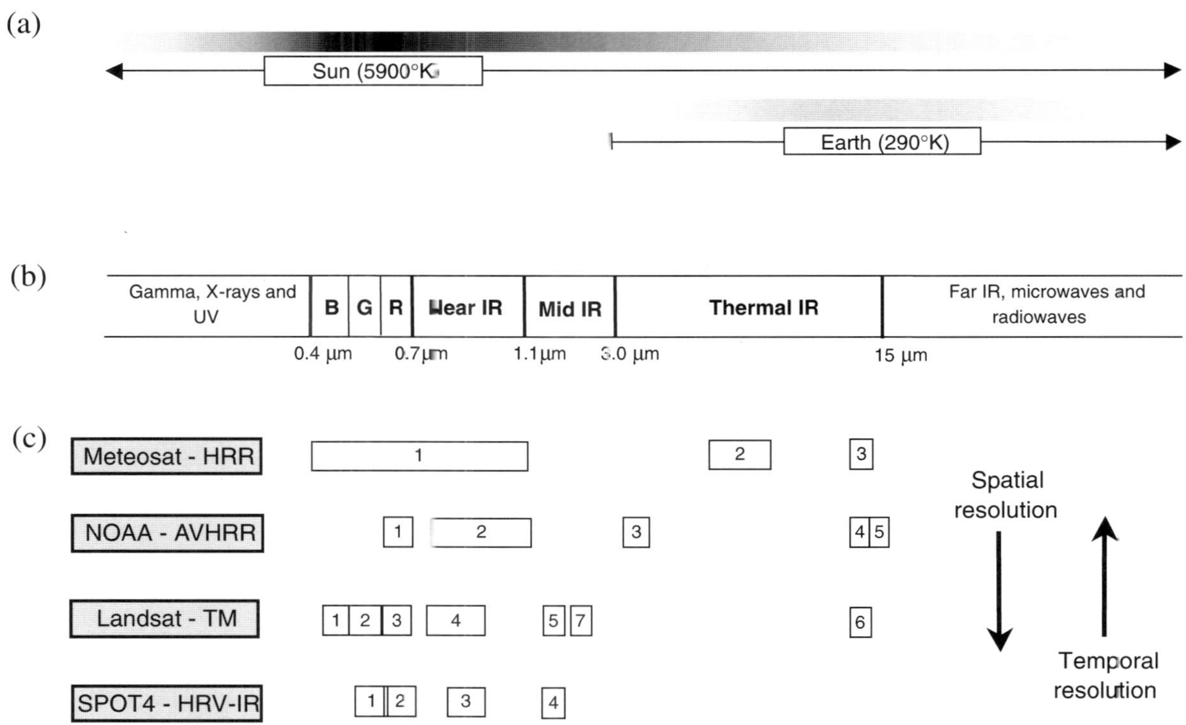

Fig. 1.11. Interrelationships between (a) the sources of radiation sensed by satellite-borne radiometers, with darker shading indicating higher relative emittance, (b) the electromagnetic spectrum in the region sensed by these radiometers (note the log scale), and (c) the bands (numbered) within this spectrum which are sensed by four radiometers carried on board the satellites NOAA-17, Landsat-7, SPOT-4 and Meteosat. UV, ultraviolet; B, blue; G, green; R, red; IR, infrared.

series, such as the Thematic Mapper (TM), have a high spatial resolution, of about 30 m^2 when the satellite is directly overhead. Although spatial resolution falls off at the margins, this resolution means that individual fields can be identified, and makes it ideal for comparing different types of vegetation cover. However, the Landsat satellites only achieve this high spatial resolution by sensing a narrow part of the earth at each pass (about 185 km), which means that the return time to a particular point is of the order of 16 days. By contrast, the main radiometers that have been carried on board the NOAA series, the Advanced Very High Resolution Radiometer (AVHRR), have a much greater field of view, with a swath width of around 2400 km. This gives a maximum spatial resolution of 1.1 km^2, though in practice over much of the sensed area the resolution is much lower, at around 7 km^2. However, this is compensated for by a much greater temporal resolution, the NOAA satellites returning to a position above the same point on the earth every day. This revisit frequency has an immense advantage in overcoming one of the greatest problems with satellite remote sensing – that of loss of useful data when an area is obscured by cloud cover. This is particularly important in humid areas, where many passes may be needed to build up cloud-free composite images. The problem with such Landsat composites is that they may represent different seasons, and the vegetation land-cover may have change substantially with the seasons. For diseases that have a strong seasonal component, as is the case with many vector-borne diseases, such as trypanosomiasis and East Coast fever (see Chapter 6), the need to obtain information about seasonal changes generally outweighs the need for high spatial resolution. The situation becomes more problematic when both high spatial and high temporal resolution are required, and the only solution is to use two or more sources of remotely sensed imagery. However, each image set tends to have a number of individual quirks, which can make direct comparison difficult.

While spatial and temporal resolution are properties determined in large part by the satellites, a third key property, that of spectral resolution, is intrinsic to the sensing instrument – the on-board radiometer. The operating principles of radiometers are very similar to those of digital cameras; both record the amount of electromagnetic radiation (EMR) sensed at a given pixel. In a digital camera, EMR in the visible spectrum (i.e. light) is reflected off a surface (e.g. a person's face) and then enters the camera's shutter, where the intensity (brightness) and the colour are recorded, different colours corresponding to different wavelengths. The same principles apply in a space-borne radiometer, except that the source of radiation may be the earth for the longer wavelengths, in the thermal and far infrared parts of the EMR spectrum (Fig. 11a and b). In addition, each radiometer 'sees' different parts of the EM spectrum, the number of bands and their widths defining its spectral resolution. Thus the Landsat-TM radiometer has a high spectral resolution in the visible and near infrared, while the meteorological radiometers (NOAA–AVHRR and Meteosat) have better resolution in the thermal infrared part of the spectrum. The choice of a radiometer's spectral resolution is thus conditioned by the main purpose for which the remote sensing system has been developed. With systems for observing the land surface, the most important parts of the EM spectrum are the visible and the near infrared, because by examining reflection properties in these bands it is possible to discriminate land-cover classes, such as vegetation, water, soil and built-up areas. The ideal is that each of these classes and subclasses, such as deep and shallow water or coniferous and evergreen forests, has its own unique response to solar radiation (i.e. a spectral 'signature') and thus can be easily recognized and discriminated when the image is processed. However, in practice this is rarely achieved, as many complex factors, such as the variation of the spectral response with the angle of the sun, make image interpretation as much an art as a hard science.

The idea of using the spectral response to determine land cover can be illustrated in the following example. In the wet–dry tropics, a common landscape is the gallery forest, which is characterized by a band of evergreen trees alongside permanent watercourses, particularly rivers. At a distance, the vegetation is not sufficient to maintain a closed forest, and the landscape becomes one of a typical savannah, with single trees interspersed amongst groundcover of seasonal grass. From an aeroplane, such a landscape may resemble that shown in Colour Plate 4a to the human eye, the visible colour and reflected intensity being combined (processed) in the brain to make identifiable the three dominant kinds of land cover making up this landscape. To a radiometer aboard a satellite with the capacity to record in the red and near-infrared (NIR) wavebands, the same scene might look like Colour Plate 4b. In the red channel, all three types of land cover appear dark, as the radiation is strongly absorbed, with typical reflectance values of only 5–10%. There is a section in the middle that has a lower reflectance and an experienced remote sensing specialist may well suspect that this is a watercourse. This would be confirmed by an examination of the NIR channel, as one of the signature features of water is that it has minimal reflectance for this waveband. The river is now easily picked out from the vegetation, which typically reflects infrared radiation strongly. However, we do not yet have unique signatures for the two types of vegetation, and for this we must use a common image-processing technique whereby each pixel in two co-registered images is subjected to an arithmetic transformation. In this case we will use the normalized difference vegetation index (NDVI), which is calculated as the NIR value minus the red, which is then divided by the NIR value plus the red. The logic of such spectral vegetation indices, of which there are a large number, is that stressed vegetation absorbs slightly more NIR and red radiation than unstressed vegetation. Although this difference is not always obvious when either band is examined separately, when they are looked at together the difference becomes more apparent. Thus, the NDVI in our example clearly distinguishes the gallery forest from the savannah grassland (Colour Plate 4c). Nevertheless, we already know how to interpret the NDVI as we are familiar with the landscape from Colour Plate 4a, but this is not the usual case for most image analysts. What then needs to happen is that he or she needs to consult paper maps or vegetation experts, or even undertake a 'ground truthing' survey to associate the images with the separate types of land-cover (Colour Plate 4d). This is often the most difficult step and may not be entirely successful, as few land-cover classes have such clearly defined signatures as in our example.

To make practical the above brief introduction to the basic principles of remote sensing, we will turn to yet another example from the veterinary literature of a mapped disease. In Algeria, sheep-pox is a serious disease that can cause high mortality rates in flocks. Attempts to control the disease more efficiently have been constrained by a lack of understanding of many basic epidemiological parameters, such as the exact means of transmission. During the period 1984–1997, a descriptive epidemiological study was undertaken in which the incidence of the disease was estimated for each province of the country (Achour and Bouguedour, 1999). The study showed that the incidence was highest in parts of the coastal region (Fig. 1.12) and in the autumn, although there was a complex dynamic with the timing of vaccination. Having successfully established the basic pattern of the disease, a follow-up study might be one in which we attempt to define more precisely the role of several possible risk factors. For example, what exactly is causing the seasonality of the outbreaks? Might it be the congregation of the animals following their pasturage in the mountains in the summer months, or could it be the effect of biting insects transmitting the disease between animals?

To answer such questions, much more data will be required than was necessary in the first study, particularly as we now require a lot of information about the physical environment. However, this is more complex than it might seem at first sight. Unlike the case of liver fluke in Victoria, where we had prior research to direct us to collate rainfall estimates for our analysis, we do not know exactly what we need to measure. In an ideal world, in which scientific research is not limited by resources, we could of course undertake field studies to measure many variables of possible interest, from climate parameters through vegetation to animal densities. In reality we have no such luxury, and what we need to do is to use as many indirect sources of information as possible in order to direct our fieldwork to specific parameters and the key areas. This is precisely the situation in which remote sensing can be of immense practical use to veterinary epidemiologists.

The first step is to determine which remote sensing system may be of most use. The choropleth maps recording the data collected by

Achour and Bouguedour were at the provincial level, which is a very coarse spatial scale of resolution, with a mean area of 48,000 km^2. This indicates that the remotely sensed images from the meteorological satellites are adequate, and we will use data from NOAA–AVHRR because a number of environmental indicators can be derived. As an example of how this imagery looks, we have downloaded an area over northern Algeria from NOAA's Satellite Active Archive (http://www.saa.noaa.gov) (Colour Plate 5). While this imagery is already registered to the earth's surface, it must still go through a number of preprocessing steps that allow geometric and radiometric correction. After these it is then aggregated with other images to form a continuous, 'stitched' image with minimum cloud interference. As is obvious in this image, cloud cover is a particular problem for remote sensing in the visible and near-infrared channel. To allow for this, standard practice is to take maximum values over a 10- or 30-day period ('maximum value composites'), on the assumption that these values are the closest possible to those of a cloud-free image. All these steps are necessary if we are to use the downloaded image in real time; however, because image preprocessing is a skilled task, most epidemiologists have tended to use preprocessed AVHRR image sets for their analyses (see Chapter 11).

For this work, we used 30-day maximum value composites for the entire year 1994, and from the download of channel 1 and 2 the NDVI was calculated [(channel 2 − channel 1)/(channel 2 + channel 1)]. The north coast of Algeria, where the great majority of the sheep (and human) population is found, has a typical Mediterranean climate. The seasonality of the rainfall is clearly shown when the autumn and spring NDVIs are compared, as is the lack of rainfall in the Sahara desert to the south (Colour Plate 6). AVHRR data may also be used to obtain a measure of temperature, using the split-window approach, which compares adjusted radiation levels in the two thermal infrared channels (channels 4 and 5), and is termed the 'land surface temperature' (LST). The LST [channel 4 + 3.33 (channel 5 − channel 4)] is the temperature just above ground level and does not equate to the air temperature as measured by a meteorological screen; nevertheless it is a good surrogate, especially to gauge variability between sites and seasons (Hay and Lennon, 1999).

Having now accumulated a large data set for some of the key environmental determinants of animal disease for the whole country, we are in the position to use it to examine possible correlates of high incidence of sheep-pox. Yet it should be clear that we are beginning to face another difficulty – how to manage such a large data set in any resulting analysis, having 12 monthly variables for NDVI and LST per year. If we extend the period and involve other remote sensing-derived variables, such as the cold cloud duration, a surrogate of rainfall using Meteosat images, we quickly accumulate excessive data. The problem here is not that a model cannot be fitted, but rather that it becomes very difficult to interpret the model. For example, how could we give sensible biological meaning to a regression model that showed higher incidence for a given month to be modelled best by the LST of the previous month and NDVIs in 3 different months in the past year? This problem of interpretation is not unique to remote sensing, but its sheer capacity to generate large volumes of spatiotemporal data makes it more serious.

A statistical solution to this difficulty arises from the fact that, although we may have large amounts of spatiotemporal data, the actual amount of information is much less. This is because there is a considerable temporal autocorrelation, the value of one variable, such as the June NDVI for a given area, being very similar to that of the May and July values. In addition, these variables are likely to be strongly correlated with others, such that high-rainfall months are likely to be associated with lower-temperature months and vice versa. The solution, therefore, is to use multivariate statistical techniques that reduce the data set to a small number of manageable variables that capture the key information. In fact, the problem of excess data is a very familiar one in the processing of remote sensing imagery, and one technique, principal components analysis (PCA), is commonly used to overcome the data redundancy between bands of multispectral images (Mather, 1999).

To reduce data redundancy when our interest is only in one band of an image, the preferred technique is Fourier transformation. This functions by decomposing an image into a series of sinusoidal waves, although only the first couple contain the majority of the relevant information. The technique was originally introduced into remote-sensing image-processing to filter out noise and other defects in single images, but it has also proved particularly useful for reducing the redundancy in data sets derived from multitemporal images. Given the intrinsic sinusoidal nature of many seasonal parameters, such as temperature and rainfall, the technique can be considered a natural choice for the problem. Applying a Fourier transformation to the Algerian data set for the NDVI and LST for 1996, this large volume of data can be summarized by a few parameters. These parameters can then be used to classify the vegetation–climate of Algeria into a meaningful number of classes (Colour Plate 7).

Having now reduced our data set to a manageable number of explanatory variables, we could potentially apply some of the spatial regression techniques discussed in Section 1.4 of this chapter to the data shown in Fig. 1.12. Nevertheless, there is a clear danger in undertaking such an analysis using transformed independent variables and a measure of disease averaged over several years. This is particularly so because the authors of the original research implied that the season climate *per se* was not the main reason for the higher incidence in autumn, but rather a combination of it and management factors, including the time of vaccination. Our previous discussion will hopefully have

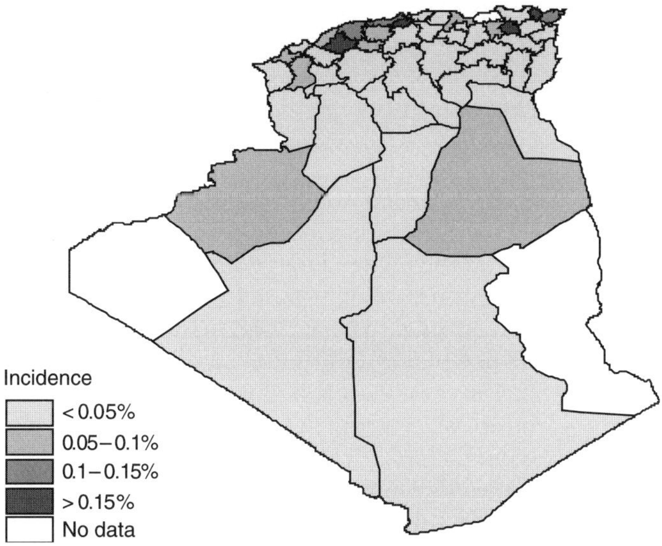

Fig. 1.12. Mean annual incidence of sheep-pox in Algeria, 1984–1997. Redrawn from Achour and Bouguedour (1999).

indicated the dangers of focusing on the methods of spatial analysis whilst being blind to the actual animal health and management. It is more appropriate to use the map of the Fourier-transformed climate surrogates for hypothesis generation and, in collaboration with local researchers, to develop a surveillance system that may help select areas for small-area, targeted studies.

1.6 Conclusion and overview

We have travelled a considerable distance in this chapter, almost circling the globe with our selected case studies. During this trip, we have at various stages pointed out many interesting features. We have seen that spatial analysis can be a useful tool in epidemiology, able to add considerable value and insight into animal health problems and their relationship with the physical environment. However, applying sophisticated spatial techniques to poor-quality data will not create an insightful investigation. We have also seen that the three components of spatial epidemiology (GIS, spatial analysis and remote sensing) can be complex and difficult tools to master. Indeed, our metaphor for these would possibly have been more apt if we had referred to them as toolboxes rather than as tools; many practitioners use only some of the contents and never require the use of any of the vast number of techniques available. This introduction to how the component parts function (and possibly interrelate) will, we hope, be of some assistance in understanding the succeeding chapters.

The chapters that follow touch on a number of the themes and issues we have introduced. In the next chapter, Peter Durr introduces some ideas from spatial epidemiology and considers their application to animal disease (Chapter 2). In particular, he considers two areas of contemporary concern in veterinary epidemiology: bovine spongiform encephalopathy (BSE) and bovine tuberculosis (TB). He also outlines some current work on multidrug-resistant *Salmonella* Newport.

Two chapters placing veterinary spatial epidemiology in its wider biomedical context constitute the next part of the book. Thus, Tony Gatrell reflects on the use of GIS and spatial analysis in a human health context (Chapter 3). He reviews a number of problems, studies and methods, some – but not all – of which have been raised by veterinary scientists. In the second chapter, Peter Diggle, who has been at the forefront of methodological developments in spatial statistics, considers some aspects of this field as applied to the biomedical sciences (Chapter 4). Diggle considers both exploratory and model-based methods and applications. Among the former he considers the use of kernel-smoothing to examine spatial variation in the risk of infection with particular strains (spoligotypes) of bovine TB. Among the latter, he outlines a hierarchical logistic regression model and applies this to data on the prevalence of childhood malaria in The Gambia. He also flags the importance of developing online surveillance tools in a spatial setting.

In the succeeding chapters, our colleagues consider a range of applications specific to animal health issues. First, Dirk Pfeiffer considers the use of GIS and spatial analysis in animal health (Chapter 5). He illustrates the use of empirical Bayes estimation in the mapping of rare diseases (e.g. infection of red foxes with *Echinococcus multilocularis* in Lower Saxony; Berke, 2001). Such estimates are needed in order to counteract the problems of small numbers in area data. He further illustrates an application of the smoothing of spatial point data (kernel or density estimation; for an introduction, see Bailey and Gatrell, 1995) by applying these ideas to the changing geography of BSE incidence in Britain. The detection of spatial clustering (using *K* functions) is illustrated using data on an outbreak of poultry disease in Northern Ireland. From a modelling perspective he demonstrates the power of linking GIS to statistical spatial analysis in a prediction of the incidence of theileriosis in Zimbabwe; here, a logistic regression model with spatial effects is employed, in which covariates include land-use and environmental factors.

Parasitology has a long history of using GIS and remote sensing, and this is reviewed by Guy Hendrickx and his colleagues, who place current trends in the historical context of relevant work done in the pre-GIS era (Chapter 6). They look at three areas of application: tsetse-transmitted trypanosomiasis, liver fluke and East Coast fever. In each case, issues relating to the collection of covariate data are discussed and the use of various analytical techniques is illustrated. Particular attention is given to the temporal domain and to the emergence of spatial decision support systems.

Nigel French and Piran White consider the use of GIS in developing simulation models of the spatial and temporal spread of animal diseases (Chapter 7). After summarizing different modelling approaches, three case studies are used to illustrate the application of different forms of modelling and the use of GIS. The examples considered by French and White are rabies and tuberculosis in wildlife, myiasis in livestock and foot-and-mouth disease in livestock populations.

Dominic Mellor and his colleagues focus on the use of GIS in companion animal epidemiology (Chapter 8). This focus of application brings fresh challenges, since research is inhibited by the relative dearth of spatially referenced data on the distribution of such populations. Also, the nature of the distribution differs markedly from that for other animal populations; for example, companion animals tend to live close to their owners and in small groups. As the chapter shows, we know little about the distribution by owners' social class and the characteristics of the areas in which these animals live. Mellor and colleagues also discuss the data issues involved in trying to understand the spatial epidemiology of disease such as canine cancer.

Robert Sanson looks specifically at the use of GIS in epidemic disease response (Chapter 9). Like others, he considers issues of data availability and quality, and then focuses on two areas of recent concern. The first is the response to the *Varroa destructor* (Asian honeybee mite) epidemic in New Zealand in 2000. The second is the 2001 foot-and-mouth disease outbreak in the UK. Sanson discusses the importance to trained professionals of having high-quality and up-to-date data available, as well as high-performance software.

Lastly, Joanna McKenzie considers the application of GIS in the surveillance and management of wildlife diseases (Chapter 10). The logistics and expense of capturing wild animals and testing them for disease are, of course, a major challenge. Like others before her, issues of data availability and quality figure prominently in her overview of applications from a number of different contexts, and at different spatial scales. As with other applications, collecting high-quality data on environmental covariates is crucial to the success of the modelling enterprise.

We end the book with a brief overview of resources, covering the GIS and spatial statistical software environment and advice on how to obtain spatially referenced data (Chapter 11). As noted there, we have set up a 'virtual space' (http://www.gisvet.org) within which those interested in methods and applications in this broad field can interact. We hope this will prove productive.

Acknowledgements

For our deceptively simple case studies we called upon the assistance of a large number of people, and in particular we thank Nigel Tait, whose technical skill made possible the production of the more demanding maps and analyses. For the Philadelphia case study, Maurice Fine provided details of the locations of the sampling points and Martin Hugh-Jones facilitated the geocoding of the veterinary practices. The liver fluke example proved the most challenging, and we thank Peter Mansell for tracking down the thesis by Watt, and Graeme Garner for providing a digital boundary map of the old Victorian shires. Finally, we acknowledge Jan Biesemans of Avia-GIS for his assistance in using the NOAA-TOOLS freeware package, which produced Colour Plate 5.

References

Achour, H.A. and Buoguedour, R. (1999) Épidémiologie de la clavée en Algérie. *Revue Scientifique et Technique Office International des Epizooties* 18, 606–617.

Bailey, T.C. and Gatrell, A.C. (1995) *Interactive Spatial Data Analysis*. Longman, Harlow, UK.

Berke, O. (2001) Choropleth mapping of regional count data of *Echinococcus multilocularis* among red foxes in Lower Saxony, Germany. *Preventive Veterinary Medicine* 52, 119–131.

Boray, J.C. (1969) Experimental fascioliasis in Australia. *Advances in Parasitology* 7, 95–210.

Burrough, P.A. and Frank, A.U. (eds) (1996) *Geographic Objects With Indeterminate Boundaries*. Taylor and Francis, London.

Cliff, A.D. and Haggett, P. (1988) *Atlas of Disease Distribution: Analytic Approaches to Epidemiological Data*. Basil Blackwell, Oxford.

Cromley, E. and McLafferty, E. (2002) *GIS and Public Health*. Guilford Press, New York.

Foody, G.M. and Atkinson, P.M. (eds) (2002) *Uncertainty in Remote Sensing and GIS*. John Wiley & Sons, Chichester, UK.

Forer, P. and Unwin, D. (1999) Enabling progress in GIS and education. In: Longley, P.A., Goodchild, M.F., Maguire, D.J. and Rhind, D.W. (eds) *Geographical Information Systems*. John Wiley & Sons, Chichester, UK, pp. 747–756.

Gatrell, A. and Löytönen, M. (eds) (1998) *GIS and Health*. Taylor and Francis, London.

Hay, S.I. and Lennon, J.J. (1999) Deriving meteorological variables across Africa for the study and control of vector-borne disease: a comparison of remote sensing and spatial interpolation of climate. *Tropical Medicine and International Health* 4, 58–71.

Hay, S.I., Randolph, S.E. and Rogers, D.J. (eds) (2000) *Remote Sensing and Geographical Information Systems in Epidemiology*. Academic Press, London.

Hutchinson, M.F. (1995) Interpolating mean rainfall with thin plate-smoothing splines. *International Journal of Geographical Information Systems* 9, 385–403.

Jones, C. (1997) *Geographical Information Systems and Computer Cartography*. Longman, Harlow, UK.
Lawson, A.B., Browne, W.J. and Vidal Rodeiro, C.L. (2003) *Disease Mapping with WinBUGS and MLWin*. John Wiley & Sons, Chichester, UK.
Longley, P.A., Goodchild, M.F., Maguire, D.J. and Rhind, D.W. (1999) Introduction. In: Longley, P.A., Goodchild, M.F., Maguire, D.J. and Rhind, D.W. (eds) *Geographical Information Systems*. John Wiley & Sons, Chichester, UK, pp. 1–20.
MacEachren, A.M. (1995) *How Maps Work: Representation, Visualization and Design*. Guilford Press, New York.
Mather, P.M. (1999) *Computer Processing of Remotely-Sensed Images: an Introduction*, 2nd edn. John Wiley & Sons, Chichester, UK.
McHarg, I.L. (1969) *Design With Nature*. Natural History Press, New York.
Messina, J.P. and Crews-Meyer, K.A. (2000a) A historical perspective on the development of remotely sensed data as applied to medical geography. In: Albert, D.P., Gesler, W.M. and Levergood, B. (eds) *Spatial Analysis, GIS, and Remote Sensing Applications in the Health Sciences*. Ann Arbor Press, Chelsea, Michigan, pp. 129–146.
Messina, J.P. and Crews-Meyer, K.A. (2000b) The integration of remote sensing and medical geography: process and application. In: Albert, D.P., Gesler, W.M. and Levergood, B. (eds) *Spatial Analysis, GIS, and Remote Sensing Applications in the Health Sciences*. Ann Arbor Press, Chelsea, Michigan, pp. 147–168.
Monmonier, M. (1996) *How to Lie With Maps*, 2nd edn. University of Chicago Press, Chicago, Illinois.
Reif, J.S. and Cohen, D. (1970) Canine pulmonary disease. II. Retrospective radiographic analysis of pulmonary disease in rural and urban dogs. *Archives of Environmental Health* 20, 684–689.
Robinson, T.P. (2000) Spatial statistics and geographical information systems in epidemiology and public health. In: Hay, S.I., Randolph, S.E. and Rogers, D.J. (eds) *Remote Sensing and Geographical Information Systems in Epidemiology*. Academic Press, London, pp. 82–128.
Thrall, S.E. and Thrall, G. (1999) Desktop GIS software. In: Longley, P.A., Goodchild, M.F., Maguire, D.J. and Rhind, D.W. (eds) *Geographical Information Systems*. John Wiley & Sons, Chichester, UK, pp. 331–345.
Watt, G.E.L. (1980) An approach to determining the prevalence of liver fluke in a large region. In: Geering, W.A., Roe, R.T. and Chapman, L.A. (eds) *Proceedings of the 2nd International Symposium on Veterinary Epidemiology & Economics, Canberra, Australia, 7–11 May, 1979*, pp. 152–155.
Worboys, M.F. (1995) *GIS: a Computing Perspective*. Taylor and Francis, London.

Spatial Epidemiology and Animal Disease: Introduction and Overview

2

Peter A. Durr

2.1 What is spatial epidemiology?

An appropriate beginning for this overview is to define the scope and intent of spatial epidemiology as applied to animal health and disease. This is required as we are in the realm of a new subdiscipline of epidemiology, one whose subject matter is scarcely referred to in any of the standard texts (Martin *et al.*, 1987; Thrusfield, 1995). It is hard to think of an epidemiological investigation without location being at least inferred. For example, the simplest epidemiological data, such as a list of the number of foot-and-mouth disease (FMD) cases in each country of the world in a given year, provides a wealth of spatial information. The countries with cases tend to be closer to each other (i.e. there is clustering) and have environmental and socioeconomic characteristics different from those free of the disease, the latter being mostly wealthier nations in the higher latitudes. Thus, while listing 'case countries' is not spatial epidemiology, a description of the spatial pattern starts to be, and a detailed exploration of these in terms of spatial processes most definitely is.

In laying claim to spatial epidemiology being a different sort of epidemiology, we are of course indirectly asking what makes and justifies a subdiscipline. No one makes such a claim for 'temporal' epidemiology, as time is so intrinsic to epidemiology that ignoring it would make a study untenable. What makes a subdiscipline, however, is not the fact that it is used in only a small proportion of investigations; rather, the critical thing is that it has its own distinct viewpoint, terminology and methods. These are familiar to practitioners but less so to the general epidemiology community. In spatial epidemiology it is the disease map that defines this viewpoint most overtly; in modelling (mathematical epidemiology) the equivalent of the disease map is the system of equations of disease transmission between groups of susceptible, infectious and immune animals. Nevertheless, there can be more subtle differences, especially in terminology. For example, for molecular epidemiologists the term ‘cluster’ refers to genotypes with similar genetic markers, as identified by a ‘dendrogram’, which is the output of a cluster analysis from a statistical package. For spatial epidemiologists, the concept ‘cluster’ generally refers to a group of cases that, when mapped, are close together and whose investigation will involve special methods. Of course, the two types of clusters may not be mutually exclusive; genetic clusters may also be spatially clustered, and integrating the molecular and spatial subdisciplines may result in a fuller epidemiological description. This example leads us to a conceptual model of the subdisciplines of epidemiology as self-contained building blocks, each helping to form the larger discipline (Fig. 2.1a). Extending this metaphor, we can see that the structure of the parent discipline may become unstable if the subdisciplines are not bound together in some way, or if each takes on a form completely dissimilar to the others. Fortunately, epidemiology has too few practitioners at present to suffer this risk, but one can envisage a future with specialist journals of molecular epidemiology and animal health economics whose readers find each other’s subject matter incomprehensible.

The more practically minded may argue that spatial epidemiology is what spatial epidemiologists do – the materials and methods define the subject. There is something in this argument, in that spatial epidemiology has such a distinctive set of tools, which may involve a geographical information system (GIS), spatial statistical packages and remotely sensed images (Fig. 2.1b). The problem with such a functional definition is that it ignores the purpose of using these tools and the quality of what is produced. For example, most epidemiologists trained within the past 5 years are competent in using a GIS to map cases and to run a disease cluster package such as SatScan or Stat! (see Chapter 11). However, this is only the prelude to a true spatial epidemiological investigation, as the key questions of the nature of the clustering and what is causing it remain unanswered. A comparable example is the plotting of the epidemic curve by mathematical modellers, this being a starting point rather than a result. The use of the tools of GIS, spatial statistics and remote sensing is generally necessary for spatial epidemiology, but by itself not sufficient.

Using the above discussion, we can arrive at an acceptable definition of spatial epidemiology as a subdiscipline of epidemiology whose primary purpose is to describe and explain the spatial pattern of disease. This does not mean that every research study has to fulfil these

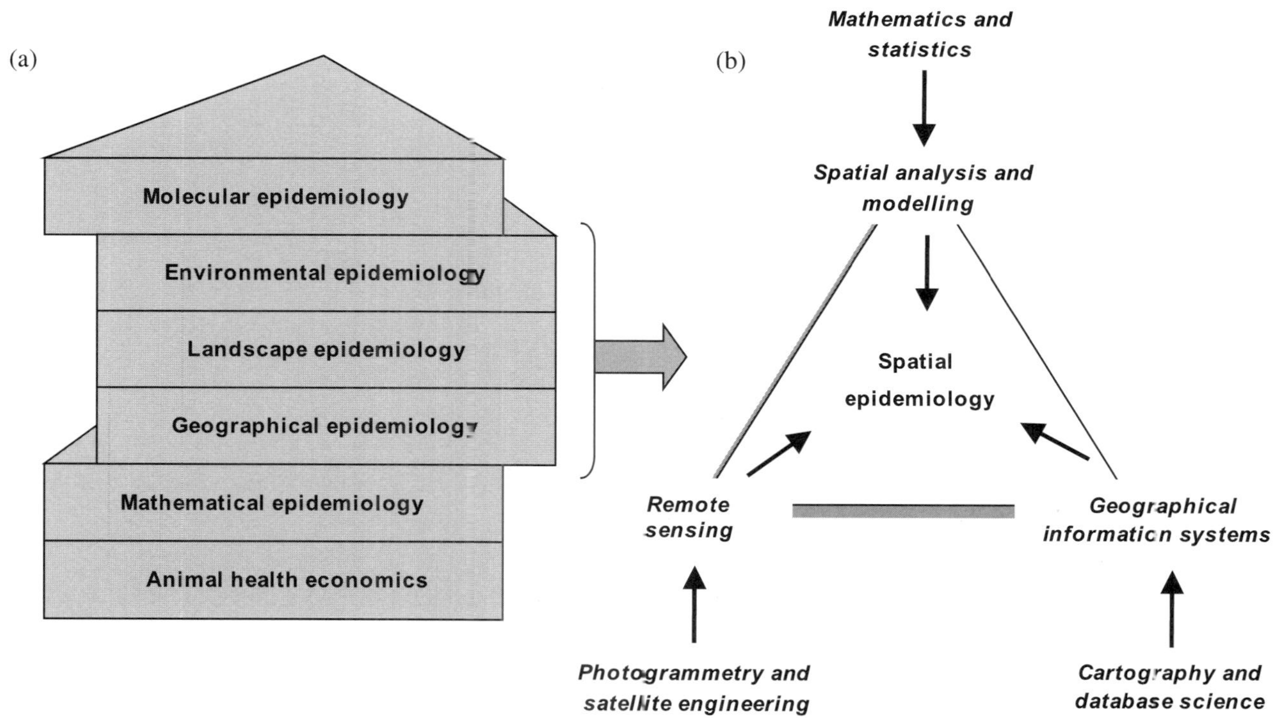

Fig. 2.1. A conceptual model for spatial epidemiology showing (a) its relationship to some other epidemiological disciplines that can be similarly defined as having a distinct viewpoint or approach, and (b) the source origins of its methodologies. Note that the list in (a) is not exhaustive.

objectives in order to be bona fide spatial epidemiology, and, as I will argue later in this chapter, the intrinsic difficulties of spatial epidemiology mean that there are very few successful case studies. Thus the destination – not the means of travel or how close we are to arrival – best defines the journey.

In the above discussion I have used the adjective 'spatial' as if it is the only one that is appropriate for the topic at hand. In fact, there are several competing terms that are used widely in the medical literature, namely 'environmental epidemiology', 'geographical epidemiology' and 'landscape epidemiology'. Each of these other spatial epidemiologies can be defined by its differing focus of research and methodology. Thus, environmental epidemiology has its foundations in toxicology and oncology and a major field of enquiry is the effect of putative sources of exposure, such as nuclear power stations and toxic waste incinerators (Hertz-Picciotto, 1998). With landscape epidemiology the parent discipline is parasitology and the concern is predominantly with vector-borne diseases, particularly the identification of areas of elevated risk, for which remote sensing is proving a key tool (Kitron, 1998). Geographical epidemiology has its roots in disease mapping (Howe, 1989), but, under the guidance of geographers, has expanded its area of concern away from spatial patterns of disease into the planning and delivery of health-care systems in a spatial context (Meade and Earickson, 2000). As each of these can be contained within our definition of spatial epidemiology, let us adopt a pragmatic approach and treat each as a component part of our preferred term, which encompasses the whole (Fig. 2.1a).

2.2 Veterinary spatial epidemiology: a short history

Up to the 1980s, it is difficult to find examples in the veterinary literature where much recognizable spatial epidemiology is evident. This is exemplified in the discussion of the spatial aspects of disease in the first major veterinary epidemiology text (Schwabe *et al.*, 1977), in which medical rather than veterinary examples were used. This probably reflects the general weakness of veterinary epidemiology in that period, when experiments rather than field observation dominated. The exception to this generalization is work undertaken by parasitologists interested in the interaction between climate and disease via its effect on vectors and intermediate hosts. One of the earliest of such studies was by Ollerenshaw, who developed a climate forecast system for predicting acute outbreaks of *Fasciola hepatica* in Wales, and later extended this to the rest of the country (Ollerenshaw, 1966). An even more impressive body of work was conducted in the 1950s in the Lake Victoria region of Tanzania in an attempt to understand sporadic outbreaks of the tick-borne disease East Coast fever (Yeoman, 1966a). By carefully mapping disease outbreaks in relation to the cattle population, it was possible to draw a line separating enzootic and epizootic areas and to map the spatial development of the epidemic (see Chapter 6). Further work attempted to define the underlying causes of these disease patterns in terms of the effects of climate and pasture ecology on tick levels on the host (Yeoman, 1966b, 1967).

During this pre-GIS era, geographers, no doubt reflecting their training in the importance of location and spatial relationships, undertook much of the more innovative research in spatial epidemiology. An early veterinary example is a study on the effect of abnormal wind currents to explain clusters of secondary outbreaks of FMD during the 1967/68 epidemic in England and Wales (Tinline, 1970). This provided a more plausible hypothesis for the spatial distribution than the official one involving the simultaneous distribution of frozen imported lamb. Another interesting example applied the concept of the spread of disease in space ('spatial diffusion') to describe a Newcastle disease epidemic, again in England and Wales (Gilg, 1973). Spatial diffusion concepts were also used by Lineback (1980) to explore why rabies persisted in wildlife in a particular area of the eastern USA.

Without doubt, the real impetus to the present growth of spatial epidemiology came as a direct result of the technical breakthroughs in computing in the 1980s, which enabled the processing of large and complex data sets on reasonably priced minicomputers and workstations. In 1981 the first commercial GIS software (ArcInfo) was released, and later in the decade, when prices began to fall, a number of researchers, particularly parasitologists, began using such packages to organize and map disease occurrences and relate them to environmental variables. Landmark work along these lines was carried out by Lessard *et al.* (1990), who collated an immense amount of data in order to visualize and explore the spatial pattern of theileriosis across the whole continent of Africa. Although this study was less successful in actually explaining the spatial pattern, to this day there are few studies that are comparable in ambition and scale.

The other major spur to the development of spatial epidemiology in the 1980s was the increasing availability of satellite imagery, particularly from the Landsat and NOAA (National Oceanic and Atmospheric Administration, USA) satellite series. The latter, carrying on board the AVHRR (Advanced Very High Resolution Radiometer) sensor, provided one of the earliest examples of the effective use of satellite imagery in veterinary science, in which areas of seasonally high risk for Rift Valley fever were detected (Linthicum *et al.*, 1987). Through the use of a spectral index (the normalized difference vegetation index, NDVI), which is correlated to the green vegetation biomass and thus indirectly to rainfall, breeding areas of the *Aedes* mosquito vector could be identified. An advance on this work was made by Rogers and Randolph (1991), who demonstrated that the NDVI could be associated not only with vector habitat but also with vector abundance, in this case for tsetse flies. This finding led to a line of research that has been expanded for a range of vector-borne diseases and continues to this day (Hay *et al.*, 2000).

In the early period of spatial epidemiology, the software needed for GIS and remotely sensed image processing was relatively complex, having command-line interfaces and proprietary programming languages. This meant that these tools were unavailable to most epidemiologists without a considerable investment in time or the employment of dedicated operators. With the emergence, in the early 1990s, of user-friendly GIS packages, such as ArcView and MapInfo, using graphic user interfaces in place of command lines, there was less need for extended training times to achieve minimum competence. These desktop GIS packages were arguably the single most important technical development in the move of spatial epidemiology from the specialist to the generalist epidemiologist. This is well illustrated by the growth in the number of papers describing work using GIS at the successive International Symposia on Veterinary Epidemiology and Economics (ISVEE) conferences in the 1990s: four at Ottawa (1991), five at Nairobi (1994), 13 at Paris (1997) and 18 at Breckenridge (2000). Just as important as having more presentations using GIS is the fact that, at the latter two conferences, most of these papers were by epidemiologists relatively new to its use. In the space of a little over 5 years GIS and spatial epidemiology have become part of mainstream veterinary epidemiology.

Looked at from this perspective, the continued growth of spatial epidemiology is assured, though many challenges remain to be overcome. One particular issue for applied veterinary epidemiologists, which became clear during its use in the 2001 FMD epidemic in Great Britain, is the need to move it away from stand-alone PCs and to integrate it closely into national animal health information systems (AHIS). This is a much more complex issue than might at first appear, as it involves fundamental decisions about the sort of locational data that should be captured in the AHIS (whether it be points or polygons; see Chapter 9) and technical issues of how best to store and retrieve these data. In this, as in so much of current computing, it is likely that the World Wide Web will play a large role, acting as the appropriate bridge between over-centralized systems represented by the vanished mainframe computer and the disconnected, almost anarchic system of the stand-alone PC running a desktop GIS.

2.3 Problems and pitfalls in spatial epidemiology

Many coming new to GIS are astounded at how easy it is to produce a disease map. All that is needed is a spreadsheet file containing, for example, location data of farms (x and y coordinates) and some attribute data, such as whether the farm is positive or negative for a particular disease. Once the three columns are imported into a GIS, a map can quickly be produced which generally shows some clustering of the disease. After a period, when the thrill of discovery drains away, some hard questions start to be asked: how were the farms located and how accurately was this done? Is the disease pattern just reflecting the distribution of the farms at risk? What is 'causing' the pattern? Each of these questions generally requires weeks, even months, to explore in depth, and only when the questions are answered can a convincing spatial epidemiological analysis be considered complete. This is a current paradox with spatial epidemiology: producing an exploratory disease map has now become one of the easiest tasks for epidemiologists, yet undertaking a rigorous spatial epidemiological analysis remains one of the hardest. Let us explore some of the reasons why this is so.

2.3.1 Obtaining spatial data

Spatial data can be defined as any data that has associated with it a set of locations on the earth's surface. However, such a definition is not really very useful, as it is difficult to think of any data without some geographical element, even in the extreme case of a bacterial gene, which has a location where the bacteria was cultured or the gene sequenced. Therefore, what we really mean by spatial data is data that permit an analysis focused upon the locational element. In practice, epidemiological spatial data fall into three classes: spatially referenced case data, population-at-risk data, and environmental or covariate data.

Spatially referenced case data are generally the easiest epidemiological data to obtain, as they arise naturally from any detailed clinical examination or on-farm disease investigation. In the case of farms, until recently this required reading a reference from a paper map, which assumes the existence of, or access to, high-resolution maps and that the user has been trained in reading them. However, the introduction of cheap hand-held global positioning systems (GPS) in the 1990s largely overcame this problem. Using a GPS, it is currently possible to obtain the latitude and longitude to within 20 m of the true location. The impact of GPS in providing spatially referenced case data is potentially greatest in those developing countries where the absence of quality paper maps means that these data are often not collectable. The other technical advance that has made obtaining spatially referenced case data increasingly easy is geocoding via postal codes. These are large databases which link all the current postal codes within an area or country to a map reference, and since the 1990s these have become widely available in many developed countries. While postal codes have limitations for georeferencing rural farms (Durr and Froggatt, 2002), they are generally very reliable for urban areas, being able (for example, in the UK) to locate a house within 10 m. This will potentially have most impact on small animal epidemiology, as clinical records invariably record postal codes. Thus, it is currently possible for a small animal practitioner who has in place a client database and access to a geocoding database to map, for example, all cases of an outbreak of distemper in dogs in the practice's catchment area. It is more than likely that the outbreak is clustered in certain areas and, using this information, the partners might decide upon a mailshot to the practice's clients in these areas, advising them to bring their pets into the clinic for booster vaccination.

While plotting case data may frequently be sufficient for operational tasks, such as defining hotspot areas for enhanced disease surveillance or control, it is inadequate – and frequently misleading – for most spatial analysis. The problem is that populations at risk – either individuals or aggregate units such as farms – are themselves spatially heterogeneous (clustered), and concentrations of populations will generally have greater numbers of cases. Therefore, meaningful spatial analysis is only possible when the case data are represented as a proportion (either incidence or prevalence) of the population at risk within the spatial area. However, true denominator data are frequently difficult to obtain. Thus, in the example of the small animal clinic and the distemper outbreak, the practitioner will have as a denominator clients within a given area, but will not have data on the true population at risk, which is the entire population of dogs. A better estimate of the denominator would be obtained by combining all the databases of the practices within an area, but this would still leave out stray animals and those whose owners do not use veterinary services, which probably represent the subpopulations most at risk. This does not mean that no analysis can be undertaken if true denominator data are absent. For example, in many countries the non-use of veterinary services and the size of the stray dog population are related to poverty, and thus it may be possible to estimate the numbers involved by statistical modelling using deprivation indices derived from socioeconomic data, when these are available (see Chapter 8).

When the effects of demography on the spatial pattern of a disease are accounted for and areas of high and low disease occurrence remain, the focus often shifts to an explanation of the distribution of these in terms of *environmental covariates*. Spatially referenced environmental data sets, especially those related to soil, climate and vegetation, are quite widely available. Nevertheless, obtaining, using and interpreting the data are rarely trouble-free. For example, the organizations owning the data will frequently charge for their use, the data sets required for a particular study may not be contemporaneous with the disease data, and the spatial resolution may not be adequate for the purposes of the study (Durr *et al.*, 2000a). Even more troublesome, data sets measuring the same variable may not be spatially compatible. For example, one hypothesis for the persistence of Johne's disease on farms relates it to soil pH (Kopecky, 1977; Reviriego *et al.*, 2000), and one would suppose that this should be easily testable by undertaking a prevalence survey and relating this to the topsoil pH. In Great Britain there are two data sets on soil acidity; one was collected at a spatial resolution of 25 km^2 (McGrath and Loveland, 1992) and the other was developed at higher resolution during a national soil mapping exercise carried out over a more extended period. While these are in broad agreement, there are significant contradictions, caused in part by sampling variability, analytical processing and changes over time, possibly induced by agriculture and pollution (Colour Plate 8). Inconsistencies such as these can be resolved by undertaking specific analyses to identify the importance of these factors, and then deciding which data set is most appropriate for the spatial pattern of the disease being investigated. However, this requires a considerable investment of time in order to understand the intricacies of the data, which leads one further away from the primary epidemiological question.

The difficulty and expense of obtaining data from ground collection and keeping it current has been one of the main motivators behind the use of satellite imagery. While the radiometers on the satellites simply record the levels of reflected and emitted radiation in certain wavelength bands, through the judicious use of image transformations, such as spectral band rationing and Fourier analysis, useful surrogates for relevant variables may be obtained. For example, Baylis and Rawlings (1998) investigated the importance of local climate on the spatial distribution of the 1987–1991 epidemic of African horse sickness in Morocco, Spain and Portugal. It was found that a spectral ratio measure of photosynthesis activity, the minimum normalized difference vegetation index, was a more useful measure of local environmental moisture than direct measurements by weather stations. However, the investigation also required a ground-sensed parameter, wind speed, to successfully fit a regression model of the distribution of the disease's insect vector, *Culicoides imicola*. In addition, the study used a coarse spatial resolution and might not have been so successful if predictions had been required at a finer spatial scale. In Britain a data set of farm-level temperature and humidity values would be ideal to test the hypothesis of the role of climate in maintaining hotspots of bovine tuberculosis in the south-west (King *et al.*, 1999). While remotely sensed surrogates for these variables have been developed (Wint *et al.*, 2002), none is currently available at the appropriate spatial scale (1 km^2), which corresponds to a mean farm size of 100 ha.

2.3.2 Spatial uncertainty and error

Anyone perusing the GIS and remote sensing literature will quickly discover that issues of error and uncertainty are major areas of research, and indeed whole books have been given over to the subject (Goodchild and Gopal, 1989). This is because the availability of large amounts of data at high spatial resolution means that error and uncertainty, which would be averaged out or largely unnoticed at a coarse spatial resolution, become explicit.

As an example, take a farm that consists of two parcels of land, one used for summer grazing and the other containing farm buildings where the animals are housed over the winter. The farmer lives in a village some distance from the farm (Fig. 2.2). The problem arises as to how best, and where, to reference the farm as a single point if the database can only store simple locational data as a coordinate pair (i.e. latitude and longitude). The issue is the choice of the point location that should be used: the farm buildings, the farmer's residence or the geometrical centre of the farm, the farm 'centroid' (Durr and Froggatt, 2002). Then there is the problem of summer grazing, which may be especially important if a disease (such as liver fluke) being investigated has a risk factor closely associated with the grazing environment. There is no single answer to these questions, and one is left with the uncomfortable feeling that any attempt to define the farm's location by a single point is inherently flawed and the data inherently uncertain. This problem of uncertainty is a common one in spatial representation. For example, how should the edge of a river with a large tidal surge be defined? Should it be its maximum, minimum or mean extent?

When first presented with problems of spatial uncertainty, the best solution may seem to collect more data: in the case of the farm, the entire boundaries. In the past this simply was not possible as storing such data would require both large computer storage capacity and a GIS linked to the animal health database. The enormous advances in computer technology in the past 10 years have now largely removed such technical constraints and the task is feasible, for example, by the use of aerial photography to establish field boundaries. However, farmers are constantly selling, renting and buying fields and changing their agricultural use from livestock to crops or even non-agricultural use. The requirement is then to keep the database up to date, but at what frequency? Monthly, annually, or when a significant change occurs? But how is 'significant' to be defined? Obviously, selling off a large part of a field for road expansion would qualify, but what about a small part? And what if a field is rented to a neighbour for 6 months, so that it functionally becomes part of the neighbour's farm for that period?

All these difficulties in georeferencing farm location could be tackled, for example, by introducing a mandatory requirement to notify

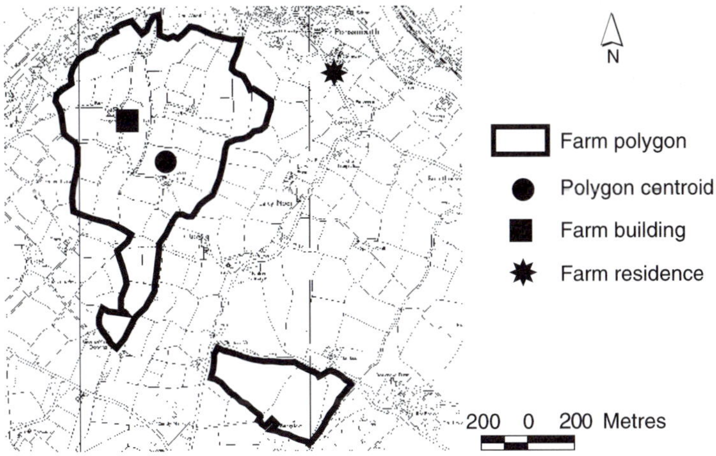

Fig. 2.2. The problem of how to spatially reference a farm as a single point, whether it be the farmer's residence in a village, the main farm building or the farm centroid. Adapted from Durr and Froggatt (2002).

the authorities when changes in ownership and usage occur, assisted by a set of rules setting the thresholds when this notification must apply. However, such a system risks an increase in database errors. At a crude level, error can be viewed as always occurring in a proportion of data points, and even an exceptionally well-maintained database would expect to have an error rate of at least 1–2% (Redman, 1992). Therefore, the absolute number of errors will, at a minimum, increase proportionally as the amount of information increases. However, this is often not the case, and moving to a more complex data capture and storage system increases the error rate substantially. More seriously, systematic errors (biases) are often introduced. For example, the system of notification of significant changes in farm boundaries and usage may not be implemented equally by all groups of farmers; for example, smallholders and those renting land may not consider that the system applies to them. One can see that without a large resource that allows regular 'ground truthing', after a period such a spatial database could become seriously degraded.

More thought along these lines soon leads to the conclusion that the problems of spatial resolution, uncertainty and error have no real answer; they involve a series of trade-offs, whereby trying to change one of the parameters inevitably affects the value of another. What is required is careful planning to establish the purpose of the spatial database and the resource that will be available to maintain it in the future. For example, if the particular study is at a low spatial resolution using data aggregated to an administrative boundary, a single point at any of the potential georeference locations for a farm (farmhouse, livestock buildings, farm centroid) would be sufficient. Conversely, for a high-resolution study investigating the spread of a disease between farms, data on the exact spatial relationships between the farms may be necessary. However, in this case it would be inadvisable to implement a system if money were available only to set up the system but not to maintain it.

The problem of error in spatial databases does not arise only at the data capture stage, but applies equally during storage and manipulation. Again, there is nothing unique about spatial data in this respect except for its volume and complexity and, therefore, the large number of processing steps it must pass though before the final output, such as a map, is produced. This is particularly a problem with desktop GIS systems, where the user may store data in a spreadsheet rather than a database and may not have been trained in systems of data integrity. The difficulty then arises that, if error is introduced it may be very hard to detect once a map has been produced, and a profound knowledge of the source data is needed in order to detect irregularities.

This problem of small data errors affecting the map and any decision that arises from it is illustrated by an example of a choropleth map of disease prevalence (Fig. 2.3a). Accompanying this is a map in which the source data have been accidentally modified by deleting one cell in the spreadsheet containing the source attribute data (Fig. 2.3b). As can be seen, the basic pattern is still there; nevertheless, a number of the areas have now been reclassified, which might have serious effects if animal disease management decisions were to be made on the basis of this classification. The problem for the end user with maps such as these, if they are produced to a high cartographic standard, is that they imply that the underlying data are of similar quality. A cliché in data science is 'garbage in–garbage out'; the trouble with GIS is 'garbage in–map out'!

2.3.3 Mapping and statistical analysis

Accepting all the difficulties involved in obtaining and maintaining reliable spatial data, it is possible with persistence to arrive at a map of the outcome of interest, this usually being either case locations (a dot map) or rates expressed on an area basis (a choropleth map). In both maps, a pattern will generally be evident, with aggregation of the cases (disease clusters) in the dot maps and areas of high rates being associated together (positive spatial autocorrelation) in the choropleth maps. Upon seeing such disease patterns, one's mind is inevitably drawn to an explanation in terms of underlying processes. This is in many ways the power of disease mapping, in that it encourages, even forces, an explanation and therefore the development of hypotheses about the causes

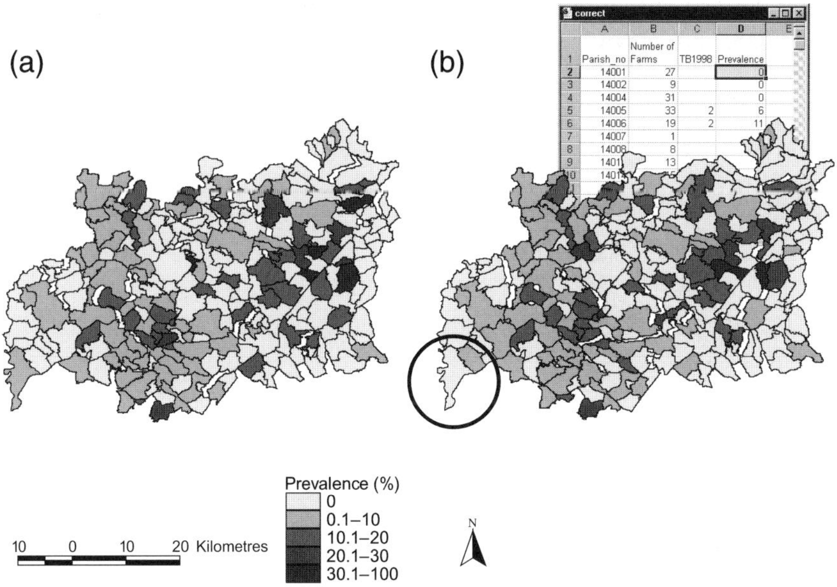

Fig. 2.3. A hypothetical example of the ease with which errors can be introduced into maps. Map (a) uses the correct data, while map (b) shows the effect of deleting a single cell in the spreadsheet containing the source data. The circled area highlights one of the regions that was misclassified after the error was made.

of the disease. However, this is one of the most difficult areas of spatial epidemiology and it contains many traps for the naive or unwary.

The key difficulty is that the human eye is highly evolved to detect pattern, even when objectively it does not exist. This phenomenon is well known to cartographers, and much of the skill in map production lies in using symbols, colour and pattern to highlight essential features of the data. Similarly, a host of different patterns can result from the aggregation and transformation of the data. There is nothing unique to maps here, and graphs can be similarly manipulated to show the data to best effect (Tufte, 1983). However, with maps it is much easier to deceive – either accidentally or deliberately – because of both our familiarity with them and the intrinsic difficulty of showing variability and uncertainty on them (Monmonier, 1996). Thus, for example, there is no agreed equivalent in cartography of the standard error bar used in a line graph to indicate the variability around the displayed averages.

These problems of map visualization can be made specific with an example: that of the FMD epidemic in Great Britain in 2001, illustrated by the maps shown in Fig. 2.4. These maps purport to show the same thing: a mapped summary of the disease situation 4 weeks after the start of the

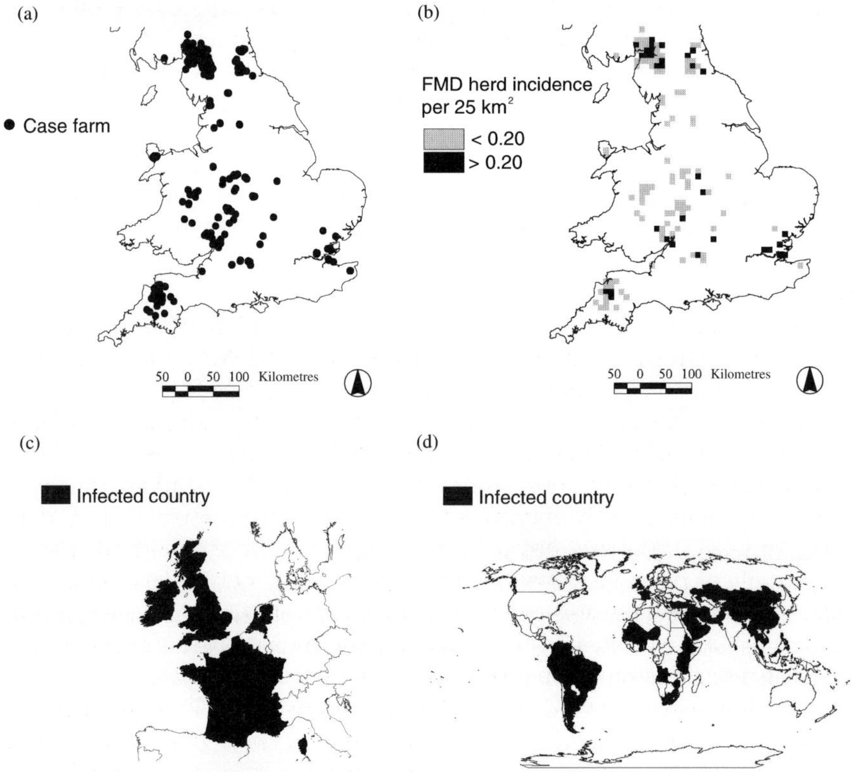

Fig. 2.4. The way in which cartographic display and data transformations can result in differing messages being given by a map, using the 2001 foot-and-mouth disease epidemic in Great Britain as an example. (a) Distribution of cases by the end of the first 4 weeks of the epidemic. (b) Calculated incidence at herd level. (c) Countries of Western Europe that were affected by the epidemic. (d) Countries reporting foot-and-mouth disease to the OIE, FAO or the World Reference Laboratory at Pirbright, UK in 2001. Data are from DEFRA and FAO.

epidemic. However, the data have been presented to show a gradient of seriousness, from the UK's point of view, from that showing an emergency situation with large clusters of case farms in hotspot areas (Fig. 2.4a) to a herd-level incidence map (Fig. 2.4b), which has been spatially smoothed with break points and colours selected to reduce visual impact. The map shown in Fig. 2.4c is problematic; although it is correct in showing that three other western European countries experienced FMD in this period, in all cases this was due to sheep exports from Great Britain, and the disease, once discovered, was quickly controlled. This map also shows the problem of comparing areas with widely different land areas. In this case, France is over-represented on the map, and distracts the eye from the main focus of the epidemic. In the final world map (Fig. 2.4d) the UK epidemic has been reduced to insignificance.

Many of the difficulties involved in map interpretation could potentially be resolved if they were accompanied by statistics that imposed objectivity on the user, such as probability levels and confidence intervals. Nevertheless, this is a troublesome area; spatial statistics, by virtue of the spatial autocorrelation, impairs the reliability of classical statistical analysis based on the assumption of independence (Legendre, 1993). In particular, positive spatial autocorrelation will reduce confidence intervals, leading to significance being declared for random associations. This phenomenon is well known to statisticians, and methods exist for both measuring it and adjusting analysis to take account of it in statistical models (Bailey and Gatrell, 1995). However, these methods require an understanding of quite advanced statistics, and an appropriate analysis frequently requires consultation with a specialist statistician, at least in the first instance of the application of a method. This is especially so because few of the methods are incorporated into standard statistical packages, and even fewer into GIS software packages, where spatial analysis extensions are currently simply a set of tools for geometric or grid cell manipulation (see Chapter 11).

To demonstrate some of the inherent complexity of spatial statistics, take the example shown in Fig. 2.5. These data were generated using a molecular typing procedure (spoligotyping) that identifies variability on a small part of the genome of the microbial cause of bovine tuberculosis, *Mycobacterium bovis* (Durr *et al.*, 2000b). During the years in question (1996–1998), as many isolates as possible were typed from infected cattle herds as well as from any badgers (a suspected wildlife reservoir) that were being trapped and autopsied as part of the then control strategy for the disease (see Chapter 10). The maps quite clearly show clustering of some types, such as spoligotype 9, but more startling is the strong spatial correlation between the types in cattle (Fig. 2.5a) and badgers (Fig. 2.5b). While this result is obvious, showing that there is a distinctive spatial association between the types in the two species, the rigorous statistical demonstration of this is a complex problem. Both the variables are multivariate (strictly, they are multinomial), making standard parametric generalized linear modelling techniques inappropriate – even those that allow for spatial dependence (see Chapter 1). An alternative is to apply non-parametric techniques, such as the extension of binary logistic regression to the multinomial case, using kernel estimation to construct risk surfaces for the variables (see Chapter 4). Nevertheless, there is a problem in the application of this technique to complex islands such as Great Britain, in that the implementation of kernel smoothing by currently available software does not recognize

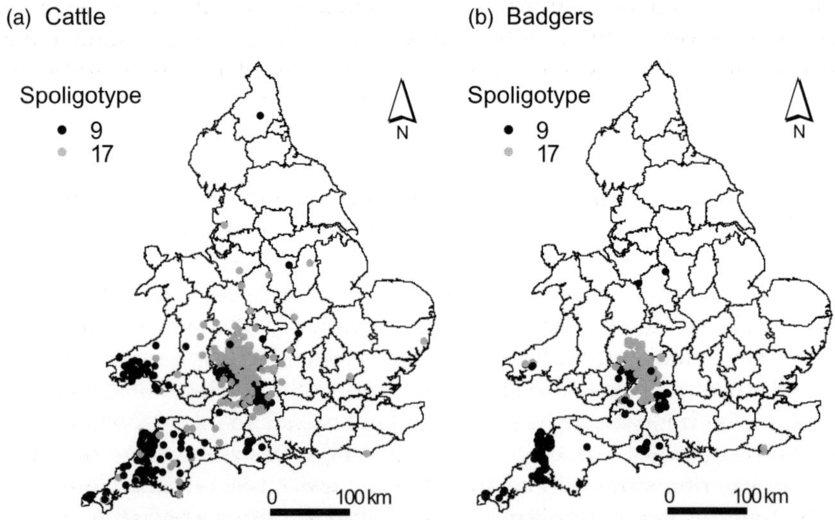

Fig. 2.5. Spatial distribution of selected *Mycobacterium bovis* spoligotypes from (a) cattle and (b) badgers in England and Wales, isolated during 1996–1998. Adapted from Durr *et al*. (2000b).

complex boundaries, in this case the coastline. This edge effect can be technically overcome with an integration algorithm, but is computationally intensive and requires software development. This example is yet another of the paradoxes of spatial statistics, wherein what is so obvious to the eye is complex to the computer.

2.3.4 Epidemiological interpretation

While statistical analyses can help reduce the subjectivity involved in simply reading a disease map, ultimately the final interpretation of any disease pattern depends upon the epidemiologist's understanding of the disease and its behaviour in the population. Where the behaviour of the disease is relatively simple and much is known about the epidemiology, as in the case of FMD, interpretation may be relatively straightforward. However, this is not the situation for the many problems in which a spatial analysis is required, and interpretation is frequently problematic. This applies to the two situations in which spatial analysis has been most frequently applied: detection of disease clusters and spatial correlation analysis.

The concept of *disease clustering* is an important one in environmental epidemiology, and arose largely out the need of public health authorities to respond to public disquiet about the effects on the incidence of cancer of putative sources of environmental contamination, such as nuclear power stations and toxic waste incinerators (Alexander and Boyle, 2000). These studies pose a large number of analytical problems, arising largely from the need to identify significant clusters from those developing by chance. More than 20 years of research have resulted in the development of sophisticated cluster analysis procedures; one of these uses the spatial scan statistic and involves the use of a moving window and adjustment for the aggregation of controls, and it generally results in the reliable identification of true clusters (Kulldorff, 1998). However, the identification of clusters has epidemiological meaning only if the clusters can be associated with a causal pathway (for example, if they are associated with areas of increased exposure), as almost all disease processes will lead to clustering to some degree (Rothman, 1990). This is most obvious in the case of infectious agents, where case clustering simply defines an agent as being contagious. Indeed, one of the pioneering studies in cluster analysis was undertaken to determine whether leukaemia in children is due to an infectious agent or to hereditary factors (Knox, 1964). Therefore, cluster identification by statistical procedures must really be considered an exploratory technique that aims to give some confidence that the clusters identified by the eye from case mapping are probably real and worthy of further attention, by further data collection and/or more detailed analysis. A problem has been that too frequently research papers have been published with disease clustering presented as the epidemiological result, as evidenced by a significant *P* value (Carpenter, 2001). Rather, it would be better to start out with the assumption that clustering will occur and to place the emphasis not so much on detecting it as on describing its nature and its causes (Rothman, 1990).

If cluster identification does lead to follow-up studies to explain their occurrence in terms of environmental covariates, this becomes an exercise in spatial association or correlation. At the crudest level, this can be done visually by simply comparing the distribution of the disease with the distribution of a measure of the purported risk factor. If this exploratory analysis indicates an association worth exploring, then this should lead on to spatial statistical modelling, for which established techniques and software are available (Bailey and Gatrell, 1995). However, equally troublesome is the epidemiological interpretation of a significant result. This problem arises because risk factors are generally always spatially correlated with other variables, which then become confounders. Thus, for example, pig farms that adopt outdoor farrowing may be geographically associated with a number of management and environmental covariates (such as being located on well-drained soils) that differ from those of farms that continue with indoor stall farrowing. If a new disease were to arise with a higher incidence in outdoor units, it would not be hard to show a spatial association with both of these soil factors, and probably a range of climatic ones as well, because soil and climate are so intricately intermingled. The epidemiologist's mantra of 'association does not equate with causation' applies as well to spatial epidemiology as to ordinary risk factor epidemiology, and what is really required is a plausible causal pathway. Even this may not be sufficient, as the chosen causal pathway may be only one of several alternatives. Such truisms, however, can easily get lost amidst high-quality mapping and sophisticated spatial statistics.

As a final note of caution in interpreting spatial association, it is particularly important to be wary of associations based upon large spatial units, as correlations typically increase with aggregation. This phenomenon is part of the 'modifiable area unit' problem (see Chapter 3), and if a spatial correlation is found at particular aggregation it is always worthwhile to establish whether it is also present at a lower level of aggregation. However, spatial error and uncertainty may increase correspondingly at this higher spatial resolution, and failure to show correlation between variables may be due to these effects rather than simply to the level of aggregation. As happens so frequently in any discussion about spatial epidemiology, the topic of concern returns to that of data quality.

2.4 A framework for using and applying spatial epidemiology

If the intrinsic difficulties of undertaking spatial epidemiology are accepted, the obvious question concerns the animal diseases for which it is most likely to be worth the effort. At one extreme, sceptics may point to the lack of examples in which spatial epidemiology has had a proven impact on understanding and controlling disease and the fact that many (even most) animal diseases were successfully investigated and controlled in the past century without recourse to a GIS or complex statistical analysis. Enthusiasts will probably counter with the reply that spatial epidemiology always provides some information, and even negative findings, such as there being no obvious spatial pattern to a disease, are useful. In this chapter a compromise position is adopted, one that provides some guidance as to when to expect the spatial element of animal disease to become important.

It is possible to define two broad end-uses of spatial epidemiology: epidemiological research and animal disease control (Fig. 2.6). The logic of this separation is not in terms of the tools and techniques used, or in either the requirement for spatial data or the control role played by disease mapping. Rather, it arises because these activities are carried out by different people working within distinct organizations with dissimilar aims and constraints. Thus, *disease control* is normally a governmental

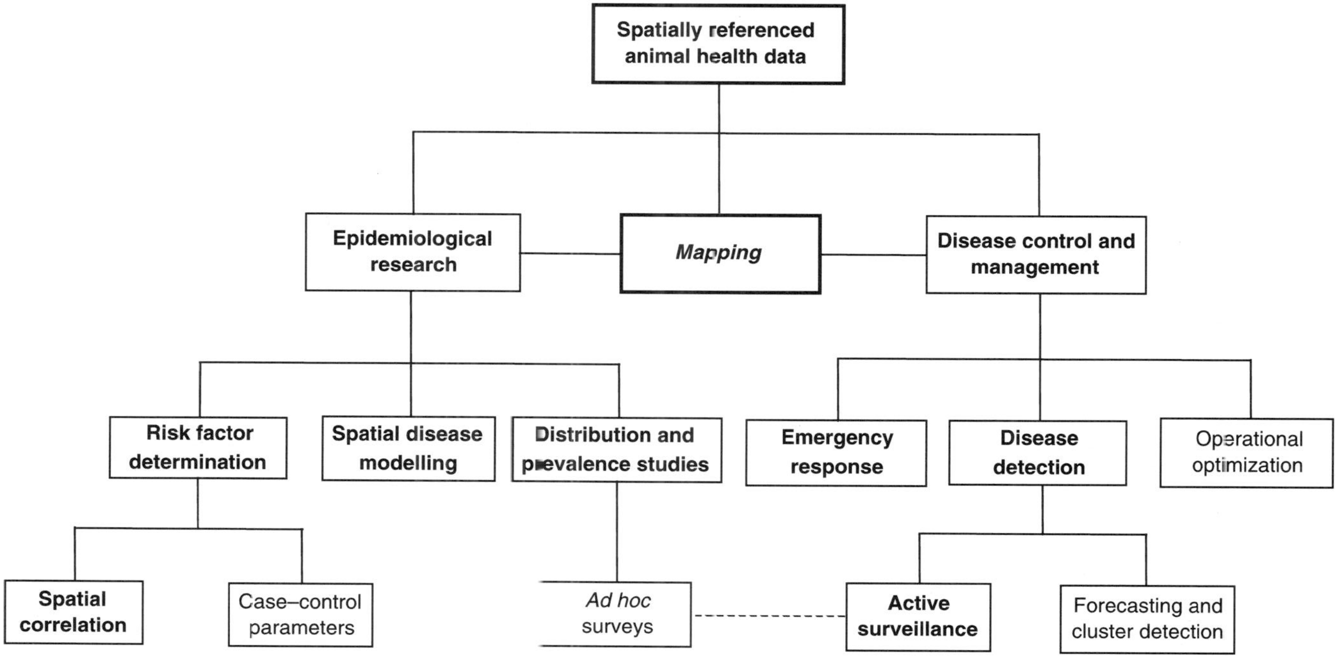

Fig. 2.6. A classification of the dominant uses of spatial epidemiology, showing a division between those of animal health managers and research workers. Note that both groups depend upon the same spatially referenced data and use the map as the key tool for exploratory data analysis.

responsibility in which the dominant aim is to minimize the economic impact of animal disease, especially those diseases that have major trade implications. By contrast, *epidemiological research* is more the activity of research institutes and universities and is generally orientated to answer specific questions about difficult problems, such as the identification of risk factors for new or emerging diseases. Although the parallels are not exact, a similar distinction between two disparate applications and user groups has long been recognized in medical geography, where the two traditions are termed 'health-care planning' and 'geographical epidemiology' (Mayer, 1982).

Some of the roles that have been identified in which GIS and an explicitly spatial approach are useful, such as theoretical modelling and emergency response, are discussed in detail in other chapters of this book (Chapters 7 and 9). Here we focus on two of the identified roles for spatial epidemiology: determining risk factors by spatial correlation and detecting disease by active surveillance. In both instances, the aim is to provide some practical guidance about when and where a spatial epidemiological approach may be appropriate.

2.4.1 GIS in epidemiological research: BSE and bovine tuberculosis in Great Britain

Bovine spongiform encephalopathy (BSE) and bovine tuberculosis (TB) have in common their seriousness for human health, their economic impact and the controversies that have surrounded their causal pathways. From a spatial epidemiological perspective, both are interesting because disease and risk factor maps have been used to argue for and against the importance of particular causal factors. Furthermore, in both instances teams of eminent scientists have investigated these causal pathways, and thus it is possible to gauge the impact of the spatial evidence presented.

BSE was identified formally in 1986, when an animal with symptoms of progressive neurological deterioration in the south-east of England underwent a rigorous post-mortem examination, the resulting histological analysis demonstrating pathology similar to that seen in scrapie in sheep (Wells *et al.*, 1987). To arrive at a better understanding of the disease, a system of case reporting was introduced, and by 1988 there was enough accumulated data to undertake an analysis (Wilesmith *et al.*, 1988). This showed that the disease outbreak was widely spread throughout the country and strongly associated with dairy farming, though with a higher herd incidence in the south-east (Fig. 2.7). This higher incidence was associated with certain feed mills and their use of meat and bone meal as a protein source for cattle feed, particularly that fed to prematurely weaned dairy calves. The hypothesis was advanced that a novel

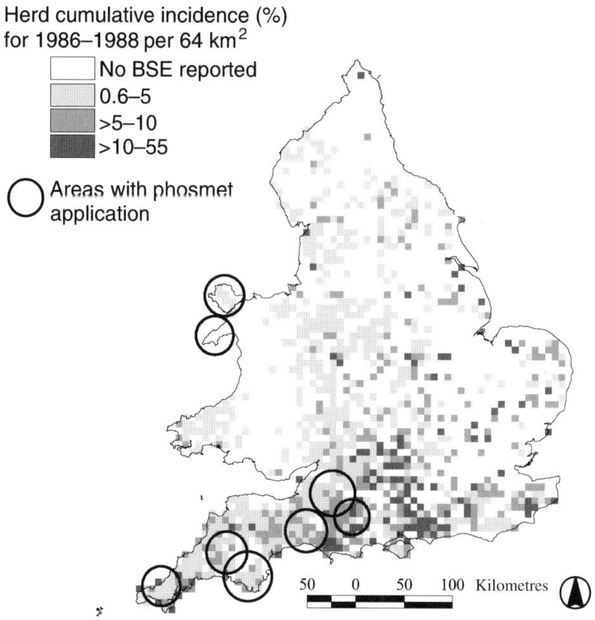

Fig. 2.7. Control areas for warble fly in the early 1980s. Areas where the insecticide phosmet was applied (circled) are superimposed on the cumulative incidence of BSE in cattle herds 1985–1988. Data are from DEFRA and CVO Reports 1981–1985.

scrapie-like organism – later identified as the prion PrP^{SC} – was infecting the calf feed, and that meat and bone meal derived from adult cattle several years earlier was responsible for the current cohort of cases.

The hypothesis of prion-contaminated cattle feed was adopted quickly by the veterinary and scientific establishment, and this led to a ban on the feeding of ruminant-derived meat and bone meal to calves in 1988. Nevertheless, alternative hypotheses about the cause of the disease were advanced, an early one being that it was associated with the use of an organophosphorus insecticide, phosmet (Purdey, 1994). This compound was used in the 1980s to treat warble fly as part of a national eradication plan. On account of its rapid degradation, this use was principally in dairy animals, in which milking could be resumed within 24 hours. In contrast, it was less frequently used in beef suckler animals, where the systemic medicine ivermectin was generally preferred.

The phosmet hypothesis received some publicity in the early stages of the BSE epidemic, but lost ground when the epidemic continued into the 1990s, despite the application of phosmet becoming minimal with the eradication of the warble fly from the national herd. However, in 1996, when a link between BSE and new variant Creutzfeldt–Jakob disease was established, there was a climate of media scepticism of established dogma about the disease and the hypothesis resurfaced. At this stage the role of the PrP^{SC} prion was generally accepted, but Purdey (1996) proposed that the use of organophosphates, aided by trace element imbalances, increased the susceptibility of the bovine brain to the effects of the prion.

The original and modified hypotheses were both sufficiently respectable to receive a mention in the report of a large public inquiry into BSE (Phillips *et al.*, 2000), and a follow-up review by a panel of scientists concerning the origin of BSE (G. Horn, M. Bobrow, M. Bruce, M. Goedert, A. McLean and J. Webster (2001) Review of the origin of BSE. Unpublished report, Department for Environment Food and Rural Affairs, London). However, the BSE Inquiry rejected the original organophosphorus hypothesis both because the epidemic continued after the use of phosmet had become minimal, and because of the spatial distribution of cases. In particular, the Channel Islands represented a natural experiment in that Guernsey, where no treatment against warble fly was carried out, had 669 cases of BSE, while Jersey had only 138 cases despite the use of the insecticide. A similar conclusion can be drawn if a comparison is made between those areas of England and Wales where phosmet was most likely used (eradication zones) for warble fly treatment and the distribution of the disease in the early years (Fig. 2.7). The modified hypothesis, linking trace element imbalances to susceptibility, similarly shows a poor spatial correlation, and a map showing this spatial mismatch was considered sufficient evidence to reject it (G. Horn, M. Bobrow, M. Bruce, M. Goedert, A. McLean and J. Webster (2001) Review of the origin of BSE. Unpublished report, Department for Environment Food and Rural Affairs, London).

While the example of phosmet and BSE is relatively straightforward, the opposite can be said concerning the role of the Eurasian badger (*Meles meles*) as a cause of infection of cattle with TB. As in the rest of Europe, the disease was widespread in the cattle population in Great Britain, but by the 1960s it had been successfully reduced by an eradication campaign to a very low prevalence. However, it persisted in two counties, Cornwall and Gloucestershire. This spatial patterning did not have a plausible explanation until 1971, when a severely infected badger was found on a farm with the problem (Muirhead *et al.*, 1974). The hypothesis that the badger was a source of disease for cattle was strengthened by subsequent trapping in high-incidence areas, supplemented by a national road traffic accident survey (Evans and Thompson, 1981; Cheeseman *et al.*, 1989). In all the years studied, a strong spatial association is evident between those areas where the disease was most prevalent in badgers and those where the problem in cattle persisted (Fig. 2.8). More recently, a spatial association has been shown between the genetic types of *Mycobacterium bovis* isolates in the two species (Fig. 2.5).

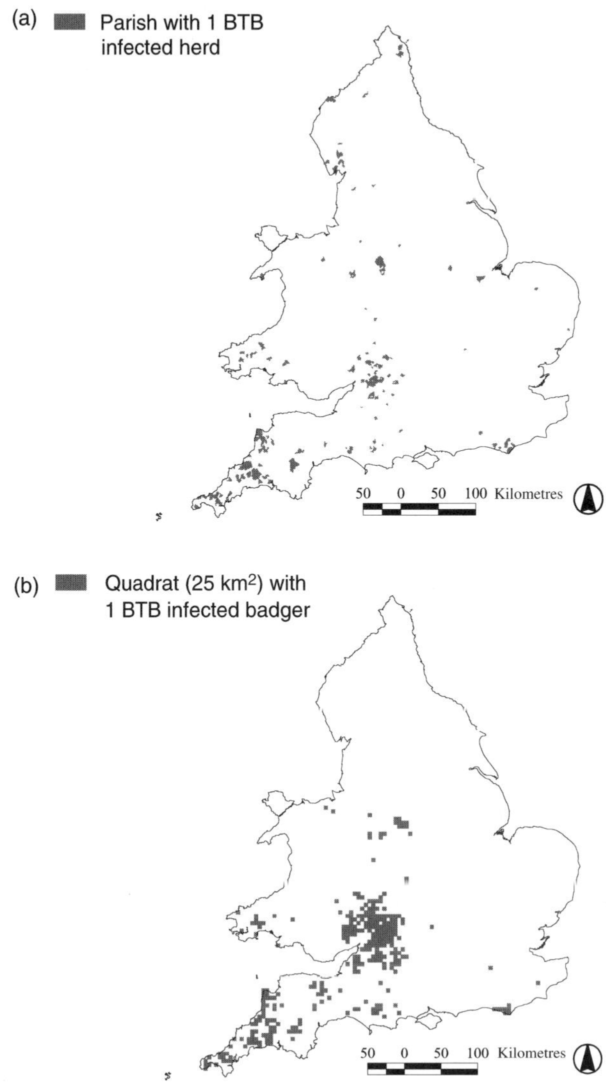

Fig. 2.8. The spatial association between bovine tuberculosis (BTB) in cattle herds and badgers as demonstrated by (a) parishes where at least one cattle herd was confirmed to have BTB in 1989/90, and (b) quadrats (25 km^2) where at least one infected badger was found between 1980 and 1989 during a national road traffic accident survey. Data are from DEFRA.

To many, maps such as these provide overwhelming evidence that badgers are a wildlife reservoir and the predominant cause of the continuing problem in cattle. However, there are flaws in such reasoning, as the pattern could equally be explained by transmission in the opposite direction, namely from cattle to badgers. Furthermore, it is plausible that a third species, such as deer, is acting as the true reservoir, infecting both cattle and badgers. What is required for an informed spatial epidemiological study is a long-term, properly structured survey that will be able to map the space–time dynamic of the disease in the main host species. If this were to show that, in each case, disease in one species is always (or mostly) preceded by disease in the others, then the spatial analysis could be shown to be (probably) causative. However, such a national surveillance strategy involving all purported wildlife reservoirs would be an extremely difficult and expensive undertaking. Not surprisingly, in the most recent review of the bovine TB problem a decision was made by the scientific review team to adopt an experimental approach, focused solely on the areas of high prevalence (Krebs *et al.*, 1997).

What lessons can be learnt for spatial epidemiology from these two examples? In general, disease and risk factor mapping was more successful in disproving a hypothesis than the reverse. Thus, the Purdey hypothesis was dismissed on the evidence of a spatial mismatch between a purported risk factor and the disease, despite some experimental evidence to support it. By contrast, when a good match was found, as in the case of the disease in cattle and badgers, this was considered not sufficient by itself, on the grounds of correlation not being causation. By extension, this indicates that spatial epidemiology may have an important role in screening purported risk factors, and in focusing research attention on factors for which the spatial patterning indicates that they may be plausible components of the causal pathway.

However, there are several important caveats to consider before making any recommendation to use spatial epidemiology in this way. First, because of the problem of multiple spatial associations, it is important to question the biological plausibility of a spatial correlation between disease and risk factor. For example, in the case of BSE it is possible to show a negative association between the incidence of the disease and altitude, and, presented with this 'fact', a number of contributory causes to the disease may be hypothesized. However, in this instance the association is spurious, arising from the spatial partitioning of beef suckler herds, which had few homebred cases of the disease, in the uplands and the dairy farms in the lowlands. Secondly, it is important to bear in mind the effects of aggregation on any maps in assessing spatial correlation and, in particular, the fact that spatial correlations may exist at one level of aggregation but disappear at another. It is interesting to note that Purdey (1994) used a map of data similar to that of Fig. 2.7 as evidence for his hypothesis, although his map was aggregated to a county level. It is one of the great strengths of GIS that it has made exploratory analysis of spatial data at differing resolutions and aggregations a relatively easy task, and this capacity should be used fully in any thorough spatial analysis designed to explore the role of epidemiological risk factors.

2.4.2 GIS in animal disease control: multidrug-resistant *Salmonella* Newport

The potential of GIS as a tool for animal disease control and management was first indicated for emergency responses to diseases, and in particular for dealing with the introduction of an exotic disease into a country (Sanson *et al.*, 1991). This proved to be the case in the massive epidemic of FMD in Great Britain in 2001, when GIS played a key role in both local operational activities and in deciding national strategy (see Chapter 9; Morris *et al.*, 2002). Nevertheless, this situation was exceptional because, in response to the seriousness of the emergency, resources were essentially not limiting and all attention was focused on the disease. Establishing a role for GIS in peacetime is more difficult, as a large number of endemic diseases potentially need to be managed or controlled, and laboratory and veterinary resources will always be insufficient for all the tasks at hand.

To illustrate the use of GIS in ordinary surveillance, I will use a topical example: that of an emerging organism, multidrug-resistant *Salmonella enterica* serotype Newport (MRSN). This bacterium is important mainly to the human population, in which it can cause serious enteric illness, and in susceptible groups (young children, the elderly and the immunocompromised) it may even be fatal. MRSN was first identified in 1984 (Holmberg *et al.*, 1984), and since that time has spread throughout North America (Anon., 2002). The bacterium has been isolated from a range of animals and from the environment, but is particularly prevalent in dairy cattle. Clinical outbreaks have been reported but, as with other salmonellae, asymptomatic infection can occur. Their importance lies in their capacity to multiply and become widely disseminated, particularly through the contamination of watercourses by slurry.

In 2002, a detailed risk assessment concluded that the most probable scenario for the introduction of this organism into Britain was via tourists from North America (E. Snary, A. Hill and M. Woolridge (2002) A qualitative risk assessment for multidrug-resistant *Salmonella* Newport. Unpublished report, Veterinary Laboratories Agency, Weybridge). The problem faced by disease control managers was how to implement a surveillance strategy to detect infection in the cattle population at the earliest possible stage and how to enable action to minimize environmental contamination and the spread of the organism. Developing such a strategy poses several problems: its exact epidemiological behaviour in Britain is uncertain; because it can be asymptomatic in cattle it may not be detected though clinical submissions; and only limited resources are available for enhanced surveillance. A more specific question is whether GIS might have a role in developing a cost-effective surveillance strategy.

In response, I proposed a GIS strategy with three tiers, which could

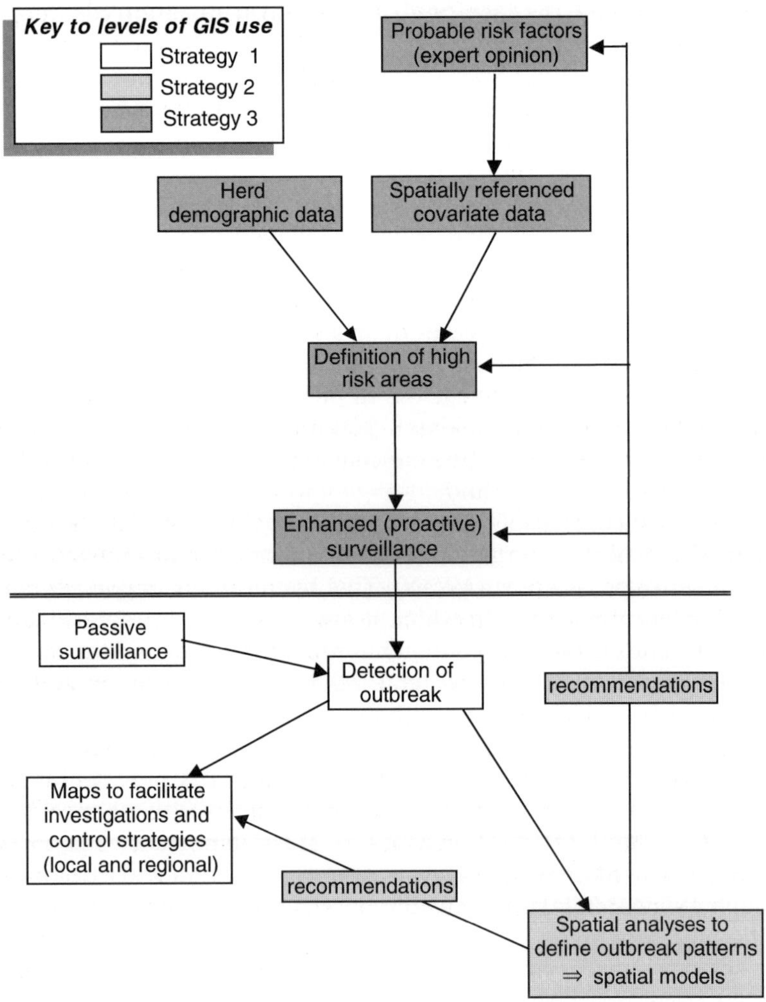

Fig. 2.9. A conceptual framework for applying spatial epidemiology to the problem of detection and control of multidrug-resistant *Salmonella* Newport in Great Britain.

be adopted successively depending upon the resources available for the problem (Fig. 2.9). The simplest (and cheapest) option would be to depend upon passive surveillance, in which no specific action for early detection would be undertaken apart from raising awareness of the organism among the veterinary profession, thus encouraging them to submit samples from cattle exhibiting typical clinical signs. Once MRSN was confirmed, an intensive epidemiological investigation of the affected farms would take place, in which GIS would have a key role. For example, mapping the farm and its natural features would help the investigators gain an overview and help visualize the relations between key epidemiological factors, such as the location of the infected cattle in relation to neighbouring farms, and the potential for contamination of watercourses by slurry. This strategy is considered technically feasible, because during the 2001 FMD epidemic veterinary and administrative staff in Great Britain gained considerable experience in the use of GIS.

While simple visualization of the local outbreak is considered the most cost-effective use of GIS, a better understanding of the disease would be possible by a spatial analysis, focusing particularly on the space–time dynamic of the disease. Although, like the first strategy, this would essentially be reactive once the infection had been identified, its implementation would require more planning, to ensure a sufficient skills base to carry out such analyses. Ideally, only epidemiologists with pre-existing experience with the techniques would undertake the analysis. However, this would entail the risk of these epidemiologists being overwhelmed if multiple outbreaks occurred. An alternative would be to develop specific analytical routines that could be implemented by trained local veterinary officers, the results of which would be incorporated into the outbreak investigation report. This would aid in understanding the behaviour of the epidemiology of the infection and could assist in improved surveillance in other areas.

The third option for the use of GIS for the MRSN problem would be its use to develop a surveillance strategy of on-farm visits and sampling. This differs from the previous two strategies in being proactive, in that it would put in place a system of national surveillance to try to detect this organism in the British cattle herd as early as possible, or alternatively to be confident that it had not already arrived. To achieve this, and in the absence of more specific information, it is assumed that MRSN would behave as a typical *Salmonella* serotype. A number of observational studies have been conducted on salmonellosis in cattle, the most recent being a longitudinal survey of a random sample of dairy herds in 2000, which aimed to identify risk factors for another multidrug-resistant salmonella, *S. typhimurium* DT104 (Davison *et al*., 2003). Only dairy farms were visited, as previous work had shown that these have a much greater risk of becoming infected than cattle at pasture (Evans and Davies, 1996). During the survey for DT104, other *Salmonella* species were cultured, generally from healthy or subclinically infected animals. Using the total *Salmonella* isolates as the response variable, the data were reanalysed to determine what factors were associated with farms having dairy cows that harboured the organism. A simple statistical model was developed which related this risk to herd size and the Ministry of Agriculture's six regional divisions (these are surrogates for unquantified environmental variables, such as rodent populations or

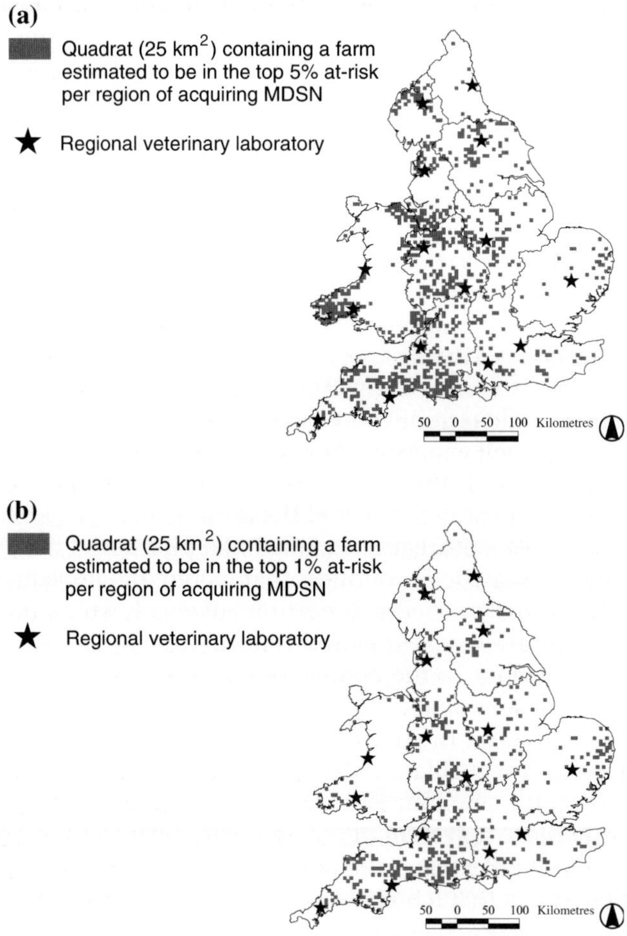

Fig. 2.10. Distribution of 25 km^2 quadrats containing at least one dairy farm hypothesized to be at a high risk of acquiring multidrug-resistant *Salmonella* Newport. (a) Top 5% of at-risk farms by Ministry of Agriculture region. (b) Top 1% of at-risk farms by region. Data are from DEFRA.

environmental survival of the bacteria). Using a GIS, it was possible to assign each dairy farm in the country a value of this risk function. Within each region, the top five percentiles of dairy farms with the highest risk ranking were then allocated to a 25 km^2 grid and those areas having at least one of these dairy farms were targeted for active surveillance (Fig. 2.10), and farmers and veterinarians were encouraged to submit samples from ill cattle with diarrhoea. Thus, the essence of the surveillance strategy was to replace single farms with a defined spatial area as the surveillance unit. This is a more cost-effective approach because for a highly contagious disease such as MRSN each farm can act as a sentinel for infection in its neighbours.

The benefit of such a GIS-based approach is that it makes explicit the costs and benefits of any proposed surveillance, and focuses upon the compromises that may have to be made to achieve this. For example, it may be decided that resource limitations mean that it is possible to visit not 5% but only 1% of the spatial areas containing dairy farms at risk, and the probability of detecting disease can be assessed under various scenarios. Accordingly, it may be concluded that the best strategy would be to combine elements of the existing passive surveillance for salmonellosis, whereby isolates of public health concern from clinically affected animals currently generate an advisory farm visit. Thus, high-risk quadrats might be visited as a system of supplementary active surveillance if no submission for *Salmonella* is reported from the passive surveillance within a defined period, such as the previous 3–6 months.

Ultimately, these decisions are not strictly epidemiological but rather managerial, as only a limited amount of resource (time, people, laboratory capacity) is available, and implementing a complex surveillance system for a disease not yet present in a country would be resisted if it had an adverse effect on other activities. GIS-based modelling has potential for managing this situation, as one of the biggest costs in active surveillance systems is the time needed to travel to the farms. For example, the farms within quadrats to be visited may be divided among laboratories or animal health offices by working out the travel time according to distance and the mean car speeds for different road classes within the network. Once all the data are accumulated (locations of offices and farms, and travel times), the actual calculations are readily undertaken in a GIS. The problem of needing to achieve multiple goals within the context of limiting resources is currently a topic of active GIS-based research ('multicriteria decision-making') and may well have a major impact on the design of animal health surveillance systems in the future (Robinson *et al.*, 2002).

2.5 Conclusion

Starting with a definition of spatial epidemiology, in this chapter I argue that this is a new and distinct subclass of epidemiology and briefly review its application to animal health problems. A 'spatial is special' argument is then followed, focusing upon the unique nature of spatial data and the complexities it adds to data collation, organization and analysis. In this context, I discuss the reasons why few spatial epidemiological projects properly bear fruit. However, there are practical examples of instances in which spatial epidemiology has successfully contributed real insight to animal health problems, and these are made specific in a discussion of two important diseases: BSE and bovine TB. I also attempt to provide, albeit somewhat indirectly, a conceptual framework for the use of spatial epidemiology in terms of the availability of resources, data, analytical skills and experience. According to this schema, the tools of spatial epidemiology, particularly GIS, can – and should – be used by all epidemiologists, in particular to visualize and explore the data. Nevertheless, true spatial epidemiology will remain a specialist subdiscipline, requiring a long-term commitment to data collection, a good understanding of geographical and ecological concepts and advanced statistical skills. The argument for multidisciplinary and even multi-institutional collaboration is strong if spatial epidemiology is to fulfil its potential.

Acknowledgements

Thanks are extended to Nigel Tait and Alice Froggatt for assistance in the production of the maps, John Wilesmith for useful discussions on the early years of the BSE epidemic, Robin Sayers for reanalysing the longitudinal study of *Salmonella* in dairy herds, and Sarah Evans for insight into the epidemiology of salmonellosis. This review was funded by DEFRA and VLA under three interrelated projects investigating the use of GIS for animal disease control (SE3001, SC0084 and SE3020).

References

Alexander, F.E. and Boyle, P. (2000) Do cancers cluster? In: Elliott, P., Wakefield, J.C., Best, N.G. and Briggs, D.J. (eds) *Spatial Epidemiology: Methods and Applications*. Oxford University Press, Oxford, pp. 302–316.

Anon. (2002) Outbreak of multidrug-resistant *Salmonella* Newport – United States, January–April 2002. *Morbidity and Mortality Weekly Report* 51, 545–548.

Bailey, T.C. and Gatrell, A.C. (1995) *Interactive Spatial Data Analysis*. Longman, Harlow, UK.

Baylis, M. and Rawlings, P. (1998) Modelling the distribution and abundance of *Culicoides imicola* in Morocco and Iberia using climatic data and satellite imagery. *Archives of Virology* Supplement 14, 137–153.

Carpenter, T.E. (2001) Methods to investigate spatial and temporal clustering in veterinary epidemiology. *Preventive Veterinary Medicine* 48, 303–320.

Cheeseman, C.L., Wilesmith, J.W. and Stuart, F.A. (1989) Tuberculosis: the disease and its epidemiology in the badger, a review. *Epidemiology and Infection* 103, 113–125.

Davison, H.C., Smith, R.P., Sayers, A.R., Pascoe, S.J.S., Davies, R.H. and Evans, S.J. (2003) Identification of risk factors associated with the *Salmonella* status of dairy herds in England and Wales. *Research in Veterinary Science* 74 (Supplement A), 2.

Durr, P.A. and Froggatt, A.E.A. (2002) How best to geo-reference farms? A case study from Cornwall, England. *Preventive Veterinary Medicine* 56, 51–62.

Durr, P.A., Argyraki, A., Ramsey, M. and Clifton-Hadley, R.S. (2000a) Agro-ecological databases for spatial correlation studies: methodological issues. In: Thrusfield, M.V. and Goodall, E.A. (eds) *Proceedings of the Society for Veterinary Epidemiology & Preventive Medicine, University of Edinburgh, 29th – 31st March, 2000*, pp. 225–235.

Durr, P.A., Clifton-Hadley, R.S. and Hewinson, R.G. (2000b) Molecular epidemiology of bovine tuberculosis: II. Applications of genotyping. *Revue Scientifique et Technique Office International des Epizooties* 19, 689–701.

Evans, H.T.J. and Thompson, H.V. (1981) Bovine tuberculosis in cattle in Great Britain. 1: Eradication of the disease from cattle and the role of the badger (*Meles meles*) as a source of *Mycobacterium bovis* for cattle. *Animal Regulation Studies* 3, 191–216.

Evans, S. and Davies, R. (1996) Case control study of multiple-resistant *Salmonella typhimurium* DT104 infection of cattle in Great Britain. *Veterinary Record* 139, 557–558.

Gilg, A.W. (1973) A study in agricultural disease diffusion: the case of the 1970–71 fowl-pest disease. *Transactions of the Institute of British Geographers* 59, 77–97.

Goodchild, M.F. and Gopal, S. (eds) (1989) *The Accuracy of Spatial Databases.* Taylor and Francis, London.

Hay, S.I., Randolph, S.E. and Rogers, D.J. (eds) (2000) *Remote Sensing and Geographical Information Systems in Epidemiology*. Academic Press, London.

Hertz-Picciotto, I. (1998) Environmental epidemiology. In: Rothman, K.J. and Greenland, S. (eds) *Modern Epidemiology,* 2nd edn. Lippincott Williams and Wilkins, Philadelphia, Pennsylvania, pp. 555–583.

Holmberg, S.D., Osterholm, M.T., Senger, K.A. and Cohen, M.L. (1984) Drug-resistant *Salmonella* from animals fed anitmicrobials. *New England Journal of Medicine* 311, 617–622.

Howe, G.M. (1989) Historical evolution of disease mapping in general and specifically of cancer mapping. *Recent Results In Cancer Research* 114, 1–21.

King, E.J., Lovell, D.J. and Harris, S. (1999) Effect of climate on the survival of *Mycobacterium bovis* and its transmission to cattle herds in south-west Britain. In: Cowan, D.P. and Fear, C.J. (eds) *Proceedings of the 1st European vertebrate management conference, University of York, 1–3 September, 1997.* Filander Verlag, Fürth, Germany, pp. 147–161.

Kitron, U. (1998) Landscape ecology and epidemiology of vector-borne diseases: tools for spatial analysis. *Journal of Medical Entomology* 35, 435–445.

Knox, E.G. (1964) Epidemiology of childhood leukemia in Northumberland and Durham. *British Journal of Preventive and Social Medicine* 18, 17–24.

Kopecky, K. (1977) Distribution of paratuberculosis in Wisconsin, by soil regions. *Journal of the American Veterinary Medical Association* 170, 320–324.

Krebs, J.R., Anderson, R., Clutton-Brock, T., Morrison, I., Young, D. and Donnelly, C. (1997) *Bovine tuberculosis in cattle and badgers. Report to the Rt Hon Dr Jack Cunningham MP.* MAFF Publications, London.

Kulldorff, M. (1998) Statistical methods for spatial epidemiology: tests for randomness. In: Gatrell, A. and Löytönen, M. (eds) *GIS and Health.* Taylor and Francis, London, pp. 49–62.

Legendre, P. (1993) Spatial autocorrelation: trouble or new paradigm? *Ecology* 74, 1659–1673.
Lessard, P., L'Eplattenier, R., Norval, R.A.I., Kundert, K., Dolan, T.T., Croze, H., Walker, J.B., Irvin, A.D. and Perry, B.D. (1990) Geographical information systems for studying the epidemiology of cattle diseases caused by *Theileria parva*. *Veterinary Record* 126, 255–262.
Lineback, N.G. (1980) A model of rabies diffusion. *Southeastern Geographer* 20, 1–15.
Linthicum, K.J., Bailey, C.L., Davies, F.G. and Tucker, C.J. (1987) Detection of Rift Valley fever viral activity in Kenya by satellite remote sensing imagery. *Science* 235, 1656–1659.
Martin, S.W., Meek, A.H. and Willeberg, P. (1987) *Veterinary Epidemiology: Principles and Methods*. Iowa State University Press, Ames, Iowa.
Mayer, J.D. (1982) Relationships between two traditions of medical geography: health systems planning and geographical epidemiology. *Progress in Human Geography* 16, 216–230.
McGrath, S.P. and Loveland, P.J. (1992) *Soil Geochemical Atlas of England and Wales*. Blackie, Glasgow, UK.
Meade, M.S. and Earickson, R. (2000) *Medical Geography*. Guilford Press, New York.
Monmonier, M. (1996) *How to Lie With Maps*, 2nd edn. University of Chicago Press, Chicago, Illinois.
Morris, R.S., Sanson, R.L., Stern, M.W., Stevenson, M. and Wilesmith, J.W. (2002) Decision-support tools for foot and mouth disease control. *Revue Scientifique et Technique Office International des Epizooties* 21, 557–567.
Muirhead, R.H., Gallagher, J. and Burn, K.J. (1974) Tuberculosis in wild badgers in Gloucestershire: epidemiology. *Veterinary Record* 95, 552–555.
Ollerenshaw, C.B. (1966) The approach to forecasting the incidence of fascioliasis over England and Wales 1958–1962. *Agricultural Meteorology* 3, 35–53.
Phillips, L., Bridgeman, J. and Ferguson-Smith, M. (2000) *The BSE Inquiry. Volume 2: Science*. The Stationery Office, London, pp. 89–91. http://www.bseinquiry.gov.uk/
Purdey, M. (1994) Are organophosphate pesticides involved in the causation of bovine spongiform encephalopathy (BSE)? *Journal of Nutritional Medicine* 4, 43–82.
Purdey, M. (1996) The UK epidemic of BSE: slow virus or chronic pesticide-initiated modification of the prion protein? Part 2: An epidemiological perspective. *Medical Hypotheses* 46, 445–454.
Redman, T.C. (1992) *Data Quality: Management and Technology*. Bantam Books, New York.
Reviriego, F., Moreno, M. and Dominguez, L. (2000) Soil type as a putative risk factor of ovine and caprine paratuberculosis seropositivity in Spain. *Preventive Veterinary Medicine* 43, 43–51.
Robinson, T.P., Harris, R.S., Hopkins, J.S. and Williams, B.G. (2002) An example of decision support for trypanosomiasis control using a geographical information system in eastern Zambia. *International Journal of Geographical Information Science* 16, 345–360.
Rogers, D.J. and Randolph, S.E. (1991) Mortality rates and population density of tsetse flies correlated with satellite imagery. *Nature* 351, 739–741.

Rothman, K.J. (1990) A sobering start for the cluster busters' conference. *American Journal of Epidemiology* 132, S6–S13.

Sanson, R.L., Pfeiffer, D.U. and Morris, R.S. (1991) Geographic information systems: their application in animal disease control. *Revue Scientifique et Technique Office International des Epizooties* 10, 179–195.

Schwabe, C.W., Riemann, H.P. and Franti, C.E. (1977) *Epidemiology in Veterinary Practice*. Lea and Febiger, Philadelphia, Pennsylvania, pp. 114–131.

Thrusfield, M. (1995) *Veterinary Epidemiology*, 2nd edn. Blackwell Science, Oxford.

Tinline, R.R. (1970) Lee wave hypothesis for the initial pattern of spread during the 1967–8 foot and mouth epizootic. *Nature* 227, 860–862.

Tufte, E.R. (1983) *The Visual Display of Quantitative Information*. Graphics Press, Cheshire, Connecticut.

Wells, G.A.H., Scott, A.C., Johnson, C.T., Gunning, R.F., Hancock, R.D., Jeffrey, M., Dawson, M. and Bradley, R. (1987) A novel progressive spongiform encephalopathy in cattle. *Veterinary Record* 121, 419–420.

Wilesmith, J.W., Wells, G.A.H., Cranwell, M.P. and Ryan, J.B.M. (1988) Bovine spongiform encephalopathy: epidemiological studies. *Veterinary Record* 123, 638–644.

Wint, G.R.W., Robinson, T.P., Bourn, D.B., Durr, P.A., Hay, S.I., Randolph, S.E. and Rogers, D.J. (2002) Mapping bovine tuberculosis in Great Britain using environmental data. *Trends in Microbiology* 10, 441–444.

Yeoman, G.H. (1966a) Field vector studies of epizootic East Coast fever. I. A quantitative relationship between *R. appendiculatus* and the epizooticity of East Coast fever. *Bulletin of Epizootic Diseases of Africa* 14, 5–27.

Yeoman, G.H. (1966b) Field vector studies of epizootic East Coast fever. II. Seasonal studies of *R. appendiculatus* on bovine and non-bovine hosts in East Coast fever enzootic, epizootic and free areas. *Bulletin of Epizootic Diseases of Africa* 14, 113–140.

Yeoman, G.H. (1967) Field vector studies of epizootic East Coast fever. III. Pasture ecology in relation to *R. appendiculatus* infestation rates on cattle. *Bulletin of Epizootic Diseases of Africa* 15, 89–113.

3 Geographical Information Science and Spatial Analysis in Human Health: Parallels and Issues for Animal Health Research

Anthony C. Gatrell

3.1 Introduction

My aim here is to identify some of the issues, of a representational and analytical nature, with which geographers wrestle when seeking to understand and model the distribution of human disease or ill-health in a spatial setting. I do so in order to see what common ground there is, or might be, between geographical epidemiologists dealing with human disease and ill-health and colleagues whose research interests lie in the animal world. Of course, the two interests intersect, as there is a common concern with vector-borne disease.

I structure my account using three broad headings. First, I consider the area of visualization, where we seek some graphical or visual representation of health or disease data. Included in this section is a discussion of issues of spatial representation and spatial referencing of the objects of enquiry, and I also introduce to veterinary scientists what may be a novel and potentially useful map transformation. Next, I consider exploratory spatial data analysis, in which visual and statistical methods are combined in order to gain insights into disease distribution. Here, we lack explicit hypotheses to test; rather, we search for structure and pattern in our data, with a view, perhaps, to deriving hypotheses that may be tested elsewhere. Lastly, I turn to modelling, where we do have one or more explicit hypotheses to test. In this section I consider four areas of modelling. First, I examine spatial diffusion modelling, an area to which geographers have made highly original contributions (some of which have attracted the attention of veterinary scientists). Next, I consider the relatively new method of multilevel modelling, in which explanation of a health problem requires information from different hierarchical levels. Thirdly, I wish to say something about the broad area of environmental modelling, in particular the sense in which we might model the relationship between disease and environment, with a view to assessing the health consequences of large-scale environmental change. Lastly, and in a very different context, I draw attention to modelling the location of health facilities to serve a population or to deal with a public health problem. An excellent overview of many of these ideas, couched within a geographical information system (GIS) framework, is provided by Cromley and McLafferty (2002); see also the collection of papers edited by Gatrell and Löytönen (1998).

I refer in the title to geographical information *science* rather than geographical information *systems*. This is to suggest that my interest is less in software aspects and more in the underlying conceptual issues, many of which are shared in veterinary epidemiology (see Chapters 1 and 2).

3.2 Visualization

3.2.1 Spatial representation and georeferencing

In any geographical analysis of the distribution of human disease or illness we have to ask ourselves what the objects of analysis are. In a sense, this is unproblematic; people, not areas, get ill, and so a group of people with the same disease form the object of analysis. Yet this is deeply problematic in practice. For one thing, unless we work closely with those undertaking a diagnosis we shall rarely have access to individual data and the addresses of individual cases. Even if we did, then for entirely appropriate reasons of patient confidentiality we would not wish to map them as point objects, unless we could undertake some random 'jittering' of the point locations so as to mask the correct addresses (a procedure proposed by Rushton (1998, pp. 65–66) and other authors). From a more conceptual point of view, we ask ourselves whether the address at diagnosis is an appropriate form of spatial representation. In the case of diseases with lengthy latency periods, when exposure to some environmental insult may have occurred years earlier, this may be quite uninformative (a point I return to later). In the case of some adult populations, the residential address may be uninformative for other reasons, since people do not remain at home 24 hours a day waiting to be exposed to some pathogen or pollutant; rather, they have daily and weekly 'activity spaces', comprising locations (workplaces, leisure centres, shops, and the like), the set of which for any individual will overlap, to a greater or lesser extent, with those of others (Schærstrom, 1996). With few exceptions, rather little progress has been made in getting to grips with the fluidity of human behaviour and its consequences for understanding disease distribution or diffusion. Rather than conceiving 'location' as a single, fixed-point framework for the analysis of disease events, perhaps we should be exploring the feasibility of multiple, overlapping sets of points. In terms of spatial relationships between individual cases (typically measured by the Euclidean distance between pairs of point locations), should we be devising new metrics that reflect social interactions between pairs of people? Put simply, if their activity spaces do not intersect, the direct distance from one individual to another is infinity, though they may well come into contact via some intermediary source. Clearly, there are similar issues in companion veterinary epidemiology, where simply georeferencing a dog-owner's home address is not necessarily informative if we want to look at its risk of developing respiratory disease (see Chapter 1).

As an alternative to using individual place of residence, health or medical geographers use systems of spatial or areal units of varying levels of resolution. These are much more common in published work, since, as noted above, confidentiality may prevent either the release or the use of individual data.

The problems with area data are several. Usually, there is a preference to have the areas as small as possible, since if we wish to examine local variations in disease risk we are more likely to detect such variation at a fine level or resolution. On the other hand, data for small areas will be subject to considerable Poisson variation; counts will typically be small, making any estimate of disease risk highly unstable. There are statistical methods for dealing with the problem of small numbers, or alternative strategies of simply extending the data collection period (Bailey and Gatrell, 1995; see also pp. 124–127).

One issue that has not yet benefited from sufficient research concerns the relevance of the underlying space for the variable being mapped. *Choropleth maps* shade the zone or areal unit uniformly according to value. Yet the variable being mapped may relate to something that can only occupy a fraction of the space. For example, if we have a zone that comprises 95% forest and 5% built-up area and we are mapping a disease, it surely makes most sense to restrict the shading of incidence to the built-up area. Cartographers refer to this as 'dasymetric mapping'. It does not seem yet to have been widely implemented in GISystems (Martin, 1991, pp. 146–148).

A major problem with area data is that the zones are usually rather arbitrary in nature. Whether the data concern communes, counties, electoral districts, health areas or some other system, the boundaries frequently have little meaning and the zoning system itself is inherently arbitrary (Fig. 3.1). This has led researchers to speak of the 'modifiable areal unit problem' (MAUP), on which a considerable volume of research

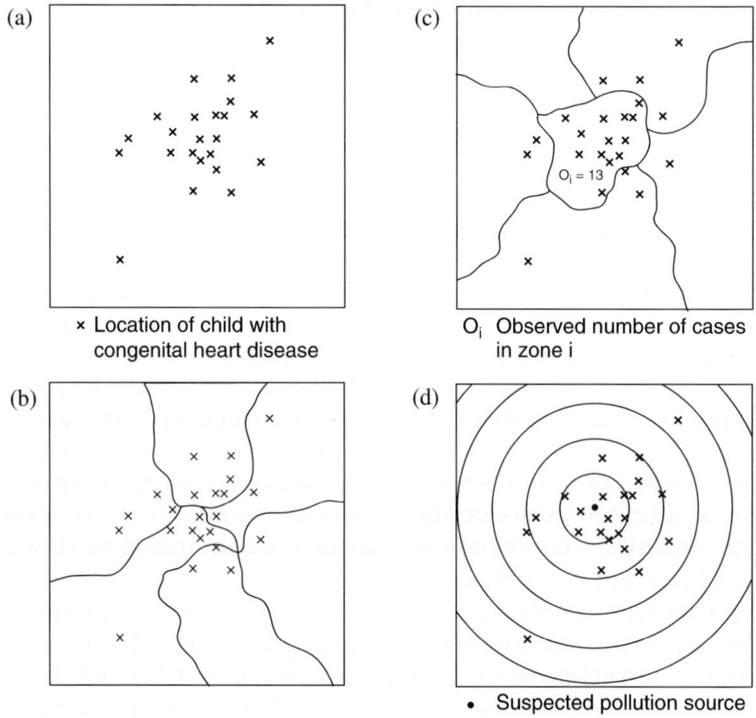

Fig. 3.1. The modifiable areal unit problem. From Gatrell (2002).

activity has been expended (see, for example, Alvanides *et al.*, 2002; Gatrell, 2002, pp. 53–54). Such research shows that the results of analysis are strongly dependent on the system of areal units deployed; change this and the results alter.

A further problem is that the small areas invariably form a patchwork quilt of zones, of irregular size and shape. Typically, the largest zones are the most sparsely populated, rural ones, so that if we produce a shaded choropleth map with the shade or colour relating to disease rate or risk, our eye may well be drawn to those large zones that, in fact, carry a lower disease burden than the much smaller urban ones. One solution is to forgo the blanket shading of areas and to simply locate a small symbol in the less densely populated areas. Another is to transform the underlying geography. It is to this strategy that we now turn, though not without noting that conventional choropleth maps demand considerable care and thought in terms of the selection of class intervals and shading and colour schemes (Monmonier, 1996).

3.2.2 Cartograms: new maps for old problems

Rather than represent 'container space' as a set of areal units whose size represents land area, we might prefer to have the size of the units proportional to the underlying population at risk. This kind of (iso)demographic base map or population cartogram (also known as a density-equalizing map projection) has been in use, though hardly in common currency, for many years (for an early epidemiological application see Raisz, 1934; Forster, 1966). Before the advent of modern computing environments cartograms were produced by hand and, because graph paper was used, they had a blocky appearance; a unit square on this represented a fixed population. Most examples seek to preserve adjacency or contiguity, though this is not a simple matter and the resulting distortion may render the map unintelligible to the lay reader. As a result, some authors forgo the requirement for strict contiguity between areal units and derive non-contiguous cartograms, using circles or other symbols to represent the areal units, packing them together in such a way as to maintain the look of the conventional map (Dorling, 1995, 1996).

A number of techniques have been devised to automate the construction of contiguous area cartograms, though all of them work on the principle of iteratively moving the points on a digitized boundary file. The publication of an algorithm by Gusein-Zade and Tikunov (1993) breathed new life into this area. Some authors (Selvin *et al.*, 1988; Merrill *et al.*, 1996) have used various algorithms in epidemiological contexts, both transforming the base map and also simultaneously mapping point locations of disease cases onto the transformed map. Since population density is constant over the transformed map, the distribution of point events under a hypothesis of no spatial clustering should follow complete spatial randomness. This can be assessed using nearest neighbour techniques. An application to 401 cases of childhood cancer in four California counties, diagnosed between 1980 and 1988, shows some evidence of spatial clustering (Merrill *et al.*, 1996). Other methods, such as the spatial scan statistic developed by Kulldorff (for a review of this and other methods, see Kulldorff, 1998), allow us to detect the locations of clusters. The spatial scan statistic is beginning to attract a variety of epidemiological applications (e.g. Hjalmars *et al.*, 1996; Kulldorff *et al.*, 1997). Kulldorff's approach does not require the prior transformation of geographical space, since it can allow for variation in background risk.

3.3 Exploratory spatial data analysis

The distinction between visualization and exploratory analysis is becoming increasingly blurred, to the extent that some research groups (e.g. at Pennsylvania State University) speak of 'exploratory visualization'. This means the integration of tools designed to map spatial data but also to detect pattern and structure, such integration being made possible by software that permits the interactive linking of different views of the data (MacEachren *et al.*, 1997).

3.3.1 Density estimation

A number of methods have been devised for the exploratory analysis of spatial point (event) data, depending on the purpose of the investigation. For example, *K*-functions (Diggle and Chetwynd, 1991; Bailey and Gatrell, 1995) are now quite widely used to assess generalized disease clustering (see pp. 131–132). If we wish to assess instead the nature of spatial variation in disease risk (in the absence of any explicit hypothesis) there are other methods available. We noted above the spatial scan statistic, but an earlier example, devised by the geographer Stan Openshaw (Openshaw *et al.*, 1987), was the geographical analysis machine (GAM), the construction of which was motivated, like similar work, by the question of varying risk of childhood leukaemia in northern England (and, indeed, the hypothesis that this was associated with proximity to a nuclear installation).

Using point data for both cases and a population at risk (or suitable controls), we can derive an estimate of the spatial variation in disease risk using kernel or density estimation. Graphically, this amounts to superimposing a kernel function of fixed size and radius over all locations on the map and estimating the local density (weighted according to distance and depending on the shape of the kernel function). If we do this for both cases and controls we may form a relative risk surface by taking the ratio of the case and control densities at any given point. If there is no variation in relative risk we would expect the resulting surface to be uniformly flat; to the extent that it is not, we can identify hotspots or coldspots of high and low relative risk. Because of sampling fluctuation we can always expect some of these by chance, but the significance or otherwise of peaks and troughs may be assessed using Monte Carlo simulation methods. To give an example (Gatrell, 2002), consider the data on babies born with cardiovascular malformations in part of north-west England between 1985 and 1994, shown in Fig. 3.2a. Using healthy births as controls (Fig. 3.2b), the relative risk surface shows no significant spatial variation (Fig. 3.2c); in this study the sample size was very small (138 cases) and more data would be needed to detect any significant variation. In the USA, Rushton (1998) has applied similar ideas to data on infant mortality in Des Moines, Iowa, and the method is attracting attention in veterinary epidemiology (see pp. 127–129).

Interestingly, this idea can be applied to births of males and females,

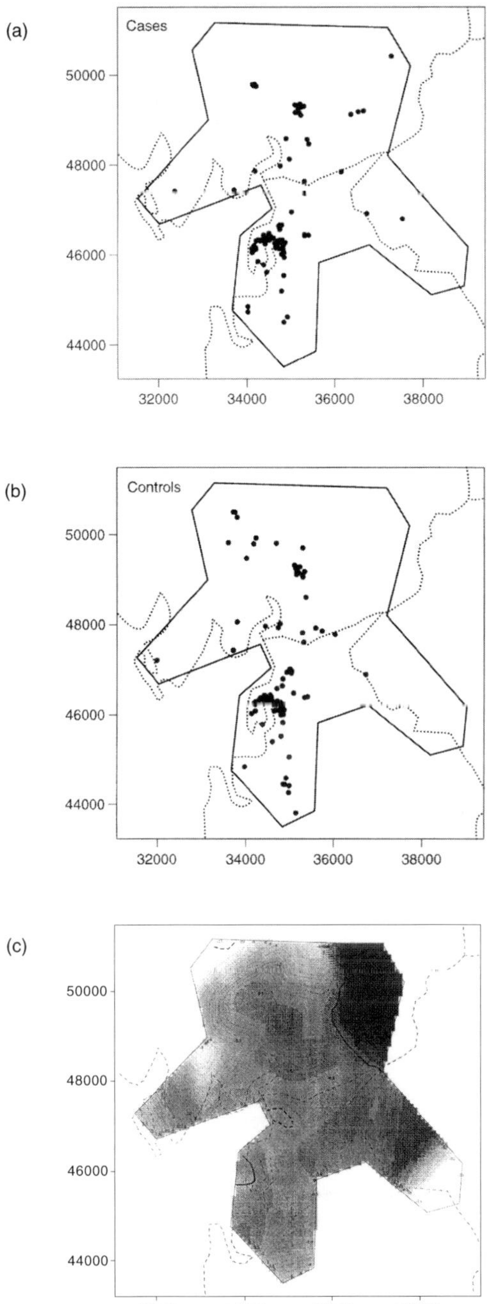

Fig. 3.2. Distribution of (a) cases of cardiac malformations and (b) controls in north Lancashire and south Cumbria, UK, and (c) a relative risk surface. From Gatrell (2002).

and the relative risk of a male compared with a female birth can be assessed. Allowing for the slight excess of male births, we would not expect spatial variation in relative risk. However, some writers (Lloyd *et al.*, 1985) have pointed to an unusual sex ratio downwind of a pollution source in Scotland and consider that this might be a marker of exposure to pollution. After the Seveso explosion in Italy in 1976, which released dioxins into the environment, research showed considerable change in the sex ratio (Mocarelli *et al.*, 1996). Following a suggestion from the author to pursue this idea further, Kelsall and Diggle (1995) took data on male and female births in the north-west of London and examined spatial variation in the ratio of male to female births; no significant variation of this kind was found.

3.2.2 Exploratory analysis of area data

Ian Bracken and David Martin (Martin, 1991, pp. 153–158; Martin, 2002) have applied similar ideas of density estimation in deriving raster-based 'surfaces' of socioeconomic data. This obviates the need for working exclusively with the 'patchwork quilts' referred to earlier, and offers interesting scope for epidemiologists whose environmental data may come only in a raster-based form. This is clearly important in environmental modelling (see Section 3.4).

Margaret Oliver (1996) has demonstrated how broadly similar ideas of density estimation may be applied to area data in an epidemiological setting. This draws on geostatistics, a field orientated more towards the handling of spatially continuous environmental data (for an introduction see Bailey and Gatrell, 1995). Oliver takes data on the incidence of childhood cancer in the West Midlands – 345 cases diagnosed between 1980 and 1984 distributed over a set of 840 electoral wards, many of which have no cases resident there. The incidence rates are used to estimate and model a variogram, a function that relates the similarity of rates between areas located at different distances or spatial lags (see also pp. 17–19). This in turn is used for spatial interpolation of cancer risk, in a procedure known as *kriging* (see Chapter 1). In Oliver's example (Fig. 3.3), rural and suburban areas are those of highest risk. Kriging also offers a map of the distribution of 'estimation variance', which highlights where observations are most sparse. Whether or not this approach offers any advantage over those which represent (and more especially, seek to model) risk by area is a moot point, but in seeking a continuous spatial representation of risk it is similar in spirit to the density estimation of point data.

As noted in Chapter 1, the variogram is closely related to a spatial autocorrelation function, which represents spatial dependence over various distances. The use of spatial autocorrelation statistics in

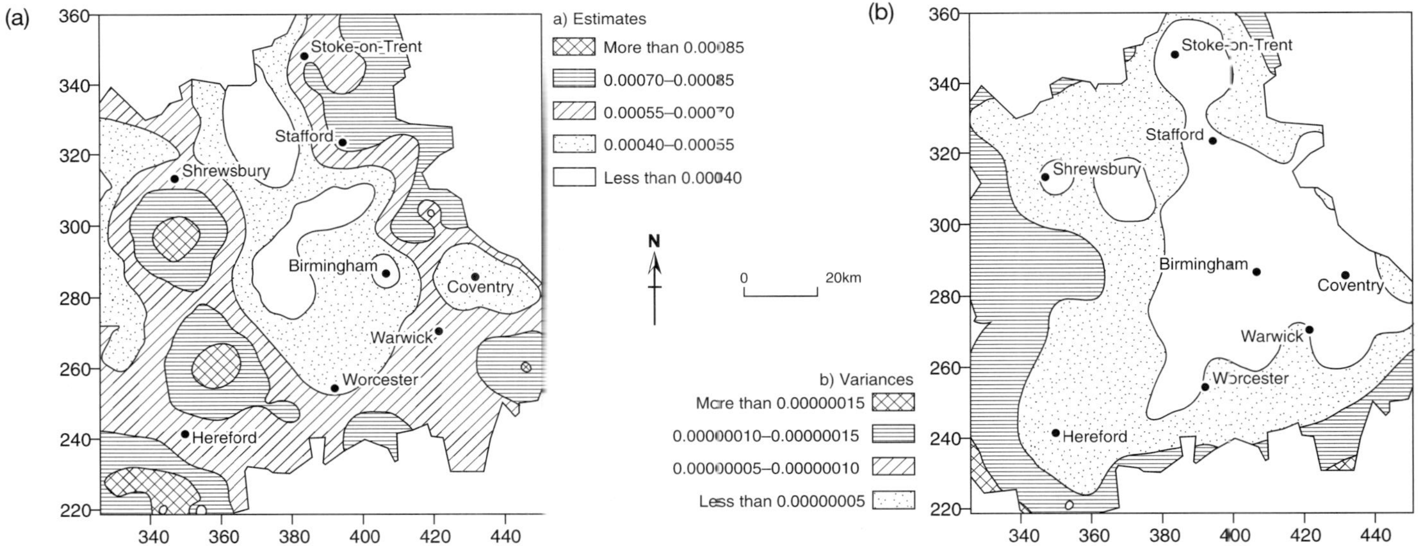

Fig. 3.3. Kriging of childhood cancer in West Midlands. (a) Kriged surface. (b) Estimation variances. Reproduced with permission from Oliver (1996).

exploring epidemiological data is long-established as a means of detecting the presence or absence of map pattern (Cliff and Haggett, 1988). Typically, we have data for a fixed set of areal units and estimate an autocorrelation coefficient according to the level of measurement of the data (join-count statistics for binary or nominal data, and a Moran statistic where the data are continuous). Note that a single statistic characterizes the whole map (although correlograms representing dependence at various lags are sometimes estimated). Some authors feel that this is rather unsatisfactory, and have developed 'local' indicators of spatial autocorrelation or association (see Chapter 1, pp. 16–17). Here, we examine the association between a disease rate in one location and rates in neighbouring locations, up to a specified distance. This might reveal clusters of high and low values: regions where, for example, high values are surrounded by other high values, or areas where low rates are surrounded by areas with equally low rates. Applications of this idea to the study of acquired immune deficiency syndrome (AIDS) in San Francisco and breast cancer in north-west Lancashire are considered by Getis and Ord (1998) – to whom credit for the original idea is due (Getis and Ord, 1992) – and Rigby and Gatrell (2000). Kitron and his colleagues (1997) have adopted the method (as well as using the *K*-functions referred to above) in detecting clusters of Lacrosse encephalitis around the city of Peoria, Illinois.

These local statistics are becoming embedded in various software environments. Perhaps the best is SpaceStat, devised by Luc Anselin (Anselin and Bao, 1997), which permits both exploratory and very sophisticated spatial modelling of area data. Conveniently, this offers a link to the GIS ArcView. Less well known, and more specialized in its computing requirements, is SAGE (Haining, 1998).

We questioned earlier whether conventional geographical space is the appropriate space within which to represent area data, and considered cartograms as a means of deriving alternative spaces. Other methods, more particularly from exploratory data analysis rather than the visualization literature, allow further spatial representations of epidemiological data. One example is multidimensional scaling (MDS). In the simplest setting, we have a lower triangular matrix of dissimilarities between a set of objects. In a geographical setting these might be a set of towns or cities between which are estimated travel times according to some means of transport. MDS seeks a new space of minimum dimensionality in which the objects are located so as to best fit the original dissimilarities; typically, the distances in the new space would preserve as far as possible the rank order of the original dissimilarities. A monotonic regression of distance on dissimilarity produces a residual sum-of-squares statistic, known as 'stress'. This will always be lower in a space of higher dimensionality, but we trade this off against the difficulties of visualizing events in more than three dimensions.

An alternative way of representing dissimilarity is to do so indirectly, constructing it on the basis of profiles of epidemiological events. As an example, Cliff *et al.* (1998, pp. 226–231) form a matrix, the rows of which are ten world regions and the columns are monthly death rates (from all causes, and then separate causes of death) from 1888 to 1912. Constructing another matrix in which elements are unity if the rate is greater than the mean for the given region and multiplying it by its transpose yields a symmetrical similarity matrix; this forms the input to an MDS procedure. Regions with similar disease profiles cluster together in the same region of 'disease space', while those that behave very differently are pushed apart. For example, Western Europe and North America lie close together, while South America is in another region of this transformed space.

We return to the use of MDS as an exploratory method when considering the literature on disease diffusion (see Section 3.4.1).

3.3.3 Space matters . . . but time matters too

We drew attention earlier to the somewhat heroic assumption that the current place of residence was an adequate locational reference for geographical epidemiology, arguing that daily and weekly activity spaces need to be given more prominence. At a different temporal scale, those interested in understanding the spatial distribution of human disease and ill health need to get to grips with migration histories. This is because in exploring the incidence of, say, adult cancers, it may well be that a mapping and spatial analysis of incidence at diagnosis is rather unrevealing. Many cancers will have a long latent period; perhaps an individual was exposed to a source of pollution in the workplace many years earlier and had since moved home, perhaps several times. Unless we can trace people back to their former homes, we may be getting at best a very partial, even misleading, picture of disease incidence. This problem has relevance in some veterinary epidemiological contexts, where diseases may manifest themselves among animals in places to which they have (been) moved, some time after their exposure to environmental insults at other locations.

To illustrate how we might address these issues, consider two studies, both on populations in Scandinavia, where the historical records are such as to permit this kind of temporal analysis.

In the first, Riise and his colleagues (1991) studied nearly 400 people who had developed multiple sclerosis in the Norwegian county of Hordaland between 1953 and 1987. Multiple sclerosis is a disease that tends to strike adults of young to middle age. The authors examined the observed and expected numbers of pairs of patients who lived in the same community and who had been born within 1 year of each other.

Their results revealed that, until the age of about 15 years, there was little evidence of significant space–time clustering, but that between the ages of 16 and 20 (in particular at 18 years) there was clear evidence of clustering. Patients of a similar age were much more likely to have lived close by in late adolescence than pure chance would suggest. A possible explanation is that the disease is a delayed response to a viral infection (such as Epstein–Barr virus) acquired, possibly by the exchange of saliva, in the late teenage years. Simply mapping the current place of residence would not have suggested this as a possible hypothesis.

In a second study, Sabel *et al.* (2000) conducted research in Finland on geographical variation in the incidence of motor neurone disease (MND; also known as amyotrophic lateral sclerosis, or ALS). MND is a rare but progressive neurodegenerative disease, the cause of which is unknown. Data were collected on 1000 deaths from MND between 1985 and 1995, matched by age and sex to population controls. Because the Finnish authorities register all changes of address, the authors were able to explore where both cases and controls had lived since the mid-1960s. Using kernel estimation (see above) they constructed a relative risk surface according to the current place of residence, but also the former place of residence. Those subsequently diagnosed with MND had, relative to people unaffected by the disease, spent many years living in the Karelia region of Finland. Whether this is symptomatic of a localized gene pool or of some common environmental factor is something that demands further research.

Lastly, although it has not generated any spatial analytical work, it is worth drawing attention to David Barker's extensive research programme on the precursors of adult disease. Using both aggregate, ecological data and individual health records, Barker demonstrates quite convincingly that there are striking associations between low birth weight and the incidence of adult diseases such as heart disease and diabetes (Barker, 1994). Again, to gain a rich understanding of disease in later life we need to reach into the past, noting that the place of residence may well have changed several times.

3.4 Spatial modelling

3.4.1 Diffusion modelling

One of the earliest contributions to the spatial analysis tradition made by a geographer was that of Torsten Hägerstrand, a Swedish geographer who, in the early 1950s, pioneered the use of computerized simulation modelling to aid our understanding of the spread of agricultural innovations (including the uptake of subsidies for controlling bovine TB). This research spawned a new field of enquiry in geography, 'spatial diffusion modelling', which has been applied to the study of diseases by a number of writers. Applications have included the study of measles, influenza and HIV/AIDS, though some of the earliest applications were veterinary ones. For example, Tinline (1971) used a two-dimensional linear operator (identical in structure to Hägerstrand's mean information field) to predict the spread of the 1967/68 foot-and-mouth disease outbreak in Britain, while Gilg (1973) examined the wave-like spread of fowl pest disease in England and Wales.

Introductions to the entire field of spatial diffusion modelling are given in Haggett (2000, 2001) and in Gould (1993, Chapter 6), with fuller expositions and examples in Cliff *et al.* (1998, 2000) and Thomas (1992). There is a simple, yet compelling, distinction to be made between two types of spatial diffusion process. In *contagious diffusion*, a disease is considered to spread in a wave-like form, rippling out from one or more centres of infection. In *hierarchical diffusion*, however, the source of infection is likely to be a large city, from which the disease spreads to smaller cities at the next level of the urban hierarchy, and thence to smaller towns and villages. It does not respect conventional geographical space; rather, human spatial interaction structures the spread such that contact is more likely to be between those living in pairs of major cities than between pairs of small towns. In a historical setting, the seminal paper by Pyle (1969) shows how the transformation of the American transport system (specifically, the growth of the railway linking major population centres) caused cholera to spread in a hierarchical fashion in the mid-19th century, in contrast to its contagious spread in the 1830s.

We may link these ideas to others developed in a spatial analysis tradition, namely 'gravity modelling' or spatial interaction modelling, and see how to use this linkage to model spatial diffusion and to conceptualize the space within which such diffusion takes place.

In the simplest sense, as Gould (1993, Chapter 6) conveys so tellingly, human spatial interaction between a pair of centres can be represented as directly proportional to the (population) size of the centres and inversely proportional to some power of the distance separating them. These simple principles, suitably refined (see e.g. Wilson, 2000), can be applied to all forms of interaction, from migration and commuting to shopping behaviour and other forms of travel. Gould argues that we can use these ideas to compute likely interactions between places and in turn to create a new disease space that structures the spread of disease. To appreciate this, consider again the technique of multidimensional scaling (MDS) that we referred to earlier. Instead of taking dissimilarities as input to the scaling procedure, let us use predicted spatial interaction as a measure of the similarity between pairs of places. If we do so, we can see how a conventional geographical space (e.g. New Zealand; Fig. 3.4a) is transformed into a new disease space in which large

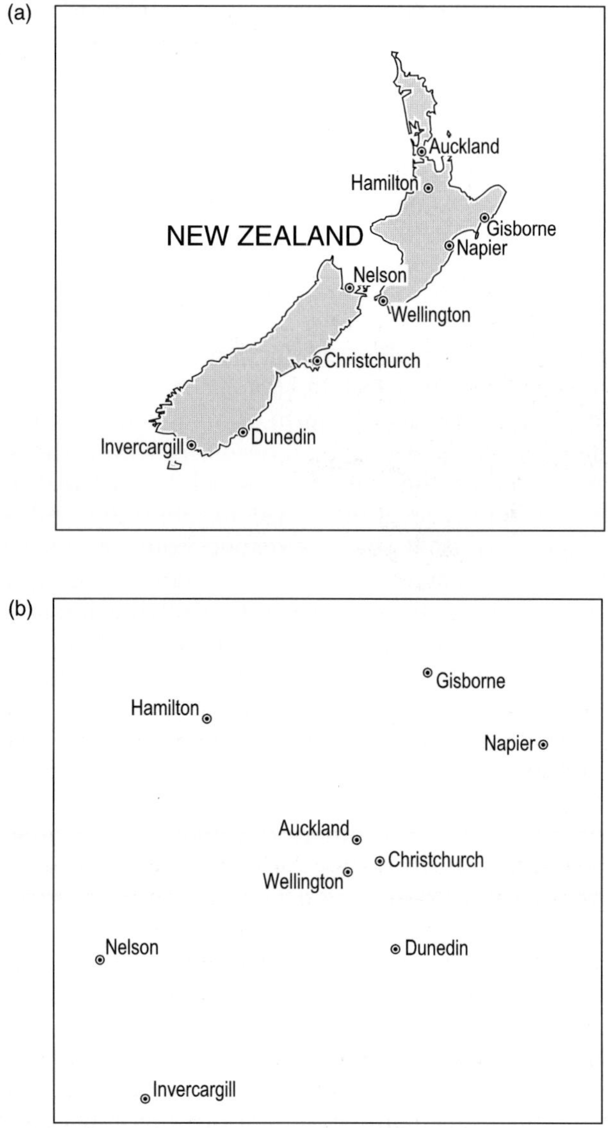

Fig. 3.4. New Zealand in (a) geographical space and (b) a hypothetical 'interaction' space (based on an idea in Gould (1993)).

cities are located close together and the smaller population centres are dispersed (Fig. 3.4b). We might therefore predict that a disease will spread contagiously away from the origin in this transformed space.

The same ideas have been exploited by Cliff *et al.* (2000) in their monumental study of disease spread in and among island populations.

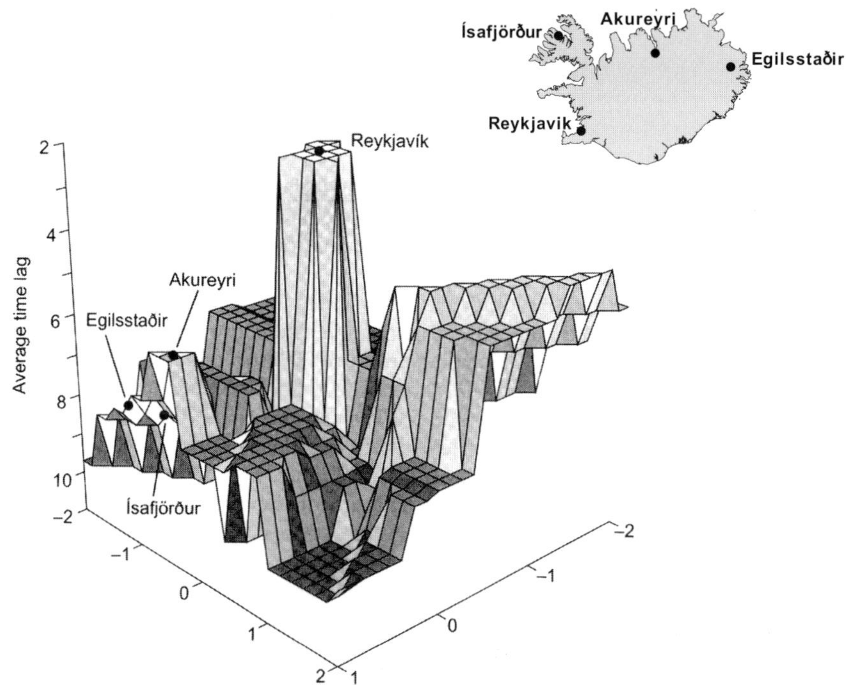

Fig. 3.5. Iceland in airline accessibility space. Average time in months taken for disease to reach medical districts, 1946–1990. Reproduced with permission from Cliff *et al.* (2000).

They constructed a matrix of airline flights from 95 islands to all of the other 199 countries and islands that they considered, and formed a similarity matrix according to the pattern of flights from one island to another. Input of this into MDS yielded an airline accessibility space, the coordinates of which were used as the locations for mapping the number of diseases recorded on each island. There was an 'outer rim of high disease counts on well-connected islands surrounding a core of fewer diseases found on islands whose relative isolation has been preserved' (Cliff *et al.*, 2000, p. 222). At a much finer spatial scale, the authors looked at Iceland's internal airline network, again constructing an airline accessibility space and then (Fig. 3.5) plotting the average time taken in months for measles to spread from the central hub, Reykjavik, to districts that are peripheral in this transformed space. 'Reykjavik is the principal point of international entry of epidemics into Iceland, and it is the epidemic diffusion pole for the rest of the country' (Cliff *et al.*, 2000, pp. 266–268).

Yet this use of MDS, attractive as it is, somewhat oversimplifies the situation. This is because spatial interaction is an asymmetrical

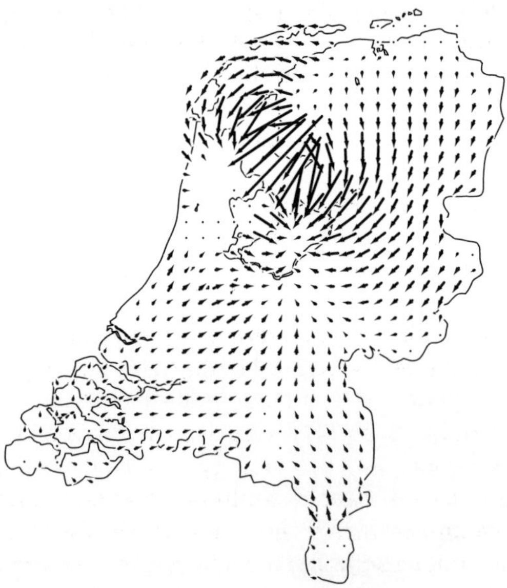

Fig. 3.6. Gradient vectors of net population flow in The Netherlands, 1985. Reproduced with permission from Clark and Koloutsou-Valakis (1992).

relationship. MDS assumes symmetry (the dissimilarity between location *i* and *j* is the same as that between *j* and *i*). Intuitively (and empirically!) there will be more movement from Lancaster to London than from London to Lancaster. Diseases tend to flow down the urban hierarchy, not upwards. How can we cope with this?

This problem was addressed over 25 years ago by Waldo Tobler (1976; see also Clark and Koloutsou-Vakakis, 1992). Tobler proposed that one could construct a vector field from the net differences in flow, and that this could be plotted as a visualization of the flow data. An example taken from data on inter-regional migration among 40 provinces in The Netherlands (Clark and Koloutsou-Vakakis, 1992, p. 118) shows how net migration is focused on Amsterdam (Fig. 3.6). Tobler further proposes, in a typically imaginative way, that one can work backwards from the field of vectors to derive what he calls a 'forcing function'; this is essentially a potential or pressure field of which the vectors are the gradient. Again, the translation from a discrete to a continuous view of the world is clear.

Thomas (1992, Chapter 4) has demonstrated very well how spatial interaction modelling can shed light on diffusion processes. We might define a set of locations and suggest that the number of contacts, *c*, between *i* and *j* is modelled as

$$c_{ij} = x_i y_j e^{-\lambda d_{ij}}$$

where x_i denotes the susceptible population in place i, y_i represents the infectives, d_{ij} is the distance between places and λ is a distance decay parameter. As λ increases, the 'friction' of distance increases. It would be interesting to examine applications of these ideas in a veterinary context, where the movement of animals from place to place is structured by a transport network in which travel time is an appropriate measure of spatial separation. Temporal change can be considered; for example, we can represent the changing numbers of infectives and susceptibles using difference equations and simulate the spatial diffusion under different assumptions.

Geographers are also rediscovering the impact that global changes in transport may have on the spread of disease. Although the concept of time–space convergence did not emerge until 1969 (Janelle, 1969), transport historians had for many years traced shrinkages in distance due to improvements in transport technology. As new modes of transport emerged, considerable distances could be traversed much more speedily, while improvements within any such mode (such as new engines developed for aircraft) also led to a convergence between places. Cliff *et al.* (2000) draw attention to a little-known book by Massey (1933) called *Epidemiology in Relation to Air Travel*, in which he points out that 'countries affected by certain major infectious diseases are brought nearer to countries which ordinarily enjoy freedom therefrom' (cited in Cliff *et al.*, 2000, p. 201). Haggett (2000, p. 616) reminds us of the epidemiological consequences. One is that there are occasional local outbreaks of tropical diseases near mid-latitude airports, such as the malaria cases that occurred near Geneva in 1989 after infected mosquitoes had survived journeys from malarial areas. A second is due to the increasing size of aircraft, whereby a doubling of capacity might quadruple the risk of any one individual infecting another. The impact of this form of globalization on disease diffusion has yet to be fully researched.

3.4.2 Multilevel modelling

As we have observed, it is common in geographical epidemiology to conduct analysis using either individual-level data or data for a set of areal units. If using individual data, we commonly fit logistic regression models in an attempt to assess which of a number of covariates increase the odds that an individual is a case rather than a control. If using area data, we fit (generalized) regression models, perhaps incorporating spatial effects if the need arises. But how do we proceed if we have data for both individuals and areas, or indeed the data at a set of scales or levels?

Consider, for example, how we might set about explaining geographical variation in childhood immunization uptake (Jones *et al.*, 1991). This might be explicable partly in terms of household variables (car ownership, education, and so on) but also in terms of the attractiveness and quality of service provided at health clinics. We might, then, want to collect data at both the individual or household level and the clinic level. The method of incorporating such data into an appropriate analysis is known as multilevel or hierarchical modelling (for a clear introductory exposition see Jones, 1991).

To fix ideas, consider a simple hypothetical example (Gatrell, 2002, pp. 67–68). Suppose we have data on smoking behaviour for a large sample of individuals who live in different towns. We believe that their age is possibly predictive of cigarette consumption. Ignoring place of residence, we might fit a model relating consumption to age, in which there is a clear linear relationship (Fig. 3.7). But this might be geographically naive; perhaps smoking behaviour varies from place to place according to local culture. Separating out the individuals according to the town in which they live yields a separate regression line for each place. It may be that the relationship between consumption and age takes the same form in each place and that it is only the overall level of smoking that varies. In this case the slopes of the regression lines are the same; only the intercepts vary. More plausibly, the intercepts and slopes will both vary, implying that the relationship between consumption and age is positive in some places, absent in others, and negative in yet others. Here, both the slopes and intercepts are said to be 'random', meaning that they come from a probability distribution.

In an interesting paper on the incidence of non-Hodgkin's lymphoma in Europe, Langford *et al.* (1998) collect data for different regions within countries (two hierarchical levels) and assess the nature of the relationship to UVB radiation. A single-level analysis masks the fact that different countries behave in different ways; for example, the association is strongly positive for the UK (though UVB values are rather low) but is negative for Italy (where values are higher).

There is a growing number of examples of multilevel modelling, ranging from predicting respiratory health from individual and neighbourhood-level variables to the prediction of low birth weight using similar hierarchical levels (e.g. Ecob, 1996; Wiggins *et al.*, 1998). Some applications are more plausible than others. The method was motivated in part by the need to predict children's school performance. Here, it seems entirely plausible that a child's success depends partly on the household environment, partly on the school environment and culture, and partly, at a third level, on the school district or education authority, which invests in education differentially from place to place. In all cases the levels 'function' or 'perform'. In health settings the levels are not always quite so natural. Many of the published applications take data from individuals and from a single further level of administrative areas that are convenient rather than meaningful. None the less, as a means of

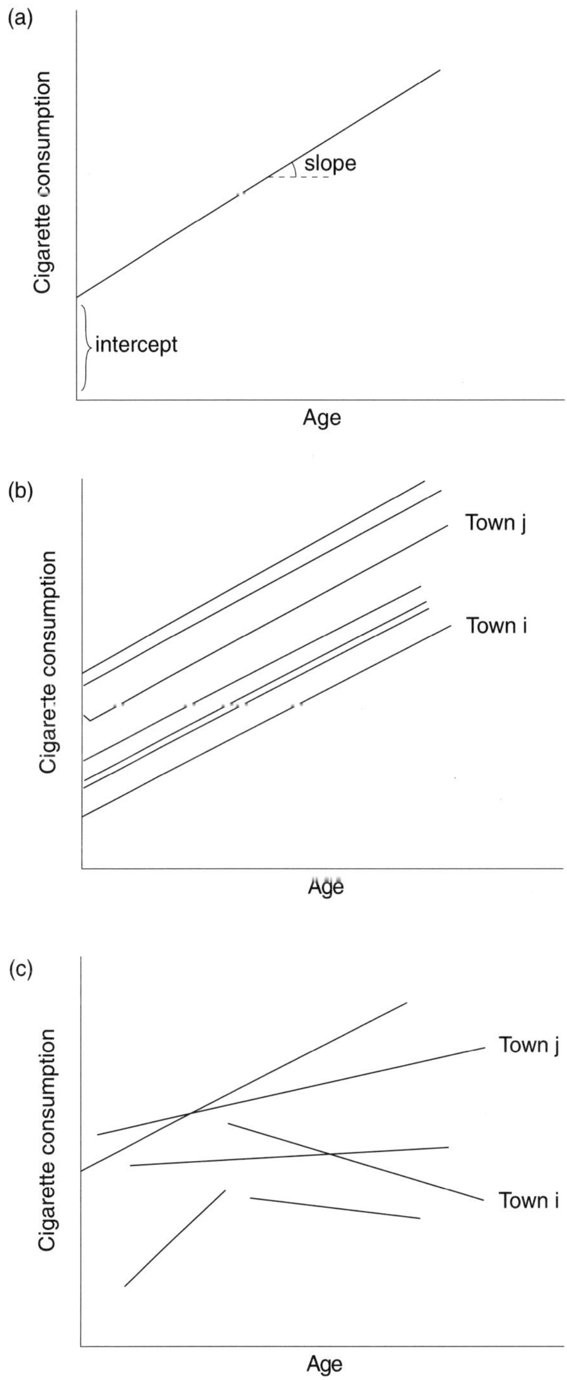

Fig. 3.7. Multilevel modelling. From Gatrell (2002).

separating out individual or 'compositional' variables from more 'contextual' influences, the method has enormous value and promise. Whether it has purchase for the veterinary epidemiologist who wishes to assess animal disease risk on the basis of individual attributes, herd or flock measures, farm-level data and perhaps influences from higher levels is a matter for further research.

3.4.3 Environmental modelling

There are problems in making associations between health and environment if these two domains draw on very different sets of spatial units. Typically, as noted already, health data either relate to individuals or are aggregated to sets of areal units. Environmental data, on the other hand, are generally sampled from a spatially continuous surface, at discrete point locations, from which interpolations are made, perhaps to a regular grid or a smoothly varying surface. How are we to relate (health) data that are collected from, or aggregated to, one system of areal units to a set of (environmental) data that have a quite different form of spatial referencing? (One solution may be to explore the surface models mentioned earlier (Martin, 1991).) The problems will be less severe if the health data are represented by point locations (places of residence), since we may then model disease risk (presence or absence) as a function of covariates that are also measured for the individuals, in addition to the estimated environmental factor(s) at the same location. For example, if we are dealing with respiratory disease we may have data on levels of smoking in the home, on the presence of pets, on housing quality – factors that might serve to predict disease risk. But allied to this we may have monitored, or modelled, data on air quality, an estimate of which we might take at the place of residence from an interpolated air quality surface. However, the problems of association would be much more severe if we only had morbidity or mortality rates for small areas, since an estimate of the burden of air pollution for any one of those small areas is difficult to secure.

We also need to be sensitive to issues of spatial scale and resolution. For example, it is well known that monitored levels of radon gas emissions vary over a very fine spatial scale; certainly, levels in neighbouring properties may be quite different depending on the characteristics of the building. There seems little point in trying to assess the relationship between, say, lung cancer and radon levels unless we have individual-level data for both, and preferably good historical data on previous residence and likely exposure there (Kohli *et al.*, 1997). Where we do have such data, there is some evidence of associations between radon exposure and childhood leukaemia; for example, in part of Sweden (Kohli *et al.*, 2000). To take another example, there is keen interest in establishing the nature of the relationship between exposure to electromagnetic fields and various cancers (especially leukaemia). However, since the field effects are highly localized and the cancers are rare, this too is a highly problematic area of research (for an estimate of likely exposure in Finland, see Valjus *et al.*, 1995).

There is a growing literature, drawn upon extensively elsewhere in this book, that uses GIS to relate the incidence of vector-borne disease (particularly malaria and Lyme disease) to the distribution of possible environmental risk factors. To give just one example, Glass and his colleagues (1995) looked at 48 cases of Lyme disease in Baltimore County, Maryland, in 1991, recording residential address and taking a random sample of 495 addresses to use as controls in a logistic regression model. A GIS database comprising five sets of variables (land use, soils, geology, elevation and watersheds) provided a set of candidate covariates, and the results suggested that residence in forested areas was associated with increasing risk (odds ratio = 3.7, 95% confidence interval = 1.2–11.8), as was loam soil.

One could argue that, since the association with forested areas is well known, there is little need for a GIS to confirm this. But this neglects the potential power of the GIS, which is to offer the possibility of simulating some alternative scenarios. Such predictive or 'what if?' modelling is important, because with it we can assess the impact of land use change on disease incidence or, as a number of authors have done (e.g. Martens, 1998), the potential impact of climate change.

The existence of spatial autocorrelation and spatial heterogeneity (non-stationarity) means that classical regression models must be adapted (see Chapter 1, pp. 14–21). One useful approach is to make use of local modelling, drawing upon the same ideas of local spatial association as those noted above (Section 3.2). Quantitative geographers at Newcastle University have introduced a method called 'geographically weighted regression', which allows the regression coefficients to vary spatially; in other words, rather than imposing a single (or global) regression model on the entire study area, the proposition is that the relationship between the response variable and the covariate(s) varies from place to place (Brunsdon *et al.*, 1996, 1999). Regression coefficients are therefore estimated for any location on the map on the basis of the values of variables in neighbouring locations. There is a close link between this idea and that of kernel smoothing. It would be productive to explore these ideas in an animal health context.

3.4.4 Location–allocation modelling

All the work reviewed above has been of an epidemiological nature, directed towards an understanding of disease distribution. But health (medical) geographers have long since had other interests, and among these is the provision of health-care facilities (Thomas, 1992). To what extent can these be provided in an optimal way? In most applications, optimality relates to minimizing the total cost of overcoming distance, resulting in an efficient distribution of facilities. However, this may not necessarily result in an equitable solution – one that ensures that there is equity of access among different population groups. The location problem is one of selecting, either on the plane or on a transport network, one or more centres to serve a population. The allocation problem seeks an optimal allocation of people to facilities. It is worth asking whether there are potential applications of this in a veterinary setting, for example where one wishes to locate centres for optimal disease control.

As with much else in the geography of health, GIS (here, geographical information *systems* as opposed to *science*) has provided a modern software environment within which to undertake forms of spatial analysis that have in reality been around for 40 years or more. This is certainly true of location–allocation modelling; Swedish geographers such as Sven Godlund were planning the location of regional hospitals using spatial analytical methods in the early 1960s (Godlund, 1961; see the discussion in Abler *et al.*, 1971). A good up-to-date review of the field is given by Church (1999).

One example of the use of GIS in reviewing the accessibility of hospital services to the populations they purport to serve is due to Walsh *et al.* (1997). Taking as their study area 16 counties in North Carolina, a set of 25 hospitals (with known bed supply), a classified road network, and data on the distribution of patients, the network modelling capabilities of a leading proprietary package are used to allocate links on the road network, and accompanying populations, to the set of hospitals. Population demand is assigned to the nearest hospital using estimated drive times, resulting in the minimization of total journey time. This yields a set of hospital catchment areas, which will of course be modified if the demand variable changes (for example, one might use demand for obstetric care instead of total population). Most importantly, the GIS can be used as a spatial decision-support system (SDSS), by simulating the impact of population change, or the closure or addition of hospital sites. Alternatively, the transport network can be modified, with new links added, others removed, or the travel times modified in specific ways.

In a recent application the author has illustrated, using MAPINFO, some of these principles with reference to the locations of hospices (centres for palliative or end-of-life care) in north-west England (Wood and Gatrell, 2002). Here, the demand for hospice care was estimated (separately for adult and child hospice care) on the basis of predicted numbers of cancers by small area (electoral wards). Data were available

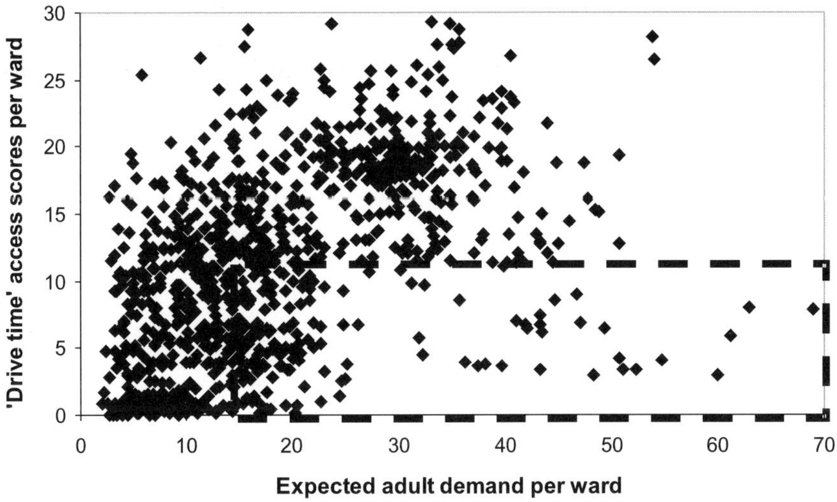

Fig. 3.8. Relationship between accessibility to hospices and expected demand for hospice care in north-west England. From Wood and Gatrell (2003).

on the locations of hospices and the numbers of beds for in-patient care (a measure of supply). The geographical accessibility of any ward to the set of hospices was estimated using a simple gravity-type model in which access is defined as the sum, over all hospices, of the numbers of beds divided by the distance between the ward and each hospice. Interest centred on those wards that had relatively high demand for hospice care (above the median) and which were relatively remote from hospices (below the median accessibility score) (Fig. 3.8). This set of wards could be mapped to show where there was a need for further hospice facilities. A further refinement selected from this set of wards those that were relatively deprived (according to socioeconomic indicators), and where access to private transport might have been poor. A map of this further subset (Fig. 3.9) is thus a useful tool for health-care providers, as an indication of where to consider locating additional supply in order to address issues of inequity of provision. Clearly, the idea can, in principle, be applied to various other health-care delivery problems.

3.5 Conclusions

Concepts from spatial analysis and geographical information science and their translation into operational tools via geographical information systems have attracted much research interest in recent years from epidemiologists dealing with human disease. As other chapters in this collection attest, there is a growing body of work that applies such

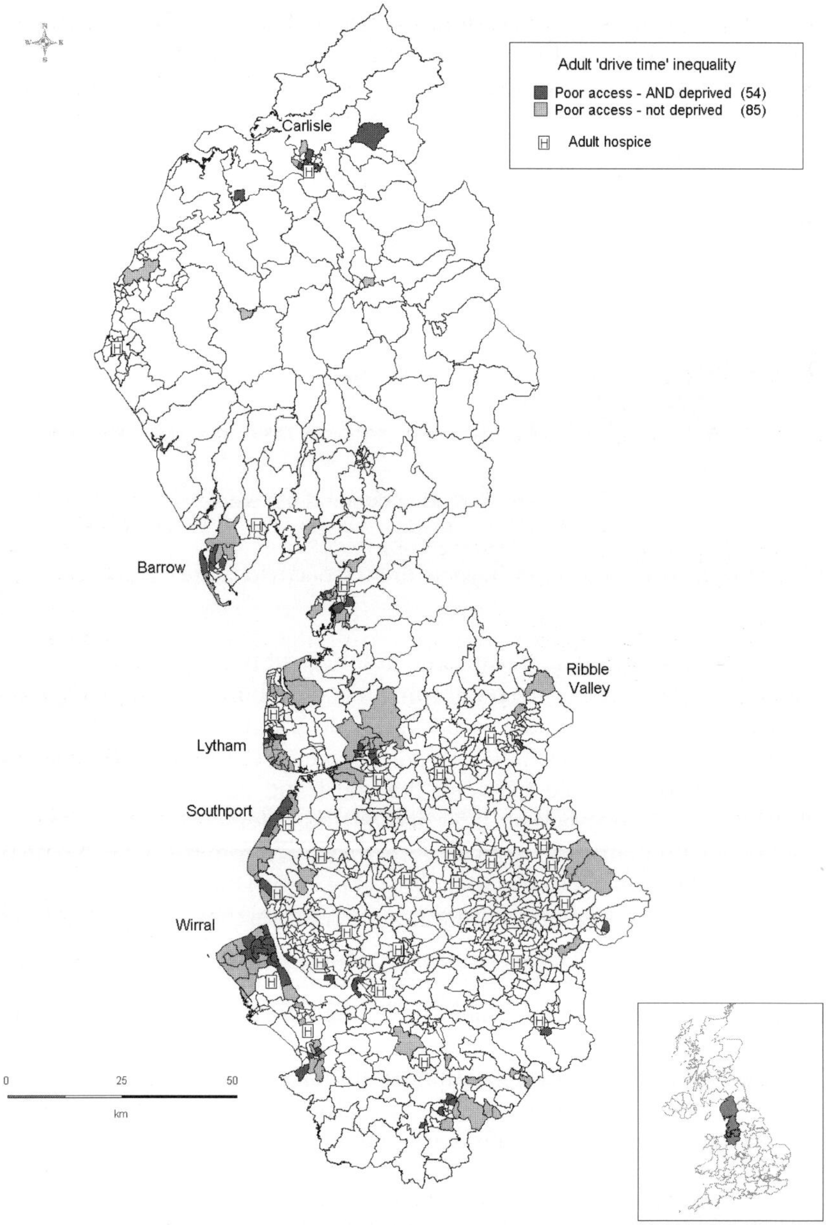

Fig. 3.9. Small areas in north-west England having inequitable access to hospice care. From Wood and Gatrell (2003).

concepts and tools in a veterinary context. There is already considerable overlap between the fields in terms of the spatial analytical tools used, in addition to the obvious overlap in dealing with vector-borne disease. I have sought here to bring to the attention of a veterinary audience some of the conceptual difficulties experienced in the human domain, and also to indicate where the research frontier in geographical epidemiology is moving. The potential for cross-fertilization has long been considerable, and remains so. I look forward to seeing these dialogues continue.

References

Abler, R., Adams, J. and Gould, P.R. (1971) *Spatial Organisation*. Prentice-Hall, New York.

Alvanides, S., Openshaw, S. and Rees, P. (2002) Designing your own geographies. In: Rees, P., Martin, D. and Williamson, P. (eds) *The Census Data System*. John Wiley & Sons, Chichester, UK, pp. 47–65.

Anselin, L. and Bao, S. (1997) Exploratory spatial data analysis: linking SpaceStat and ArcView. In: Fischer, M. and Getis, A. (eds) *Recent Developments in Spatial Analysis: Spatial Statistics, Behavioural Modelling and Neurocomputing*. Springer, Berlin, pp. 45–62.

Bailey, T.C. and Gatrell, A.C. (1995) *Interactive Spatial Data Analysis*. Longman, Harlow, UK.

Barker, D.J.P. (1994) *Mothers, Babies, and Disease in Later Life*. BMJ Publishing Group, London.

Brunsdon, C., Fotheringham, A.S. and Charlton, M. (1996) Geographically weighted regression: a method for exploring spatial nonstationarity. *Geographical Analysis* 28, 281–289.

Brunsdon, C., Aitkin, M., Fotheringham, A.S. and Charlton, M. (1999) A comparison of random coefficient modelling and geographically weighted regression for spatially non-stationary regression problems. *Geographical and Environmental Modelling* 3, 47–62.

Church, R.L. (1999) Location modelling and GIS. In: Longley, P., Goodchild, M.F., Maguire, D.J. and Rhind, D.W. (eds) *Geographical Information Systems*. John Wiley & Sons, Chichester, UK, pp. 293–303.

Clark, W.A.V. and Koloutsou-Vakakis, S. (1992) Evaluating Tobler's migration fields. *Geographical Analysis* 24, 110–120.

Cliff, A.D. and Haggett, P. (1988) *Atlas of Disease Distribution: Analytic Approaches to Epidemiological Data*. Basil Blackwell, Oxford, UK.

Cliff, A.D., Haggett, P. and Smallman-Raynor, M. (1998) *Deciphering Global Epidemics: Analytical Approaches to the Disease Records of World Cities, 1888–1912*. Cambridge University Press, Cambridge, UK.

Cliff, A.D., Haggett, P. and Smallman-Raynor, M. (2000) *Island Epidemics*. Oxford University Press, Oxford, UK.

Cromley, E. and McLafferty, E. (2002) *GIS and Public Health*. Guilford Press, New York.

Diggle, P.J. and Chetwynd, A.G. (1991) Second-order analysis of spatial clustering for inhomogenous populations. *Biometrics* 47, 1155–1163.

Dorling, D. (1995) *A New Social Atlas of Britain*. John Wiley & Sons, Chichester, UK.

Dorling, D. (1996) *Area Cartograms: Their Use and Creation*. University of East Anglia, Norwich, UK.

Ecob, R. (1996) A multilevel modelling approach to examining the effects of area of residence on health and functioning. *Journal of the Royal Statistical Society, Series A* 159, 61–75.

Forster, F. (1966) Use of a demographic base map for the presentation of areal data in epidemiology. *British Journal of Preventive and Social Medicine* 20, 165–171.

Gatrell, A.C. (2002) *Geographies of Health: an Introduction*. Blackwell, Oxford, UK.

Gatrell, A. and Löytönen, M. (eds) (1998) *GIS and Health*. Taylor and Francis, London.

Getis, A. and Ord, J.K. (1992) The analysis of spatial association by use of distance statistics. *Geographical Analysis* 24, 189–206.

Getis, A. and Ord, J.K. (1998) Spatial modelling of disease dispersion using a local statistic: the case of AIDS. In: Griffith, D.A., Amrhein, C.G. and Huriot, J.-M. (eds) *Econometric Advances in Spatial Modelling and Methodology: Essays in Honour of Jean Paelinck*. Kluwer, Dordrecht, The Netherlands, pp. 98–113.

Gilg, A.W. (1973) A study in agricultural disease diffusion: the case of the 1970–71 fowl-pest disease. *Transactions of the Institute of British Geographers* 59, 77–97.

Glass, G.E., Schwartz, B.S., Morgan, J.M., Johnson, D.T., Noy, P.M. and Israel, E. (1995) Environmental risk factors for Lyme disease identified with geographic information systems. *American Journal of Public Health* 85, 944–948.

Godlund, S. (1961) *Population, Regional Hospitals, Transportation Facilities, and Regions: Planning the Location of Regional Hospitals in Sweden*. University of Lund, Sweden.

Gould, P.R. (1993) *The Slow Plague: a Geography of the AIDS Pandemic*. Blackwell, Oxford, UK.

Gusein-Zade, S.M. and Tikunov, V.S. (1993) A new technique for constructing continuous cartograms. *Cartography and Geographic Information Systems* 20, 167–173.

Haggett, P. (2000) *The Geographical Structure of Epidemics*. Clarendon Press, Oxford, UK.

Haggett, P. (2001) *Geography: a Global Synthesis*. Prentice-Hall, London.

Haining, R. (1998) Spatial statistics and the analysis of health data. In: Gatrell, A. and Löytönen, M. (eds) *GIS and Health*. Taylor and Francis, London, pp. 29–47.

Hjalmars, U., Kulldorff, M., Gustafsson, G. and Nagarwalla, N. (1996) Childhood leukaemia in Sweden: using GIS and a spatial scan statistic for cluster detection. *Statistics in Medicine* 15, 707–715.

Janelle, D. (1969) Spatial re-organization: a model and concept. *Annals of the Association of American Geographers* 59, 348–364.

Jones, K. (1991) *Multi-Level Models for Geographical Research*. University of East Anglia, Norwich, UK.

Jones, K., Moon, G. and Clegg, A. (1991) Ecological and areal effects in childhood immunisation uptake: a multilevel approach. *Social Science and Medicine* 33, 501–508.

Kelsall, J.E. and Diggle, P.J. (1995) Non-parametric estimation of spatial variation in relative risk. *Statistics in Medicine* 14, 2335–2342.

Kitron, U., Michael, J., Swanson, J. and Haramis, L. (1997) Spatial analysis of the distribution of LaCrosse encephalitis in Illinois, using a geographic information system and local and global spatial statistics. *American Journal of Tropical Medicine and Hygiene* 57, 469–475.

Kohli, S., Brage, H.N. and Löfman, O. (2000) Childhood leukaemia in areas with different radon levels: a spatial and temporal analysis using GIS. *Journal of Epidemiology and Community Health* 54, 822–826.

Kohli, S., Sahlen, K., Löfman, O., Sivertun, A., Foldevi, M., Trell, E. and Wigertz, O. (1997) Individuals living in areas with high background radon: a GIS method to identify populations at risk. *Computer Methods and Programs in Biomedicine* 53, 105–112.

Kulldorff, M. (1998) Statistical methods for spatial epidemiology: tests for randomness. In: Gatrell, A. and Löytönen, M. (eds) *GIS and Health*. Taylor and Francis, London, pp. 49–62.

Kulldorff, M., Feuer, E.J., Miller, B.A. and Freedman, L.S. (1997) Breast cancer in northeastern United States: a geographical analysis. *American Journal of Epidemiology* 146, 161–170.

Langford, I., Bentham, G. and McDonald, A.-L. (1998) Mortality from non-Hodgkin lymphoma and UV exposure in the European Community. *Health and Place* 4, 355–364.

Lloyd, O.L., Smith, G., Lloyd, M.M., Holland, Y. and Gailey, F. (1985) Raised mortality from lung cancer and high sex ratios of births associated with industrial pollution. *British Journal of Industrial Medicine* 42, 475–480.

MacEachren, A., Polsky, C., Haug, D., Brown, D., Boscoe, F., Beedasy, J., Pickle, L. and Marrara, M. (1997) Visualising spatial relationships among health, environmental and demographic statistics: interface design issues. *Proceedings of the 18th International Cartographic Conference, Stockholm, Sweden, June 21–27, 1997*, pp. 880–887.

Martens, P. (1998) *Health and Climate Change: Modelling the Impacts of Global Warming and Ozone Depletion*. Earthscan Publications, London.

Martin, D. (1991) *Geographic Information Systems and Their Socioeconomic Applications*. Routledge, London.

Martin, D. (2002) Census population surface. In: Rees, P., Martin, D. and Williamson, P. (eds) *The Census Data System*. John Wiley & Sons, Chichester, UK, pp. 139–148.

Massey, A. (1993) *Epidemiology in Relation to Air Travel*. H.K. Lewis, London.

Merrill, D.W., Selvin, S., Close, E.R. and Holmes, H.H. (1996) Use of density equalizing map projections (DEMP) in the analysis of childhood cancer in four California counties. *Statistics in Medicine* 15, 1837–1848.

Mocarelli, P., Brambilla, P., Gerthoux, P.M., Patterson, D.G. and Needham, L.L. (1996) Change in sex ratio with exposure to dioxin. *The Lancet* 348, 409.

Monmonier, M. (1996) *How to Lie With Maps*, 2nd edn. University of Chicago Press, Chicago, Illinois.

Oliver, M. (1996) Geostatistics, rare disease, and the environment. In: Fischer, M., Scholten, H.J. and Unwin, D. (eds) *Spatial Analytical Perspectives on GIS*. Taylor and Francis, London, pp. 67–85.

Openshaw, S., Charlton, M., Wymer, C. and Craft, A. (1987) A Mark I geographical analysis machine for the automated analysis of point data sets. *International Journal of Geographical Information Systems* 1, 335–358.

Pyle, G.F. (1969) The diffusion of cholera in the United States in the nineteenth century. *Geographical Analysis* 1, 59–75.

Raisz, E. (1934) The rectangular statistical cartogram. *Geographical Review* 24, 292–296.

Rigby, J.E. and Gatrell, A.C. (2000) Spatial patterns in breast cancer incidence in north-west Lancashire. *Area* 32, 71–78.

Riise, T., Grønning, M., Klauber, M.R., Barrett-Connor, E., Nyland, H. and Albrektsen, G. (1991) Clustering of residence of multiple sclerosis patients at age 13 to 20 years in Hordaland, Norway. *American Journal of Epidemiology* 133, 932–939.

Rushton, G. (1998) Improving the geographic basis of health surveillance using GIS. In: Gatrell, A. and Löytönen, M. (eds) *GIS and Health*. Taylor and Francis, London, pp. 63–79.

Sabel, C.E., Gatrell, A.C., Löytönen, M., Maasilta, P. and Jokelinen, M. (2000) Modeling exposure opportunities: estimating relative risk for motor neurone disease in Finland. *Social Science and Medicine* 50, 1121–1137.

Schærstrom, A. (1996) *Pathogenic Paths? A Time Geographical Approach in Medical Geography*. Lund University Press, Lund, Sweden.

Selvin, S., Merill, D. and Sacks, S. (1988) Transformations of maps to investigate clusters of disease. *Social Science and Medicine* 26, 215–221.

Thomas, R.W. (1993) *Geomedical Systems: Intervention and Control*. Routledge, London.

Tinline, R. (1971) Linear operators in diffusion research. In: Chisolm, M.D.I., Frey, A.E. and Haggett, P. (eds) *Regional Forecasting*. Butterworth, London, pp. 135–161.

Tobler, W. (1976) Spatial interaction patterns. *Journal of Environmental Systems* 6, 271–301.

Valjus, J., Hongisto, M., Verkasalo, P., Jarvinen, P., Heikkila, K. and Koskenvuo, M. (1995) Residential exposure to magnetic fields generated by 100–400kV power lines in Finland. *Bioelectromagnetics* 16, 365–376.

Walsh, S.J., Page, P.H. and Gesler, W.M. (1997) Normative models and healthcare planning: network-based simulations within a geographic information system environment. *Health Services Research* 32, 243–260.

Wiggins, R.D., Bartley, M., Gleave, S., Joshi, H., Lynch, J. and Mitchell, R. (1998) Limiting long-term illness: a question of where you live or who you are? A multilevel analysis of the 1971–1991 ONS longitudinal study. *Risk Decision and Policy* 3, 181–198.

Wilson, A.G. (2000) *Complex Spatial Systems*. Prentice-Hall, London.

Wood, D.J. and Gatrell, A.C. (2003) *Equity of Geographical Access to Inpatient Hospice Care within North West England: a Geographical Information Systems (GIS) Approach*. North West Public Health Observatory, Lancaster University, Lancaster, UK. http://www.nwpho.org.uk/documents

Spatial Statistics in the Biomedical Sciences: Future Directions

4

Peter J. Diggle

4.1 Introduction

The term 'spatial statistics' refers to the collection of statistical methods in which spatial location plays an explicit role in study design or data analysis. An example of the former is the design of agricultural field trials to compare two or more different treatments. A number of experimental plots are laid out in a field and the design problem is to allocate treatments to plots in such a way as to allow efficient comparison of treatment effects. Spatial considerations then arise, for example, in defining blocks of spatially adjacent plots with a view to minimizing variability within a block, or in balancing the numbers of spatial adjacencies for different pairs of treatments to allow adjustment for competitive effects between adjacent plots.

Traditionally, the subsequent analysis of field-trial data is not explicitly spatial. By this, we mean that plot yields Y_i: $i = 1, \ldots, n$ are assumed to follow the model

$$Y_i = \mu_i + W_i \quad (1)$$

in which $\mu_i = E(Y_i)$ is defined by the design, including treatment, block and covariate effects as appropriate, and the W_i are mutually independent random variables. The mutual independence implies that at the analysis stage the physical locations of the plots within the field are irrelevant. Another way to express this is that the plot locations influence the deterministic part of the model, μ_i, but not the stochastic part, W_i.

In complicated designs, there may be advantages in considering block effects as random rather than fixed. To accommodate this, we

 GIS and Spatial Analysis in Veterinary Science (eds P.A. Durr and A.C. Gatrell)

modify model (1) as follows. Denote the plot-yields by Y_{ij}, where now i identifies blocks and j identifies plots within blocks. Then, the model becomes

$$Y_{ij} = \mu_{ij} + U_i + Z_{ij} \tag{2}$$

where $\mu_{ij} = \mathrm{E}(Y_{ij})$ as before, but now U_i and Z_{ij} are mutually independent random variables with variances $\upsilon^2 = \mathrm{Var}(U_i)$ and $\tau^2 = \mathrm{Var}(Z_{ij})$. This model induces a positive correlation, $\rho = \upsilon^2/(\upsilon^2 + \tau^2)$, between the yields from any two plots within the same block. If, as is often the case, blocks constitute sets of spatially contiguous plots, the resulting analysis is implicitly spatial in the sense that the joint distribution of Y_{ij} reflects, albeit somewhat crudely, the physical locations of the plots.

The rationale behind the definition of a block as a set of spatially contiguous plots is that plots which are spatially close should also be similar in respect of characteristics which will influence their subsequent yields (an example of the so-called first law of geography), hence spatial closeness achieves the goal of minimizing variation between plots within blocks. If we accept this argument, it is a short step from (2) to an explicitly spatial stochastic model for field-trial data.

To see this, consider the following re-expression of (2). Reverting to our earlier notation for yields as Y_i: $i = 1, \ldots, n$, we can write (2) as

$$Y_i = \mu_i + W_i \tag{3}$$

where, in contrast to (1), the W_i are no longer mutually independent. Specifically,

$$\mathrm{Corr}(W_i, W_{ij}) = \begin{cases} \rho\text{: } i, j \text{ in the same block} \\ 0\text{: otherwise} \end{cases} \tag{4}$$

More generally, an explicitly spatial model is simply a model of the form (3) in which the covariance structure, $\gamma_{ij} = \mathrm{Cov}(W_i, W_j)$, is determined by the plot locations. Formally, $\gamma_{ij} = \gamma(x_i, x_j, \theta)$, where $\gamma(.)$ is a specified function, x_i is the location of plot i and θ is a set of model parameters. In this particular example, $\gamma(.)$ is a step function and $\theta = (\upsilon^2, \tau^2)$.

The use of spatial stochastic models for field trials has its origins in the work of Papadakis (1937), who considered the possible advantage of using residuals from neighbouring plots as a covariate adjustment for each plot yield. The connection between this early work and explicit spatial stochastic models was noted by Cox (1974) in discussion of Besag (1974). Subsequent major developments include the discussion papers by Bartlett (1978), Wilkinson *et al.* (1983), Besag and Kempton (1986) and Besag and Higdon (1999). Spatial stochastic models are now well accepted in some areas of agricultural experimentation, although not universally so. In particular, the discussion of Besag and Higdon (1999) well illustrates the contrasting views held by proponents of model-based and design-based inference in this area.

Within the biomedical sciences, applications of spatial statistical methods are now widespread in at least three disparate fields. In *epidemiology*, disease registers nowadays usually include spatial information, either at the individual subject level in the form of the postcode of each subject's place of residence, or at a spatially aggregated level by the assignment of subjects to administrative subregions within a study area. Risk factor data may similarly be spatially referenced, either to the level of specific locations (e.g. air pollution measurements from a network of monitoring stations) or at a spatially aggregated level (e.g. demographic or socioeconomic data recorded from census enumeration districts). For a recent review, see Elliott *et al.* (2000).

In *medical imaging*, an image of body tissue is typically pixellated into a regular grid of locations, and the response from each pixel is stored either as a real value (greyscale image) or as one of a number of discrete categories. Image analysis has a substantial literature in its own right, some of which intersects with mainstream spatial statistics. See, for example, Glasbey and Horgan (1995).

In *neuroanatomy*, the data record the spatial arrangement of material within microscopic tissue sections. For example, the locations of cell nuclei within a tissue section define a spatial point process. Stochastic models and statistical methods for point process data are reviewed in Diggle (2003). Examples of neuroanatomical applications include Diggle (1986), Diggle *et al.* (1991) and Baddeley *et al.* (1993). Other kinds of neuroanatomical structure include networks of fibres and tessellations of cellular material. Models for structures of this kind are described by Stoyan *et al.* (1987).

In this chapter, I will discuss the use of spatial statistical methods within the context of environmental epidemiology, which is the study of disease distribution in relation to environmental and other risk factors. One reason for choosing this substantive focus is that it gives abundant scope for the combined application of spatial statistical and GIS methodologies. Another is that it generates a sufficient variety of data structures to embrace all of the main branches of spatial statistical methods.

In Section 4.2 I review spatial statistical methods, using a hypothetical epidemiological study as a motivating example. In Section 4.3 I describe three non-hypothetical examples which, in different ways, illustrate the scope of spatial statistics to contribute to substantive science and highlight a number of areas of current methodological research. In Section 4.4 I draw brief conclusions concerning future research directions and the role of spatial statistical methods in scientific research.

4.2 A taxonomy of spatial statistics

In this review of spatial statistics, I will take a model-based approach, classifying different branches of the subject according to the classes of stochastic model which they use. However, it is important to remember that models are no more than tools to help us address scientific questions. A good model is not a correct model (such a thing rarely exists). Rather, it is a model which addresses the relevant scientific questions as economically as possible whilst providing an adequate fit to the data. The thinking behind this philosophy is that, on the one hand, a demonstrably bad fit between model and data risks invalid inferences, whereas an over-elaborate model risks inefficient inferences (Altham, 1984). Elaborate models also tend to be fragile to departure from underlying assumptions, which in turn can be difficult to validate from sparse data.

Consider the following hypothetical example. Our aim is to describe the geographical variation in the risk of a particular disease over a predefined study region and period of time, with a particular focus on the possible role of air pollution as a risk factor; disease risk is known to be associated with age, sex and general socioeconomic status. Possible data sources are the following: a register of individual cases in which the information recorded for each case includes age, sex and postcoded place of residence; census information, which includes demographic and socioeconomic data from each census enumeration district within the study region; and air pollution measurements from a network of monitoring stations within the study region. This scenario embraces all three of the major branches of spatial statistics, which are: continuous spatial variation; discrete spatial variation; and spatial point processes (Cressie, 1991; Diggle, 1996). These three branches are distinguished by the basic classes of stochastic model that they use. We now describe these, initially suppressing possible structural complications, which can lead to hybrid modelling requirements in some applications.

We use the following notational conventions, with variations as necessary in specific settings. The study region is denoted A and is assumed to be a continuous region of the infinite plane, denoted IR^2. A location in two-dimensional space is denoted by the letter x. We use Y for a random variable associated with a particular location x, W for a spatial stochastic process and Z for an independent error process. Greek letters denote model parameters. A typical data set consists of a set of locations and associated random variables, hence (x_i, Y_i): $i = 1, \ldots, n$.

A model for *continuous spatial variation* is characterized by the inclusion in the model of a stochastic process, $\{W(\mathrm{x}): \mathrm{x} \in \mathrm{IR}^2\}$. Thus, at least in principle, $W(\mathrm{x})$ exists and could be measured anywhere within the study region A. In practice, each measured value Y_i is a noisy version of $W(\mathrm{x}_i)$, the value of $W(\mathrm{x})$ at the corresponding location x_i. A simple and widely used model is

$$Y_i = W(\mathrm{x}_i) + Z_i \tag{5}$$

in which the process $W(\mathrm{x})$ has mean μ, variance σ^2 and a correlation structure that is a specified function of location. For example, we might assume that the correlation between two values of $W(\mathrm{x})$ that are separated by distance of u is given by $\rho(u) = \exp\{-(u/\phi)\}$, which embodies the notion that observations at sufficiently close locations are strongly correlated whilst allowing flexibility in the strength of the relationship between correlation and distance through the parameter ϕ. Models of this kind provide a foundation for the branch of spatial statistics known as *geostatistics* (Chiles and Delfiner, 1999; Webster and Oliver, 2001).

A common use of models like (5) is for spatial prediction, by which we mean interpolation of the data to estimate values of $W(\mathrm{x})$ at arbitrary locations within A. Put more strongly, a continuous spatial variation model is indicated only if the phenomenon of interest exists throughout the study region *and* its values at unmeasured locations x are of scientific interest. For example, in our hypothetical example we might use a continuous spatial variation model to construct a continuous spatial map of air pollution values from the discrete array of measured values at monitoring stations (see Chapter 1). The resulting map might then be compared with a map of disease incidence to explore possible association between air pollution and disease risk.

In contrast, a model for *discrete spatial variation* only specifies a stochastic process W_i: $i = 1, \ldots, n$ on a predefined set of locations x_i. In this setting, the model need only define a valid and sensible distribution for the finite-dimensional random vector $W = (W_i, \ldots, W_n)$. How should such a model be constructed? The general approach is to specify what are called the *full conditional* distributions of the model, namely the n univariate distributions of each W_i, given all other W_j. From a mathematical perspective, an immediate problem is that non-obvious constraints must be imposed on the full conditionals to ensure that the implied joint distribution is valid; the general solution is given by the Hammersley–Clifford theorem, as discussed, for example, by Besag (1974). From a modelling perspective, there are distinct advantages to working with the full conditionals rather than directly with the joint distribution of W. First, outside the framework of the multivariate normal, flexible classes of directly specified joint distribution are hard to come by. Secondly, in some contexts it seems natural to formulate a model for spatial dependence by considering, for each location in turn, which other locations would directly influence the value of W_i for the location in question. Thirdly, it turns out that access to the full conditionals is central to efficient implementation of methods of inference for these models.

Any discrete spatial variation model induces a valid model for the subvector of W associated with any subset of the x_i, but validity is not necessarily preserved if further locations are added to the data. This reinforces the fundamental conceptual difference between continuous and discrete spatial variation models. Another way to emphasize this distinction is to note that, in discrete spatial variation models, the locations formally act as reference points only rather than as literal locations. In our hypothetical example we could, for example, consider the W_i to represent a level of social deprivation for each census enumeration district. We might then notionally associate each W_i with the centroid of the corresponding enumeration district, and define a model for W by allowing the full conditional for W_i to depend only on the values of W_j from enumeration districts whose boundaries touch the ith enumeration district; for example,

$$W_i \mid W_j, j \neq i \sim N(\alpha + \Sigma\beta_j W_j, \sigma^2) \tag{6}$$

where $\beta_j = 0$ unless enumeration districts i and j have contiguous boundaries. If measured deprivation, say Y_i, were thought to be a randomly perturbed version of W_i, then equations (5), with W_i replacing $W(x_i)$, and (6) could then be combined to define a model for the measured values Y_i: $i = 1, \ldots, n$, in which the difference between W_i and Y_i either represents measurement error in the determination of social deprivation or, more pragmatically, recognizes that variation in social deprivation can be explained only partly by an underlying spatially dependent process like (6).

It is important to emphasize that we are distinguishing between continuous and discrete spatial variation *models*, not data, and that the acid test of a model is its fitness for purpose rather than its absolute correctness. For example, in our hypothetical application to social deprivation data at enumeration district level we may (or may not) prefer to specify an unobserved, continuous spatial process $W(x)$ and model the measured deprivation Y_i in the ith enumeration district as

$$Y_i \mid W(x): x \in A \sim N(\mu_i, \tau^2) \tag{7}$$

where

$$\mu_i = \int \mathrm{ED}_i W(x)\mathrm{d}x \tag{8}$$

in which ED_i is enumeration district i and $W(x)$ is a stochastic process of the kind specified in (5). Equations (7) and (8) define a continuous spatial variation model for the spatially discrete data Y_i: $i = 1, \ldots, n$. The model is formally different from the discrete spatial variation model specified by (5) and (6), although it may be difficult to distinguish between the two purely in terms of their ability to fit a particular set of data Y_i: $i = 1, \ldots, n$.

The third major branch of spatial statistics is *spatial point processes*, in which the locations themselves, x_i, are the data of interest, and are presumed to have been generated by a stochastic process. When locations x_i carry associated random variables Y_i, the Y_i are called *marks*, and the resulting process is called a *marked point process*. From a theoretical point of view, the marked point process construction is a very general one. From a practical point of view, point process modelling is indicated only when the mechanism which determines the locations x_i is stochastic *and* this stochasticity is relevant to the scientific problem in hand.

Sometimes the same scientific problem can be formalized in different ways. For example, in our hypothetical example the residential locations of individual cases form a point process. However, this process will usually be of very limited scientific interest in itself, since it will largely reflect the spatial distribution of the underlying population at risk, with obvious concentrations close to centres of population. The point process of case locations becomes much more interesting if it can be related either to information on the underlying population density or to a second point process of *controls*, sampled at random from the population at risk. This is because a natural starting point, at least for the study of a non-infectious disease, is to assume that disease incidence is spatially random. When the spatial variation in population density $\lambda(x)$ is known, this implies that the point process of case locations is a Poisson process with intensity proportional to $\lambda(x)$. When $\lambda(x)$ is unknown, but a random control sample is available, spatially random disease incidence implies that the binary marks which identify cases and controls in the combined point process of locations are mutually independent Bernoulli random variables. In either case, the spatially random model defines a testable hypothesis, but in the case–control setting we make no attempt to model the locations themselves; we try to model only the labelling of locations as cases or controls.

The three-way classification of spatial statistical methods into continuous variation, discrete variation and point processes is useful as a framework for modelling, but is too simple to accommodate all applications. Rather, the different types of spatial stochastic process should be viewed as building blocks for a range of possible hybrid models. For example, in our hypothetical example, and notwithstanding our earlier warning against over-elaboration, how might we examine the spatial distribution of individual cases of disease in relation to air pollution? A possible modelling framework would be the following.

Purely for illustrative purposes, we assume that the spatial variation in the population density, say $\lambda_0(x)$, is known from census information, and we ignore the possible effects of covariates other than air pollution. A possible model for disease incidence conditional on an underlying air pollution surface $W(x)$ is that disease locations form a Poisson process with intensity

$$\lambda(x) = \lambda_0(x)\exp\{\alpha + \beta W(x)\} \tag{9}$$

Furthermore, the pollution monitoring network provides data Y_i which can be linked to the surface $W(x)$ according to a model of the form (5), i.e. $Y_i = W(x_i) + Z_i$. The combination of (9) and (5) then defines a model from which all parameters of interest, and in particular the regression parameter β, which measures the association between disease risk and air pollution, can be estimated.

If $\lambda_0(x)$ is unknown, or we wish to allow for subject-specific covariate information, a feasible strategy is to supplement the case data with a random sample of controls, in which case the Poisson process model (9) can be converted to a binary regression model for the case–control labels, with subject-specific factors and air pollution as covariates. The trick that allows this is to note that if cases and controls form independent Poisson processes with respective intensities $\lambda(x)$ and $\lambda_0(x)$, then, conditional on case and control locations x_i, the binary case–control *labels*, say L_i, where $L_i = 1$ if the event at x_i is a case, are mutually independent, with case probabilities

$$p(x_i) = P(L_i = 1) = \lambda(x_i)/\{\lambda(x_i) + \lambda_0(x_i)\} \quad (10)$$

Under the assumed model (9), $\lambda(x)$ and $\lambda_0(x)$ are proportional, the unknown surface $\lambda_0(x)$ cancels from the right-hand side of (10) and the parameters of interest can be estimated from the data (L_i, Y_i): $i = 1, \ldots, n$.

More generally, models which specify the distribution of observed quantities conditional on one or more unobserved stochastic processes are called *hierarchical models*. Hierarchical models are extremely flexible, and have become tractable to formal statistical analysis with the development of Monte Carlo methods of inference, most notably Markov chain Monte Carlo implementations of Bayesian and other likelihood-based methods (Gilks *et al.*, 1996). The availability of formal methods of inference has encouraged an explosive expansion of the range of applications of spatial statistical methods to substantive scientific problems. The limiting factor in applying spatial statistical methods is now more often the availability of sufficient data to validate the underlying modelling assumptions rather than the ability to turn the inferential handle.

4.3 Examples

To indicate some of the scope for spatial statistical methods to contribute to environmental epidemiology, we now turn to specific examples. In each case, due to space constraints we give only a summary description of the problem and proposed solution, but offer pointers to the literature for more detailed accounts.

Two of our three examples concern human epidemiology and the third concerns veterinary epidemiology. However, veterinary analogues of the two human examples could easily be identified.

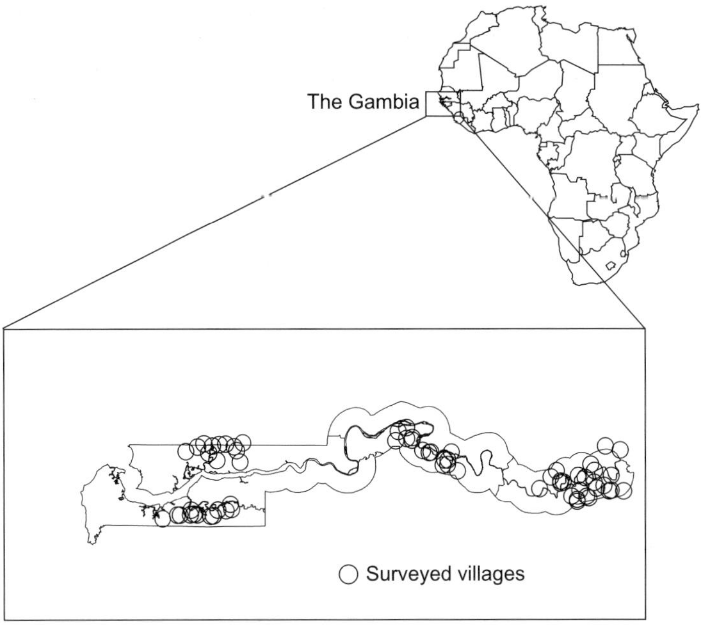

Fig. 4.1. Locations of villages in the Gambia childhood malaria survey. Adapted from Diggle *et al.* (2002).

4.3.1 Prevalence of childhood malaria in The Gambia

Our first example derives from a survey of malarial prevalence in village communities in The Gambia. The scientific background is described in D'Alessandro *et al.* (1995), Connor *et al.* (1998) and Thomson *et al.* (1999). Diggle *et al.* (2002) give a more detailed account of the data analysis summarized here. The underlying statistical methodology is due to Diggle *et al.* (1998).

The data are obtained from samples of children in each of 65 villages whose locations are shown in Fig. 4.1; these villages are themselves a small sample, chosen somewhat opportunistically, from the totality of village communities in The Gambia.

The covariate data on each child in the survey included their age, whether or not they regularly slept under a mosquito net, and, if so, whether or not the net was treated with insecticide. The binary response for each child was the presence or absence of malarial parasites in a blood sample. Additional data on each village included a satellite-derived measure of the greenness of the surrounding vegetation (see Chapter 1), which was thought likely to be predictive of the local prevalence of breeding mosquitoes, and whether or not the village belonged to the primary health-care structure of the Ministry of Health.

To model the data, we define a binary response variable Y_{ij} to take the value 1 if the jth child in the ith village tests positive for malarial parasites in the blood, zero otherwise. Covariate information is denoted by a set of variables d_{ijk}: $k=1, \ldots, 5$, noting that, in the case of the village-level covariates, all children in a given village share a common value of the corresponding d_{ijk}. The location of the ith village is denoted by x_i.

An obvious non-spatial model would be a logistic regression model for the binary responses Y_{ij}. Writing $p_{ij}=P(Y_{ij}=1)$, the logistic regression model assumes that

$$\log\{p_{ij}/(1-p_{ij})\}=\alpha+\sum_{k=1}^{5} B_k d_{ijk} \tag{11}$$

and that the Y_{ij} are mutually independent. Evidence that this simple model is inadequate, and pointers towards a better-fitting model, can be obtained from an analysis of residuals, as follows. Let $\hat{p}_{ij}$ denote the estimated value of p_{ij} and $r_{ij}=(Y_{ij}-\hat{p}_{ij})/\sqrt{\{\hat{p}_{ij}(1-\hat{p}_{ij})\}}$. Then, the *village-level residuals* from (11) are given by

$$r_i=m_i^{-0.5}\sum_{j=1}^{m_i} r_{ij} \tag{12}$$

where m_i is the number of children sampled in the ith village. If the model (11) is adequate, the village-level residuals should behave like an independent random sample from a distribution with mean zero and variance 1.

In addition to standard regression diagnostics, such as a plot of residuals r_i against corresponding fitted values $f_i=\Sigma_j\hat{p}_{ij}$, a spatial diagnostic is the *residual variogram*. The residual variogram plots half-squared differences, $v_{ij}=0.5(r_i-r_j)^2$, against intervillage distances, $d_{ij}=\|x_i-x_j\|$. The interpretability of a residual variogram is usually improved by averaging the v_{ij} within distance intervals and plotting the resulting values against the midpoints of the corresponding distance intervals. If the regression equation (11) has been specified correctly and the Y_{ij} are mutually independent, then each v_{ij} has approximate expectation 1. Under the weaker assumption that the residual variation is stationary, the approximate expectation of v_{ij} is $\sigma^2\{1-\rho(d_{ij})\}$, where σ^2 is the variance of r_i and $\rho(d)$ is the correlation between values of r_i associated with villages separated by distance d. Hence, the relationship between v_{ij} and d_{ij} can suggest what kind of model might give a reasonable description of the residual spatial variation.

Figure 4.2 shows the residual variogram for the Gambia malaria data in which the variogram ordinates have been averaged in distance bins of width 10 km. Its two important features are that the averaged variogram ordinates are generally greater than 1 and show a rising trend with increasing distance, levelling out at sufficiently large distances. To

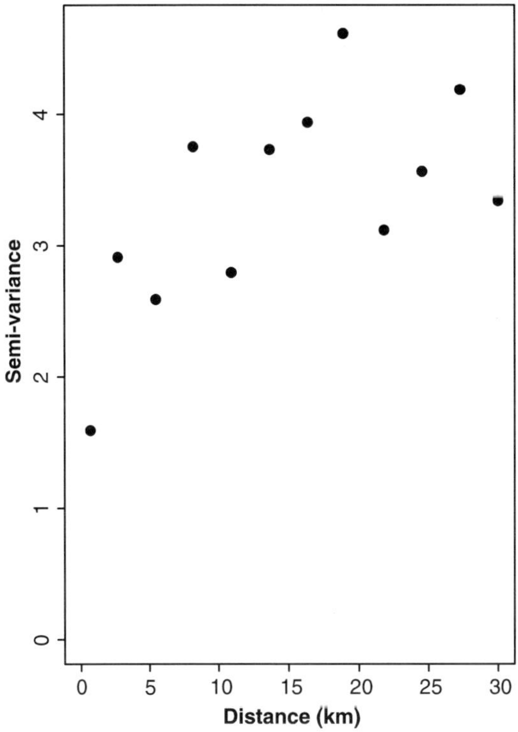

Fig. 4.2. The empirical variogram of village-level residuals from the Gambia childhood malaria survey.

account for both of these features, Diggle *et al.* (2002) extend the logistic regression model (10) to a hierarchical model

$$\log\{p_{ij}/(1-p_{ij})\} = \alpha + \sum_{k=1}^{5} B_k d_{ijk} + U_i + W(x_i) \tag{13}$$

in which the U_i are mutually independent Gaussian random variables with mean zero and variance υ^2, whilst $W(x)$ is a zero-mean Gaussian process with variance τ^2 and correlation function $\rho(d;\ \phi,\ \delta)$ of a kind proposed by Matérn (1960), in which the parameters ϕ and δ respectively determine the scale of the spatial correlation and the mean square differentiability of $W(x)$. The terms U_i and $W(x_i)$ respectively model non-spatial and spatial extra-binomial variation at the village level, the distinction between the two being that the U-values associated with two different villages are independent, whatever their respective locations, whereas the corresponding W-values will be correlated, to an extent determined by the distance between them.

Diggle *et al.* (2002) fit the model (13) using a Bayesian method, implemented by Markov chain Monte Carlo. This involves specifying *prior*

Table 4.1. 95% posterior intervals for the five logistic regression parameters.

Parameter	Posterior, Interval
Effect of age (days)	0.0004, 0.0009
Effect of untreated bednets	−0.6844, −0.0838
Additional effect of treated bednets	−0.7781, 0.0545
Effect of greenness index	−0.0397, 0.0715
Effect of PHC membership	−0.7917, 0.1807

distributions for all model parameters, and using a Monte Carlo method to simulate samples from the joint conditional distribution of all unknown quantities, namely the model parameters, the U_i and the process $W(x)$, given the observed data. This conditional distribution is the Bayesian's *posterior* distribution. Bayesian inference consists of reporting relevant summaries of the simulated samples from the posterior; for example, a Bayesian 95% posterior interval for a model parameter θ is constructed as the range of values which contains 95% of samples from the corresponding component of the posterior.

Table 4.1 summarizes the results of the analysis in terms of interval estimates of the model's regression parameters, confirming the protective effect of bed-nets. Note that the effect of the extrabinomial variation is substantially to widen these intervals; in other words, the simple logistic regression model would lead to spuriously narrow intervals and would therefore overstate the true significance of terms in the model. The other qualitative difference between the simple model (11) and its spatial extension (13) is that the extended version allows us to predict the residual variation in malarial prevalence throughout the country rather than just at the sampled villages. The final model selected by Diggle *et al.* (2002) eliminated the U_i term from (13). Figure 4.3 shows the resulting surface of predictions $W(x)$ for the whole country. With only 65 distinct locations in the data, this predicted surface is necessarily somewhat crude but is nevertheless optimal (in terms of mean square error) under the assumed model. Also, the methodology yields a posterior distribution for any property of the surface $W(x)$ which might be of scientific interest. By considering the width of the relevant posterior interval, we can therefore guard against over-interpretation of particular features in the surface of point estimates $W(x)$.

This example shows how a hierarchical logistic regression model can be combined with a model for continuous spatial variation to enable valid inference about regression parameters in the presence of unexplained spatial variation in disease prevalence, and to construct a continuous spatial interpolant as an estimate of this unexplained variation.

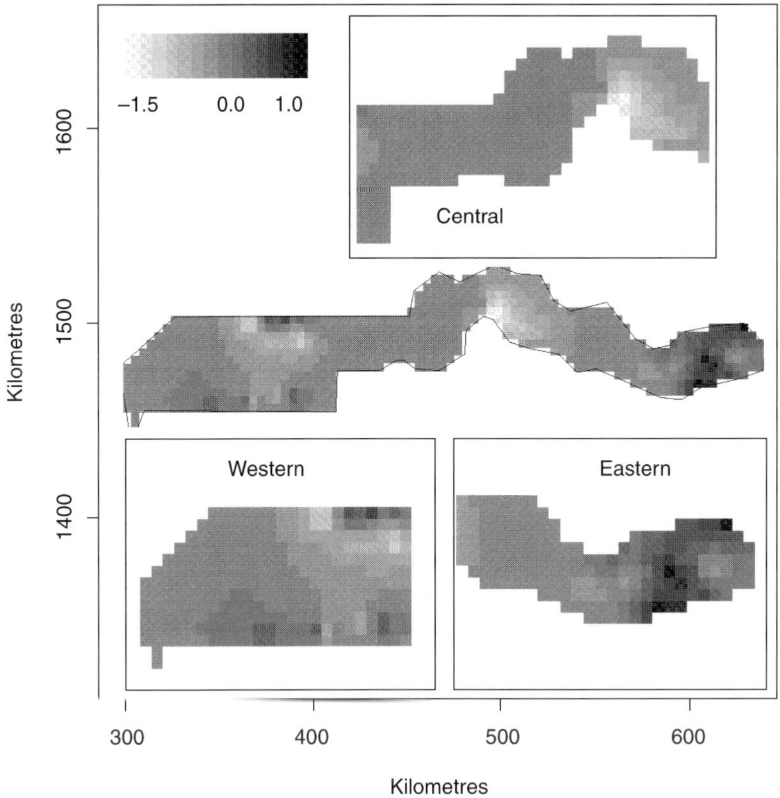

Fig. 4.3. The surface of predicted value *W*(x) for residual spatial variation of prevalence in the Gambia childhood malaria survey.

4.3.2 Spatial segregation among strains of bovine tuberculosis

An issue of some controversy in veterinary epidemiology concerns the primary mode of transmission of bovine tuberculosis, *Mycobacterium bovis*. Is the disease primarily spread within the cattle population by the movement of infected animals, or through a wildlife host such as the badger? Strain-typing of isolates of the bacterium can help to resolve whether different cases of the disease share a common source. See, for example, Collins *et al.* (1994). The kinds of genotyping methods used to investigate the relatedness of different cases are reviewed in Durr *et al.* (2000a,b). One specific application, described briefly in Durr *et al.* (2000b), is to examine the degree of spatial segregation amongst the genotypes of outbreaks in different herds of cattle. In particular, they mapped the spatial distribution of the more common genotype, using a technique known as spoligotyping (Groenen *et al.*, 1993), amongst cattle

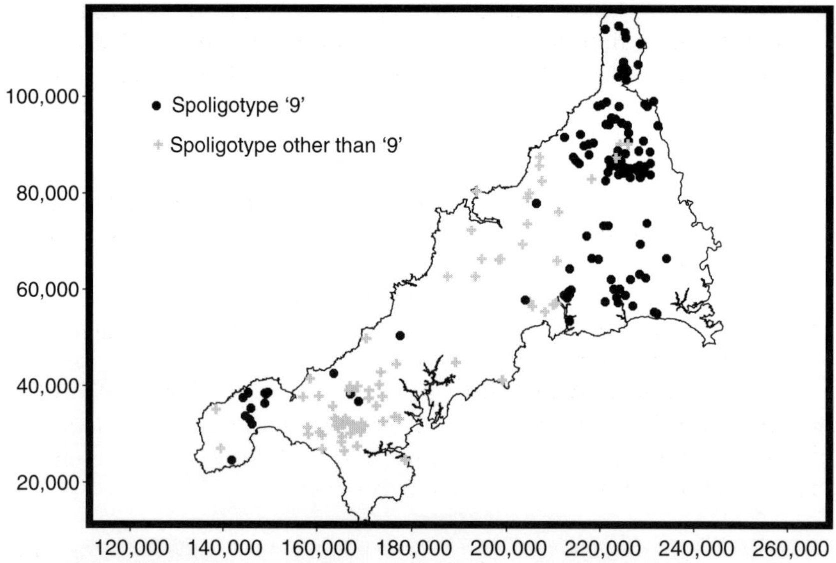

Fig. 4.4. Locations of bovine tuberculosis cases in Cornwall, UK, 1997/98. The most common genotype ('9') is indicated by a solid dot. Axes numbers refer to distance in metres from the origin point of the British National Grid.

and badgers in England and Wales during 1996/97. In the remainder of this subsection, we outline a possible method for quantifying the degree of spatial segregation in maps of this kind.

To provide a specific focus for the method we seek to develop, Fig. 4.4 shows the locations of 204 cases of bovine tuberculosis in herds in the county of Cornwall, UK, during the years 1997 and 1998. Amongst these 204 cases, ten different genotypes were identified. In Fig. 4.4 we distinguish the most common of these ('9'), accounting for 116 cases, from the remainder by using two different plotting symbols.

Let $p_j(x)$ denote the probability that, over a specified period of time, a herd at location x will experience an outbreak of type j. Then, in a *completely unsegregated process*, the value of $p_j(x)$ follows the relationship $p_j(x) = \alpha_j p(x)$, where α_j reflects the relative scarcities of the different types but the spatial variation in risk, $p(x)$, is common to all types. This results in spatially constant *relative risk surfaces*, $r_{jk}(x) = p_j(x)/p_k(x)$. In contrast, spatial variation in the surfaces $r_{jk}(x)$ is indicative of spatial segregation between spoligotypes. The extreme form of segregation arises when one of the $p_j(x)$ dominates in any given subregion, and the dominant local type varies between subregions.

One way to estimate the $p_j(x)$, and hence the $r_{jk}(x)$, is through a multivariate extension of the kernel smoothing method proposed by Kelsall and Diggle (1998) for case–control data in human epidemiology.

The adaptation of this existing, univariate method to the spatial distribution of bovine tuberculosis in Cornwall would proceed as follows.

Suppose, initially, that outbreaks within the study region are not differentiated with respect to spoligotype. Then, each herd acquires a binary label $Y_i = 1$ if herd i has suffered an outbreak during the study period; otherwise $Y_i = 0$. Let x_i denote the location of herd i. Our objective is to estimate the surface $p(x)$, where $p(x_i) = P(Y_i = 1)$. This problem could be tackled by methods similar to those used in the Gambia malaria example of Section 4.3.1 of this chapter, but, because of the larger number of distinct spatial locations involved, the kernel smoothing method of Kelsall and Diggle (1998) offers an alternative strategy and is the one we explore here.

A *kernel estimator* of $p(x)$ is simply a locally weighted spatial moving average of the Y_i. Let $w(x)$ be a *kernel function*, typically a non-negative-valued function with a single mode at $x = 0$. Then, a kernel estimator based on data (x_i, Y_i): $i = 1, \ldots, n$ takes the form

$$\hat{p}(x) = \sum_{i=1}^{n} w_i Y_i \tag{14}$$

where

$$w_i = w(x - x_i) / \sum_{i=1}^{n} w(x - x_i)$$

In practice, $w(x)$ includes a scale parameter h, called the *bandwidth*, which controls the extent to which the kernel estimator (14) takes account of data close to or remote from the target location x. Expressed algebraically, $w(x) = h^{-2} w_1(x/h)$, and the particular class of kernel estimators to be used is defined by the choice of the standardized kernel function $w_1(x)$. For example, using u to denote the distance of the point x from the origin, a simple and convenient choice is the piece-wise quartic

$$w_1(x) = \begin{cases} (1 - u^2)^2 : & 0 \le u \le 1 \\ 0 & : u > 1 \end{cases}$$

Because it depends only on distance, this kernel function has circular contours; Fig. 4.5 shows its cross-section when $h = 1$.

In general, choosing a larger value for h results in a smoother surface $\hat{p}(x)$. This is often aesthetically pleasing and reduces the variance of the estimator, but at the expense of increasing its bias. In practice, the chosen value for h will reflect a compromise between these competing considerations. One method of choosing h is to maximize a cross-validated log-likelihood, defined as follows.

The ordinary log-likelihood function is

$$L(p) = \sum_{i=1}^{n} Y_i \log p(x_i) + (1 - Y_i) \log\{1 - p(x_i)\} \tag{15}$$

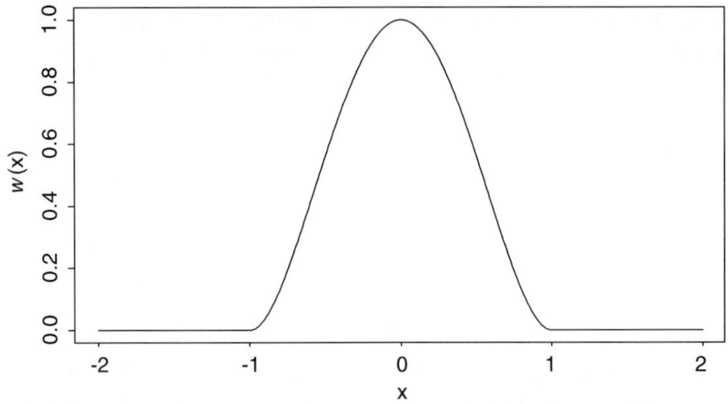

Fig. 4.5. Central cross-section of the quartic kernel function, with bandwidth $h=1$.

In a parametric model for $p(x)$, the accepted method of parameter estimation is to choose parameter values to maximize the right-hand side of (15). In the kernel setting, to do so would lead to the unhelpful bandwidth choice $h=0$, giving $\hat{p}(x_i)=1$ or 0 according to whether the corresponding $Y_i=1$ or 0. To circumvent this, the cross-validated log-likelihood function for h is defined as

$$L_c(h)=\sum_{i=1}^{n} Y_i \log \hat{p}^{(i)}(x_i)+(1-Y_i)\log\{1-\hat{p}^{(i)}(x_i)\} \quad (16)$$

where $\hat{p}^{(i)}(x)$ denotes the kernel estimator (14) based on all of the data except (x_i, Y_i). Choosing h to maximize the right-hand side of (16) is not the only, and not necessarily the best, way to choose h, but is a sensible method and has the advantage of being easily adaptable to more complicated problems.

In our case, the adaptation we seek is the estimation of a multivariate surface $\{p_1(x), \ldots, p_m(x)\}$, where $p_j(x)$ denotes the probability that a herd at location x will experience an outbreak of spoligotype j. The corresponding data are a set of categorical outcomes, Y_i: $i=1, \ldots, n$, where $Y_i=j$ denotes an outbreak of type j. Note that $j=0$ corresponds to no outbreak of any kind, and to complete the specification of the model we write $p_0(x)=1-\sum_{j=1}^{m} p_j(x)$. The log-likelihood function is then

$$L(p_1, \ldots, p_m)=\sum_{i=1}^{n} I(Y_i=j)\log p_j(x_i) \quad (17)$$

where $I(.)$ is the indicator function. Two variants of the cross-validated form of (17) could be defined, according to whether we do or do not want to choose the same bandwidth for all m components of the p-surface. The univariate theory in Kelsall and Diggle (1998) suggests that a common bandwidth might well be preferable if relative risk surfaces $r_{jk}(x) = p_j(x)/p_k(x)$ are of primary interest. Confirmation of this requires further work, which is in progress.

An altogether more challenging problem in this same substantive area is to develop a space–time model for the spread of the disease over time. If the data shown in Fig. 4.4 prove to be typical, we would expect to find a strong degree of spatial segregation. This implies that a model for the spread of disease over time would need to include a space–time diffusion component, in which cases of a particular strain spread out from an initially unidentified source. However, spoligotypes can also jump over large distances because of the movement of undiagnosed cases. Finally, the possible interaction between domestic and wild species needs to be considered.

4.3.3 Towards online disease surveillance

Our third example reports progress in the development of a surveillance system for non-specific gastrointestinal infections. In the UK, the incidence of gastrointestinal disease is increasing and there have been several well-publicized outbreaks traceable to contaminated food sources. Early detection of anomalies in the incidence pattern of cases would help to detect emerging outbreaks as quickly as possible, with potential public-health benefits. However, early detection is severely hampered by under-reporting and by delays of up to 10 days between first reporting of a case and its confirmation (Clarkson and Fine, 1987; Wheeler *et al.*, 1999). A current collaboration between the Southampton Public Health Laboratory Service, Southampton University and Lancaster University aims to put in place a system for the electronic reporting of non-specific cases, the spatiotemporal distribution of which can then be analysed daily with a view to identifying anomalies in the incidence pattern which could indicate an emerging outbreak. Cases associated with an apparent anomaly would then be followed up in detail, to establish their serotype and to look for common risk factors.

For the spatiotemporal analysis, the data on each case will consist of postcode of residence, date of onset of symptoms and an indication of recent travel history. Data will be acquired in two ways: from individual general practitioners and from NHS Direct, a region-wide, 24-hour telephone-based medical advice service that has recently been introduced in the UK. The study is based on the area of central southern England around Southampton, with a catchment population of around 2 million. It is anticipated that there could be as many as 200 incident cases per day.

We first consider how we might deal with the NHS Direct data. The postcodes and dates of onset of cases form a space–time point process. We suppose, initially, that the process is a Poisson process with space–time intensity $\lambda(x, t)$. As noted earlier, $\lambda(x, t)$ will largely reflect the distribution of the underlying population, which is of limited interest. However, if we assume a stable population then we can factorize the space–time intensity as

$$\lambda(x, t) = \lambda_0(x) r(x, t) \quad (18)$$

where $\lambda_0(x)$ is the population intensity and $r(x, t)$ the disease risk. It follows that $\lambda(x, t+1)/\lambda(x, t) = r(x, t+1)/r(x, t)$; hence, by monitoring changes in the incidence distribution we can identify changes in the underlying risk surface, as required. The assumption of a stable population is reasonable over short periods of time.

By the same token, although we cannot be sure that the pattern of usage of the NHS Direct service is geographically or demographically uniform, provided the usage pattern is stable over time the comparison between successive time-periods is valid. Monitoring the use of NHS Direct would be an interesting project in its own right.

The assumption of a Poisson process implies that cases occur independently. It cannot accommodate the kinds of spatial aggregation of related cases which we wish to detect. We therefore introduce a latent stochastic process $W(x, t)$ and model the risk surface $r(x, t)$ as

$$r(x, t) = \exp\{\alpha + W(x, t)\} \quad (19)$$

Peaks in the random surface $W(x, t)$ correspond to outbreaks of related cases. A more realistic model would replace the constant α with regression terms to account for known subject-specific or spatial risk factors, which would otherwise be attributed wrongly to $W(x, t)$.

Brix and Diggle (2001) show how to estimate the unobserved $W(x, t)$ surface in this model, using a Markov chain Monte Carlo algorithm. They allow $W(x, t)$ to have a general stationary spatial correlation structure, but assume that its temporal structure is Markovian. Specifically, if $\rho(s, u)$ denotes the correlation between values of $W(x, t)$ separated by distance s and time u, then

$$\rho(s, u) = \gamma(s; \theta) \exp(-u/\phi), \quad (20)$$

where $\gamma(.)$ is any suitable family of positive-definite functions.

Colour Plate 9 shows an application of this model to synthetic data, generated so as to mimic the anticipated structure of the gastrointestinal data and incorporating a realistic level of spatial heterogeneity based, in this case, on population data from southern Lancashire, UK. The left-hand panels of Colour Plate 9 show the true risk surfaces over three successive days, say days 5, 6 and 7, whilst the right-hand panels show the corresponding predicted surfaces. The average number of incident cases per day is 200, and the three predicted surfaces all use data from days 1–5 to predict the underlying risk surface on days 5, 6 and 7 respectively. Notice how the concurrent prediction on day 5 captures the major features of the underlying risk surface (top panels), albeit with some smoothing of peaks and troughs. The smoothing effect becomes progressively stronger as the forecast horizon increases (middle and bottom panels). This is a consequence of the modelled space–time correlation structure, specifically the decay in the temporal correlation between risk surfaces as their time separation increases.

In extending the model to accommodate general practice (GP)-based data, we need to recognize that reporting rates may vary systematically between GPs. A possible solution is to extend (19) to

$$r(\mathrm{x}, t) = \exp\{\alpha + W(\mathrm{x}, t) + U_{i(\mathrm{x}, t)}\} \tag{21}$$

where $i(\mathrm{x}, t)$ is the GP identifier for the (unique) case at location x and time t. The complete set of random variables U_i could be described by a discrete spatial variation model. However, if they are thought to arise solely through differences in the behaviour of individual GPs they might reasonably be modelled as a set of mutually independent random effects. Including both the $W(\mathrm{x}, t)$ and U_i components in the same model runs the risk of over-elaboration, leading to poor identifiability of model parameters and deterioration of predictive performance. The risk can be alleviated by identifying appropriate explanatory variables, whether at the individual patient or GP level, since inclusion of explanatory variables can account for variation which would otherwise be attributed wrongly to the $W(\mathrm{x}, t)$ or U_i terms in the model. Another possibility is that working to the spatial resolution of individual addresses will itself prove to be an over-refinement. A goal of identifying anomalies in the incidence pattern at GP level only would be less ambitious, but may lead to more robust predictions.

4.4 Conclusions

The subject of spatial statistics is now approaching maturity. Previously separate branches of the subject are being integrated in a range of substantive applications. The field of environmental epidemiology has stimulated many of the current methodological developments of spatial statistics, and veterinary epidemiology seems set to do likewise.

On the methodological side, the two most important developments of recent years have been the parallel growth of hierarchical modelling strategies and of Monte Carlo implementations of Bayesian and other likelihood-based methods of inference. More work needs to be done in both of these areas but especially, in the author's opinion, the latter with respect to the construction of algorithms which are efficient and robust, and whose convergence properties are well understood.

The ability to fit almost arbitrarily complicated models using formal, likelihood-based methods of inference is simultaneously liberating and dangerous. No longer can we justify confining ourselves to standard, simple models on the grounds that they are the only ones available. But more complicated models may rest on assumptions which are not easily validated from the available data, leading to conclusions that are assumption-driven rather than data-driven. We need to build interdisciplinary collaborations between statisticians and subject-matter scientists so that our models are soundly based and our inferences from those models are both valid and efficient. One of the great strengths of spatial statistics is its firm historical foundation in interdisciplinary collaborations of precisely this kind.

Acknowledgements

This work was supported by the European Union TMR Network in Computational and Statistical Methods for the Analysis of Spatial Data (ERB-FMRX-CT960095), The Veterinary Laboratories Agency (PU/T/PSC/00(79)) and the Department of Health AEGISS project (DH-280).

References

Altham, P.M.E. (1984) Improving the precision of estimation by fitting a model. *Journal of the Royal Statistical Society, Series B* 46, 118–119.

Baddeley, A.J., Moyeed, R.A., Howard, C.V. and Boyde, A. (1993) Analysis of a three-dimensional point pattern with replication. *Applied Statistics* 42, 641–668.

Bartlett, M.S. (1978) Nearest neighbour models in the analysis of field experiments. *Journal of the Royal Statistical Society, Series B* 40, 147–158.

Besag, J. (1974) Spatial interaction and the analysis of lattice systems (with discussion). *Journal of the Royal Statistical Society, Series B* 36, 192–225.

Besag, J. and Higdon, D. (1999) Bayesian analysis of agricultural field experiments (with discussion). *Journal of the Royal Statistical Society, Series B* 61, 691–746.

Besag, J. and Kempton, R.A. (1986) Statistical analysis of field experiments using neighbouring plots. *Biometrics* 42, 231–251.

Brix, A. and Diggle, P.J. (2001) Spatio-temporal prediction for log-Gaussian Cox processes. *Journal of the Royal Statistical Society, Series B* 63, 823–841.

Chiles, J.-P. and Delfiner, P. (1999) *Geostatistics: Modelling Spatial Uncertainty.* Wiley, New York.

Clarkson, J.A. and Fine, P.E.M. (1987) Delays in notification of infectious disease. *Health Trends* 19, 9–11.

Collins, D.M., de Lisle, G.W., Collins, J.D. and Costello, E. (1994) DNA restriction fragment typing of *Mycobacterium bovis* isolates from cattle and badgers in Ireland. *Veterinary Record* 134, 681–682.

Connor, S.J., Thomson, M.C., Flasse, S.P. and Perryman, A.H. (1998) Environmental information systems in malaria risk mapping and epidemic forecasting. *Disasters* 22, 39–56.

Cox, D.R. (1974) Contribution to the discussion of Mr Besag's paper. *Journal of the Royal Statistical Society, Series B* 36, 225.

Cressie, N.A.C. (1991) *Statistics for Spatial Data*. Wiley, New York.

D'Alessandro, U., Olaleye, B.O., McGuire, W., Langerock, P., Bennett, S., Aikins, M.K., Thomson, M.C., Cham, M.K., Cham, B.A. and Greenwood, B.M. (1995) Mortality and morbidity from malaria in Gambian children after introduction of an impregnated bednet programme. *The Lancet* 345, 479–483.

Diggle, P.J. (1986) Displaced amacrine cells in the retina of a rabbit: analysis of a bivariate spatial point pattern. *Journal of Neuroscience Methods* 18, 115–125.

Diggle, P.J. (1996) Spatial analysis in biometry. In: Armitage, P. and David, H.A. (eds) *Advances in Biometry*. Wiley, New York, pp. 363–384.

Diggle, P.J. (2003) *Statistical Analysis of Spatial Point Patterns*, 2nd edn. Edward Arnold, London.

Diggle, P.J., Lange, N. and Benes, F.M. (1991) Analysis of variance for replicated spatial point patterns in clinical neuroanatomy. *Journal of the American Statistical Association* 86, 618–625.

Diggle, P.J., Tawn, J.A. and Moyeed, R.A. (1998) Model-based geostatistics (with discussion). *Applied Statistics* 47, 299–350.

Diggle, P.J., Moyeed, R.A., Rowlingson, B.S. and Thomson, M.C. (2002) Childhood malaria in the Gambia: a case-study in model-based geostatistics. *Applied Statistics* 51, 493–506.

Durr, P.A., Hewinson, R.G. and Clifton-Hadley, R.S. (2000a) Molecular epidemiology of bovine tuberculosis: I. *Mycobacterium bovis* genotyping. *Revue Scientifique et Technique Office International des Epizooties* 19, 675–688.

Durr, P.A., Clifton-Hadley, R.S. and Hewinson, R.G. (2000b) Molecular epidemiology of bovine tuberculosis: II. Applications of genotyping. *Revue Scientifique et Technique Office International des Epizooties* 19, 689–701.

Elliott, P., Wakefield, J.C., Best, N.G. and Briggs, D.J. (eds) (2000) *Spatial Epidemiology: Methods and Applications*. Oxford University Press, Oxford, UK.

Gilks, W.R., Richardson, S. and Spiegelhalter, D.J. (eds) (1996) *Markov Chain Monte Carlo in Practice*. Chapman and Hall, London.

Glasbey, C.A. and Horgan, G.W. (1995) *Image Analysis for the Biological Science*. John Wiley & Sons, Chichester, UK.

Groenen, P.M.A., Bunschoten, A.E., van Sooligen, D. and van Embden, J.D.A. (1993) Nature of DNA polymorphism in the direct repeat cluster of *Mycobacterium tuberculosis*; application for strain differentiation by a novel typing method. *Molecular Microbiology* 10, 1057–1065.

Kelsall, J.E. and Diggle, P.J. (1998) Spatial variation in risk of disease: a nonparametric binary regression approach. *Applied Statistics* 47, 559–573.

Matérn, B. (1960) Spatial variation. *Meddelanden fran Statens Skogsforsningsinstitut* 49, 1–144.

Papadakis, J.S. (1937) *Méthode statistique pour des expériences sur champ.*

Bulletin Scientifique No. 23. Institut d'Amelioration des Plantes, Thessaloniki, Greece, pp. 12–28.

Stoyan, D., Kendall, W.S. and Mecke, J. (1987) *Stochastic Geometry and Its Applications*. Akademie-Verlag, Berlin.

Thomson, M.C., Connor, S.J., D'Alessandro, U., Rowlingson, B., Diggle, P., Creswell, M. and Greenwood, B. (1999) Predicting malaria infection in Gambian children from satellite data and bed net use surveys: the importance of spatial correlation in the interpretation of results. *American Journal of Tropical Medicine and Hygiene* 61, 2–8.

Webster, R. and Oliver, M.A. (2001) *Geostatistics for Environmental Scientists*. John Wiley & Sons, Chichester, UK.

Wheeler, J.G., Sethi, D., Cowden, J.M., Wall, P.G., Rodrigues, L.C., Tompkins, D.S., Hudson, M.J. and Roderick, P.J. (1999) Study of infectious intestinal disease in England: rates in the community presenting to general practice, and reported to national surveillance. *British Medical Journal* 318, 1046–1050.

Wilkinson, G.N., Eckert, S.R., Hancock, T.W. and Mayo, O. (1983) Nearest neighbour (NN) analysis with field experiments (with discussion). *Journal of the Royal Statistical Society, Series B* 45, 151–178.

1.

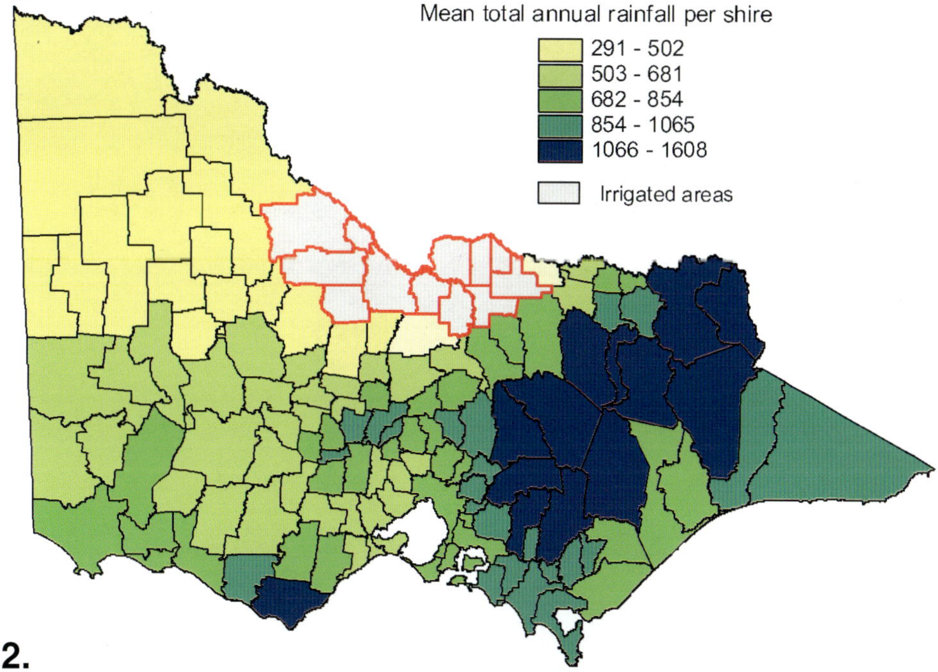

2.

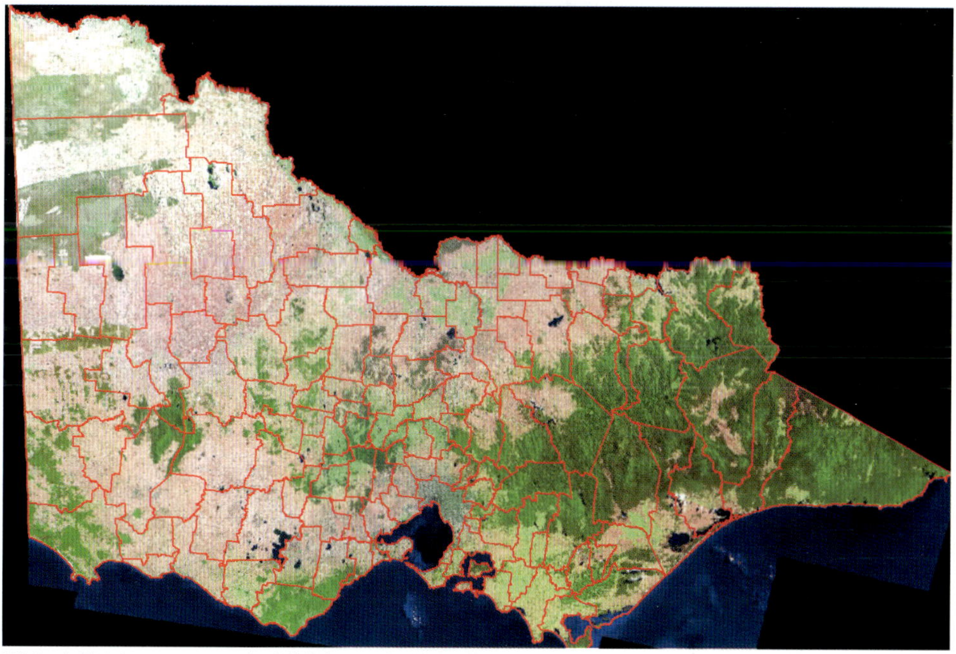

Plate 1. Total mean annual rainfall for each shire of Victoria for 1961-1990, calculated from interpolated data supplied by the Australian Bureau of Meteorology. The shaded zone indicates irrigation areas along the Murray River, as suggested by a sketch map in Watt (1977) and confirmed by satellite imagery (see Plate 2).

Plate 2. Landsat-derived satellite image of Victoria in the dry season showing the irrigated areas along the Murray River. Image contains Vicmap Information copyright The State of Victoria, Department of Sustainability and Environment, 2000; reproduced by permission of the Department of Sustainability and Environment; copyright Commonwealth of Australia - ACRES, Geoscience Australia.

3.

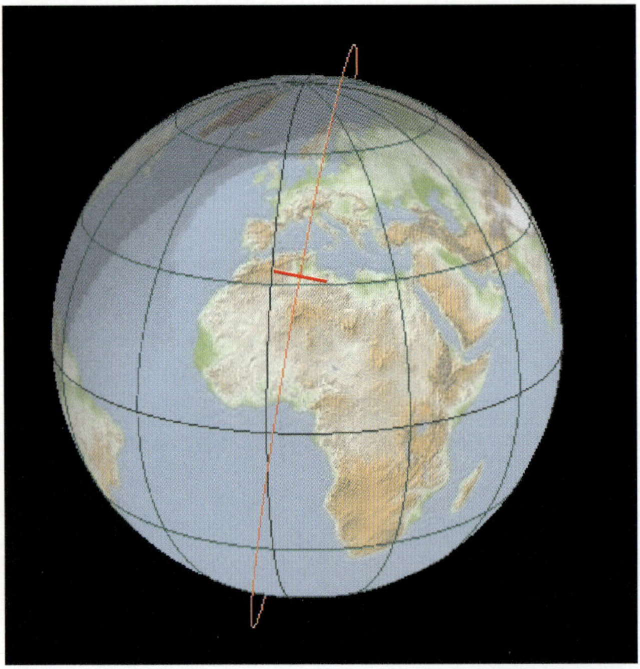

NOAA-17

20th December, 2002 10:01

5.

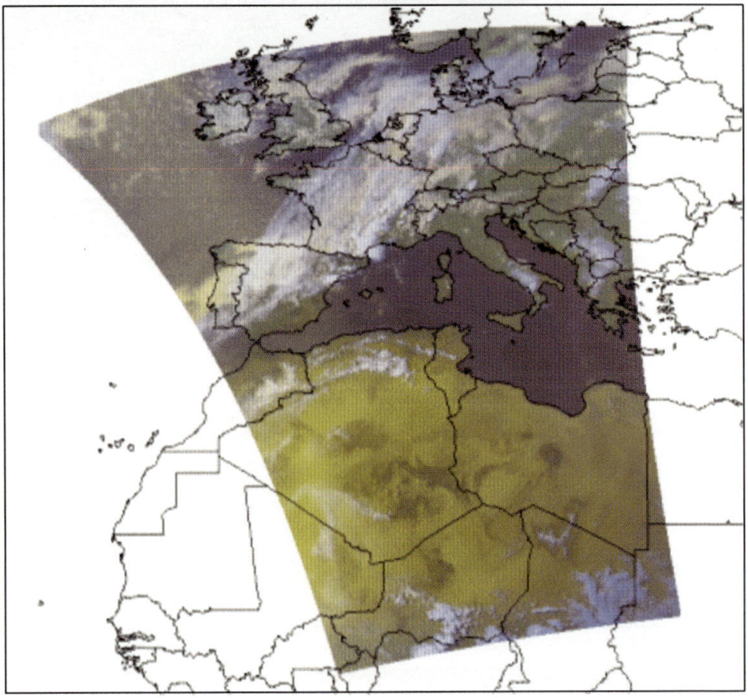

Plate 3. Orbital positions of the NOAA-17 satellite on 20 December 2002, as determined by WXtrackGL (http://www.satsignal.net).

Plate 5. AVHRR image covering part of Algeria taken in December 2002 and rectified to line up with the coast. Produced using NOAA-Tools 1.0 (http://www.avia-gis.com). Image courtesy of Dr Jan Biesemans.

4.

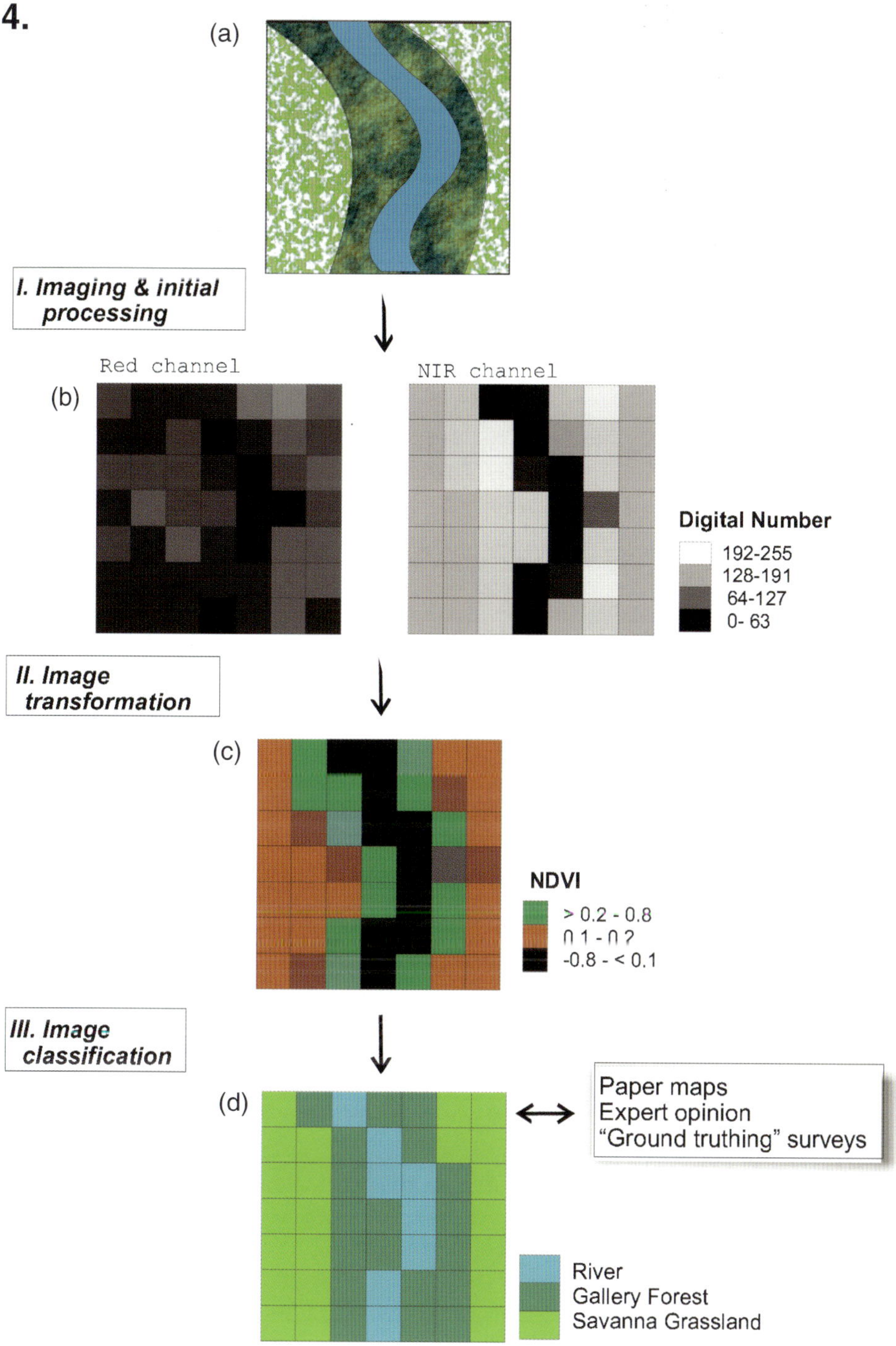

Plate 4. Schema showing the steps involved in using remotely sensed imagery to produce a land classification map of a gallery forest in a landscape in the wet/dry tropics. The panels show the landscape: (a) as it might appear to someone flying over it in an aeroplane; (b) as it would be recorded by the red and near infrared channels of a radiometer on board a satellite; (c) after the imagery had been processed to produce a vegetation index map; and (d) the final land classification map.

6.

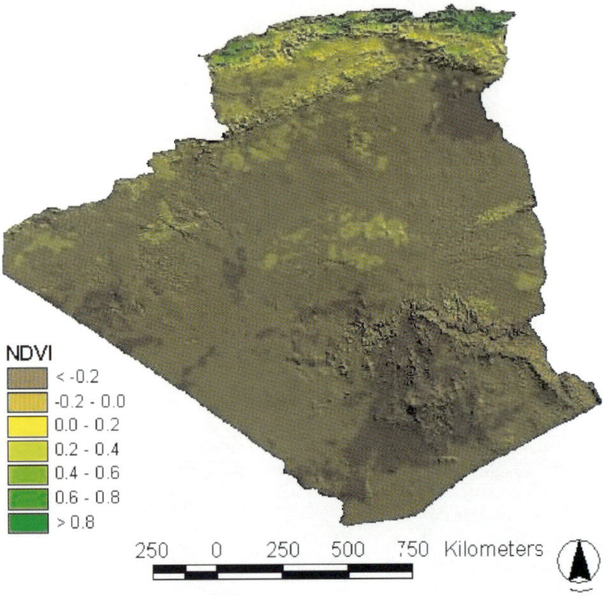

7.

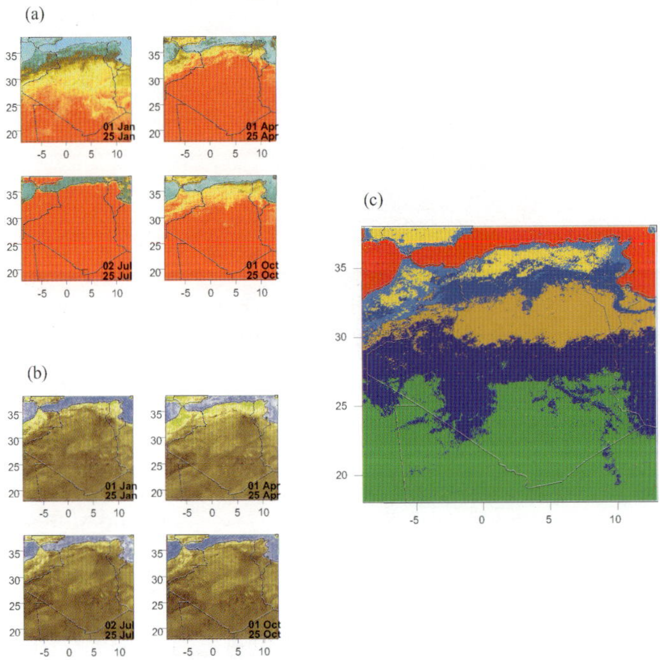

Plate 6. Normalized difference vegetation index (NDVI) for April 1994 draped over a digital terrain model of the whole of Algeria. NDVI calculated from channels 1 and 2 of the Pathfinder 64-km² data set (http://daac.gsfc.nasa.gov).

Plate 7. Examples of Fourier decomposition of seasonal channel-3 Kelvin temperature (a) and NDVI (b) for Algeria for 1996 using imagery from AVHRR NOAA-14. The complete set of temperature and NDVI maps were then used to produce a statistical ('K-means') classification of Algeria into zones of homologous ecoclimatology where similar disease processes might operate (c). Image processing by courtesy of Dr Jan Biesemans.

8.

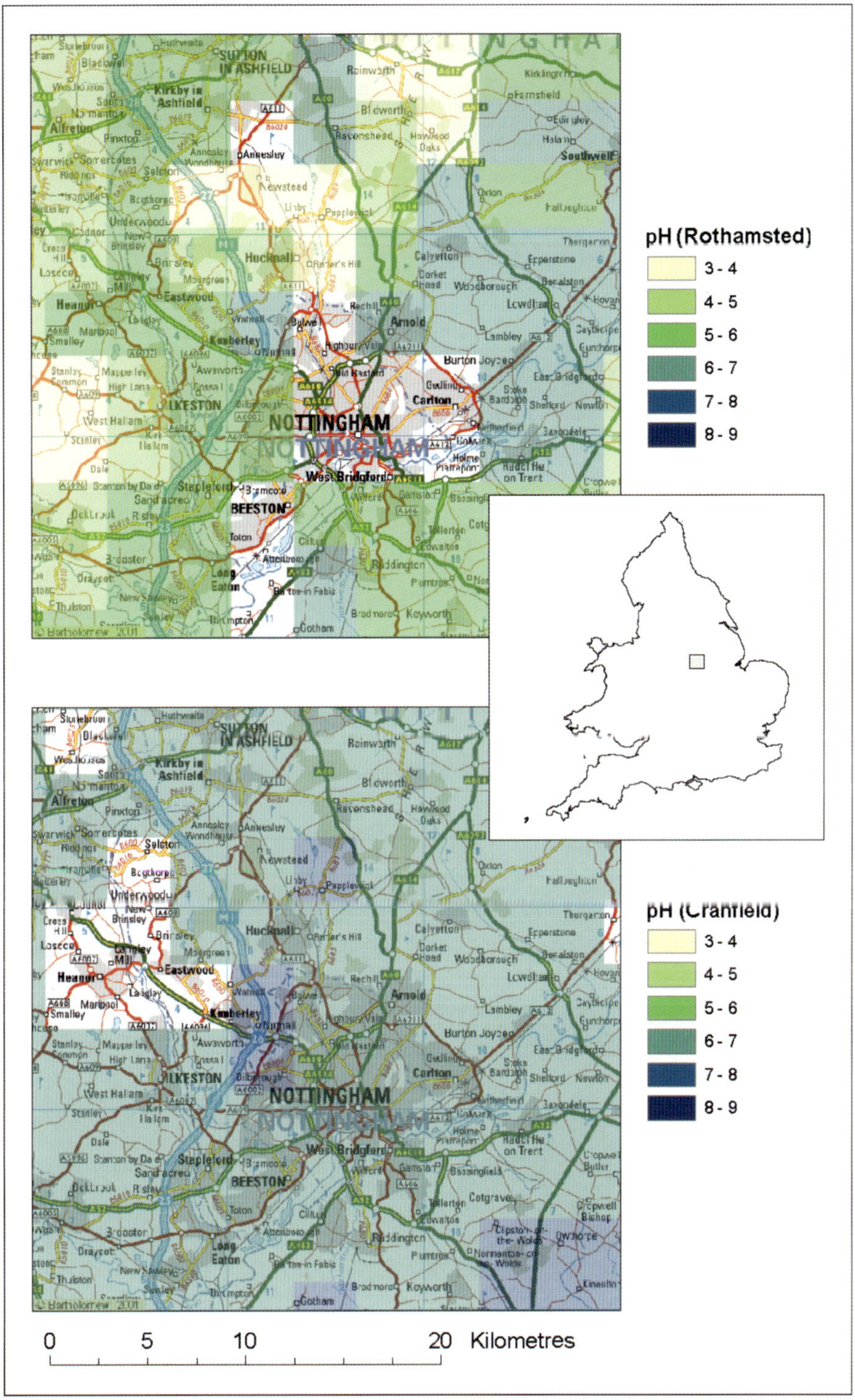

Plate 8. The variability between topsoil pH estimates from two available spatial datasets of the same location in the Midlands of England. Data are from Cranfield University and IACR-Rothamsted.

9.

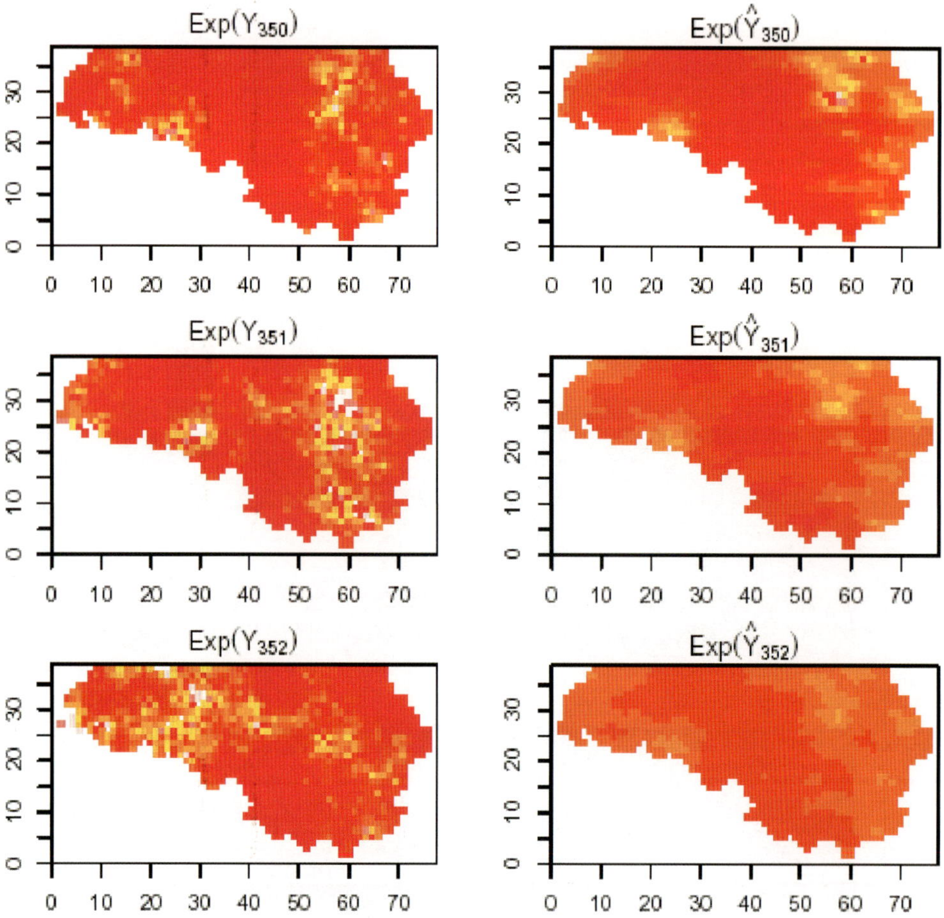

10.

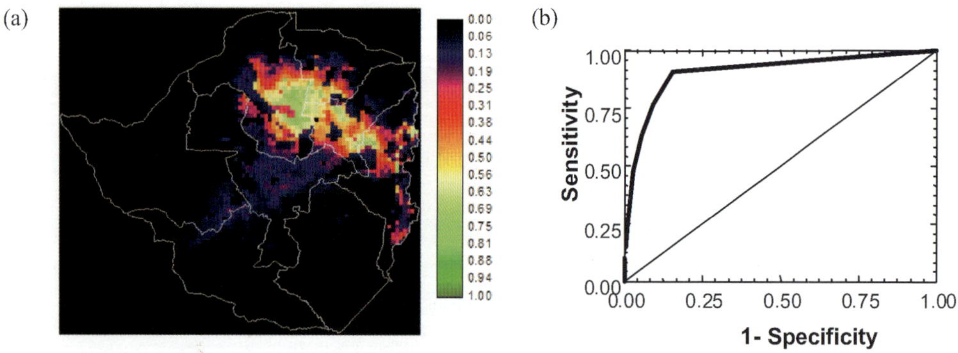

Plate 9. True (left-hand panels) and predicted (right-hand panels) surfaces W(x,t) over a 3-day period, using synthetic data based on the population distribution in southern Lancashire, UK. Reproduced from Brix and Diggle (2001), with permission.

Plate 10. (a) Logistic regression prediction of theileriosis outbreak risk in Zimbabwe. (b) ROC curve for theileriosis model. Reproduced from Pfeiffer *et al.* (1997), with permission.

11.

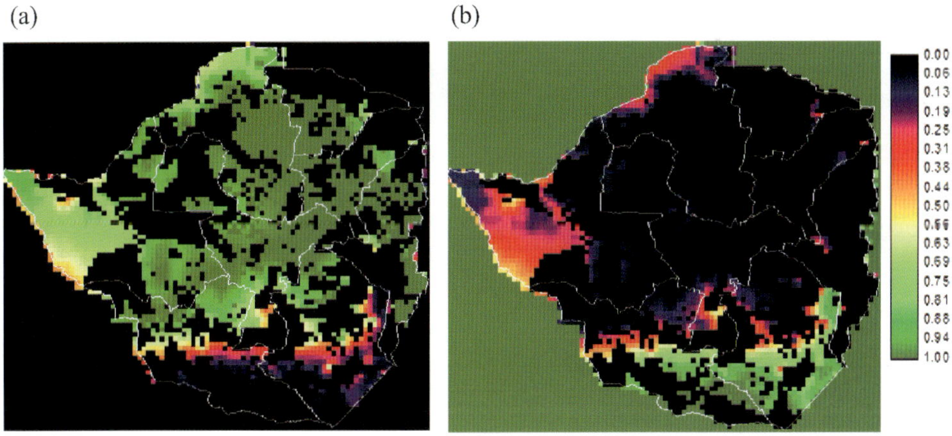

12.

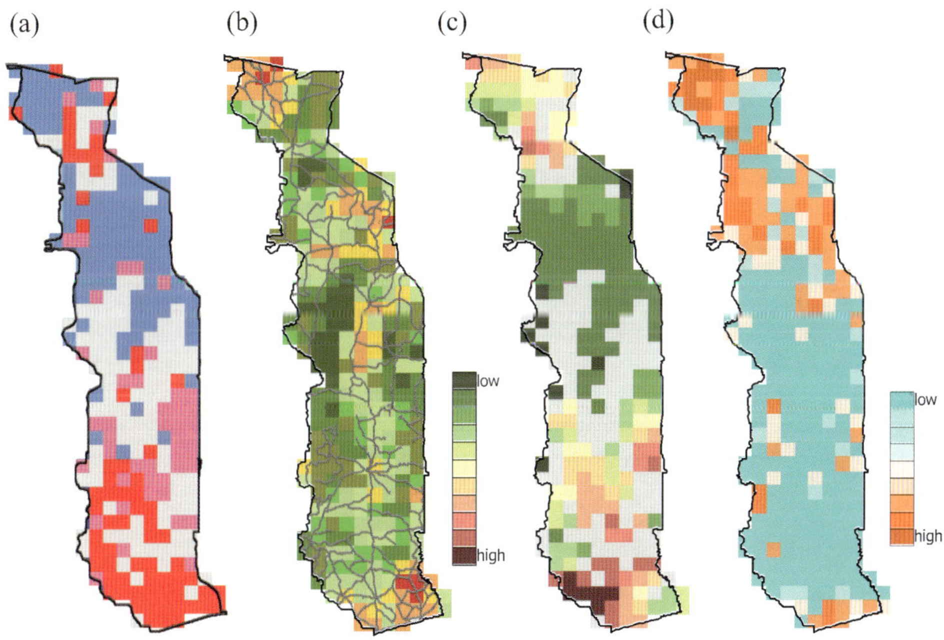

Plate 11. Maps expressing the belief and the uncertainty relating to the prediction of the presence of *Theileria parva* in Zimbabwe produced using Dempster-Shafer theory. (a) Belief map. (b) Belief interval map.

Plate 12. Togo animal husbandry systems. (a) Clustered animal husbandry systems. Blue = rural extensive systems; red = market-oriented systems; pink = intermediary systems. (b) Agriculture intensity: percentage of land included in the agricultural cycle. (c) Zebu introgression: proportion of zebu or crossbred cattle compared with indigenous trypanotolerant taurine population. Note that zebu introgression is mainly found in market-oriented and intermediary animal husbandry systems. (d) Cattle distribution.

13.

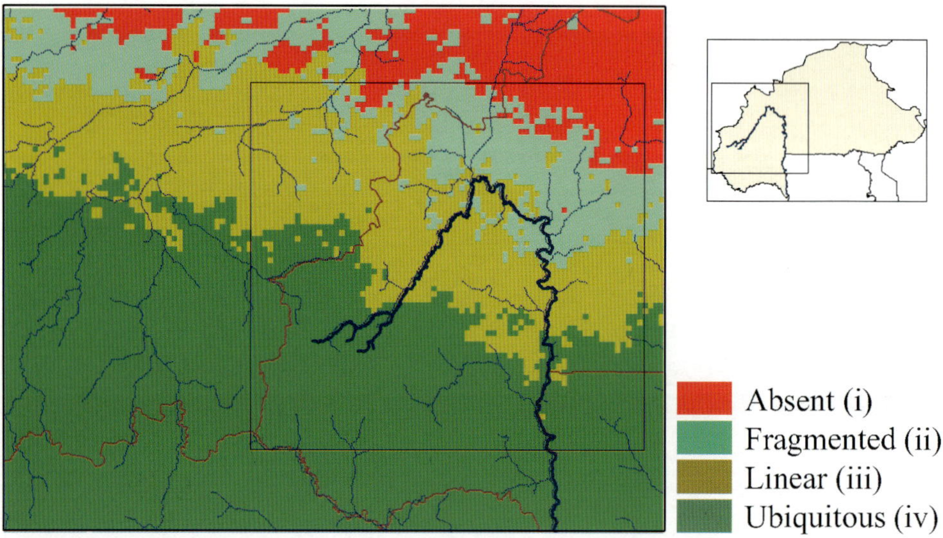

14.

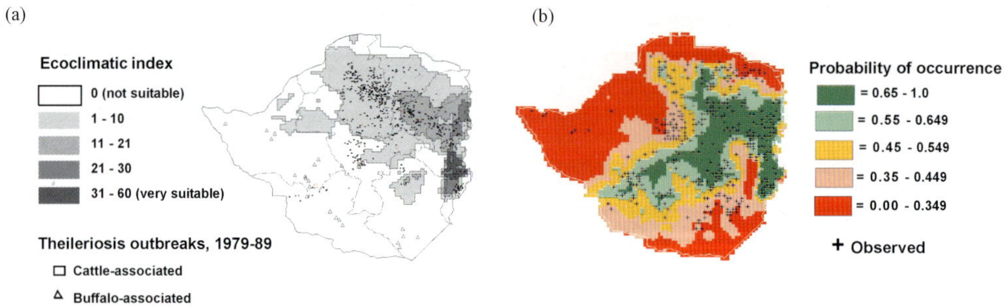

Plate 13. Predicted riverine tsetse distribution patterns in western Burkina Faso and south-eastern Mali. Four distinct classes are shown: (i) tsetse absent; (ii) fragmented tsetse populations (tsetse are present only in suitable habitat islands in otherwise hostile ecoclimatic conditions); (iii) linear tsetse populations (tsetse are found only in linear riparian habitats along mainstreams and important tributaries); (iv) ubiquitous (tsetse are present in suitable vegetation of the entire drainage system). For more detail see Hendrickx and Tamboura (2000).

Plate 14. (a) Observed locations of outbreaks of theileriosis in Zimbabwe superimposed on a suitability map for *Rhipicephalus appendiculatus* as predicted by CLIMEX. Adapted from Perry *et al.* (1991).
(b) Locations of collections of *R. appendiculatus* compared to the probability of occurrence as predicted by a discriminant analysis combining ground-measured (temperature and altitude) and remotely sensed (NDVI) data. Reprinted from Rogers and Randolph (1993), with permission from Elsevier.

15.

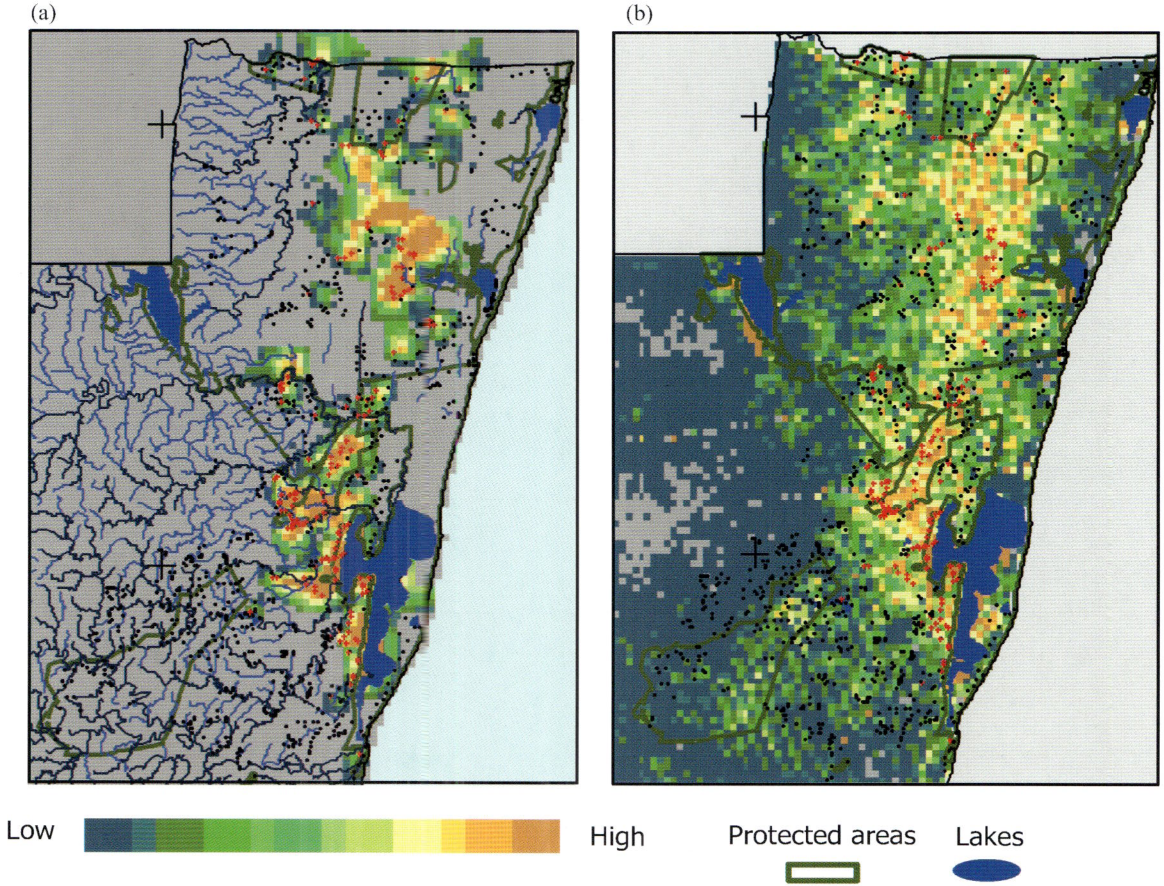

Plate 15. Spatial modelling of the distribution of *Glossina austeni* in KwaZulu Natal using geostatistics (a) and multivariate logistic regression (b). Key to (a) indicates the probability of occurrence of *G. austeni*.

16.

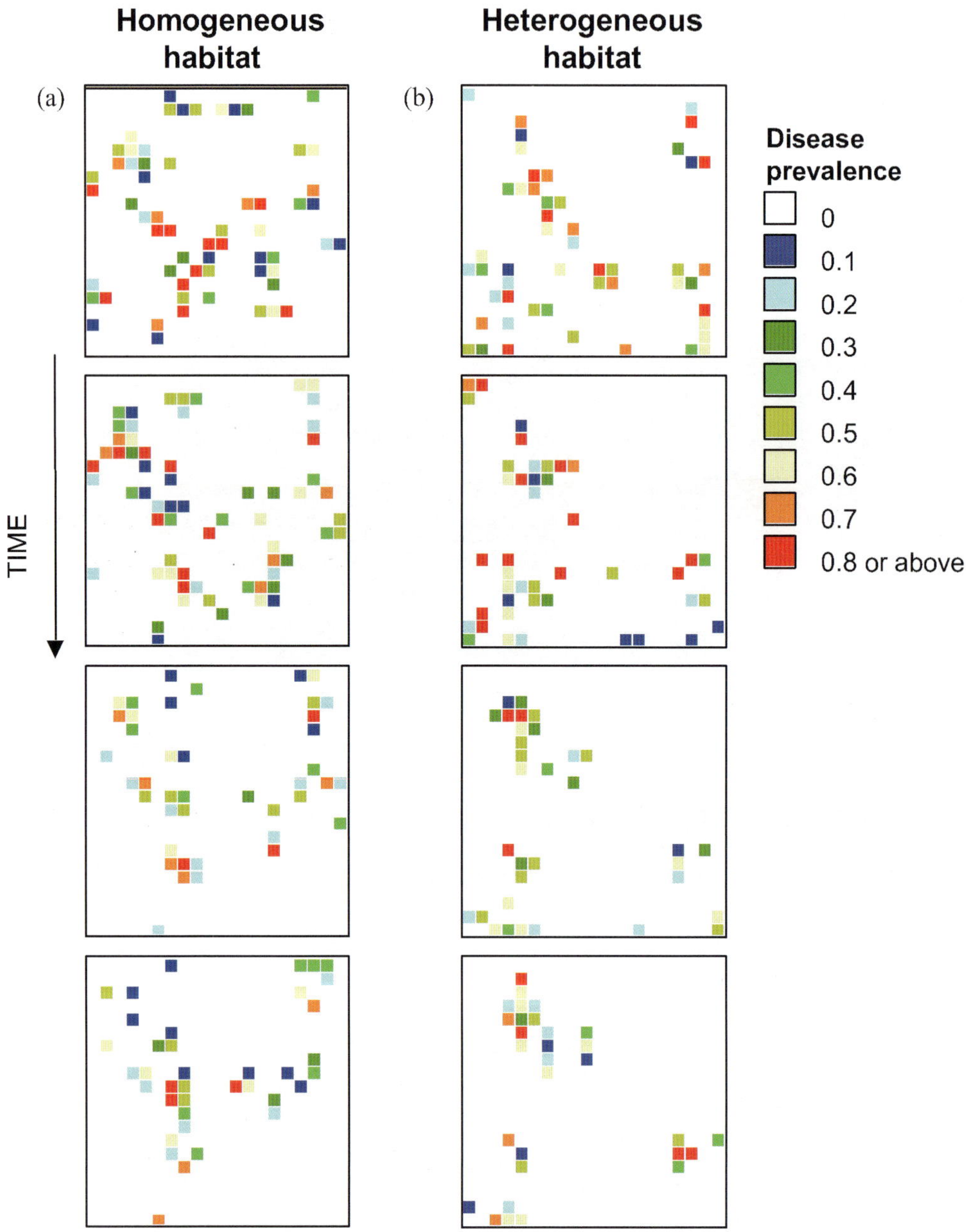

Plate 16. A spatiotemporal view of prevalence levels of TB in badgers from a simulation model with (a) a homogeneous habitat area and (b) a heterogeneous habitat area, based on GIS interpretation of remote sensing reflectance data. The homogeneous and heterogeneous habitat areas both had overall mean carrying capacities of eight adult and yearling badgers per territory. Successive images down the page are separated from each other by a 10-year period.

17.

(a)

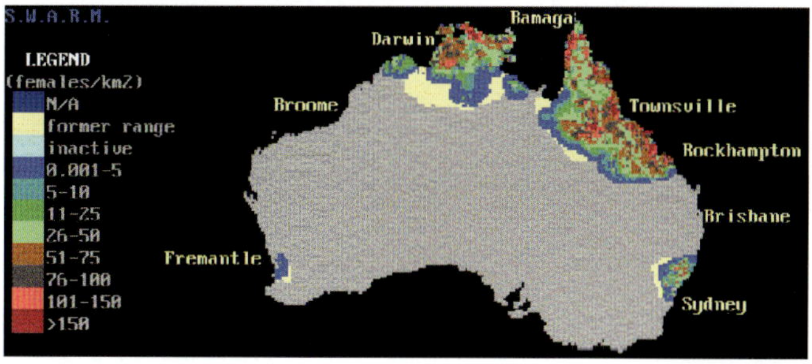

(b)

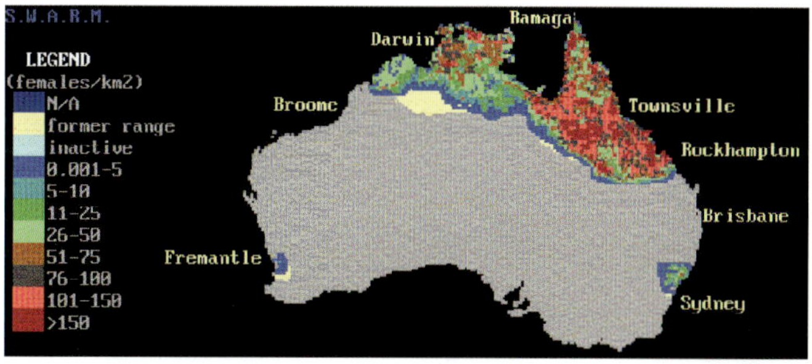

(c)

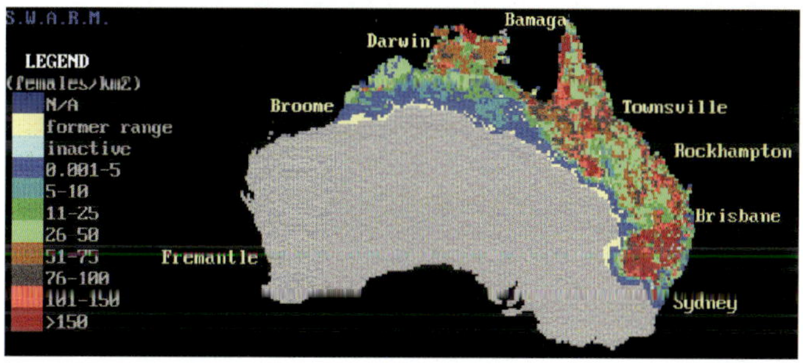

(d)

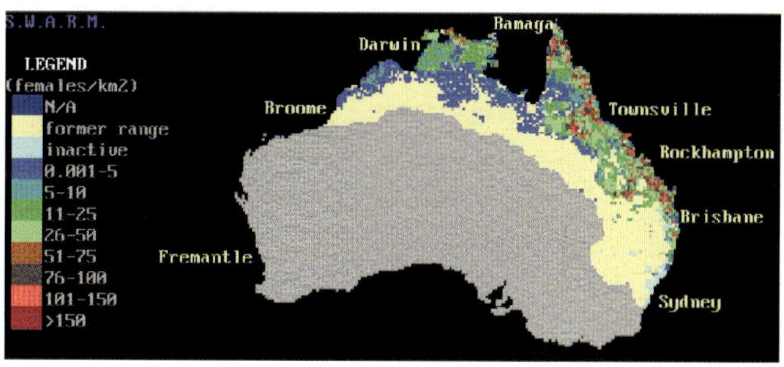

Plate 17. Output from the screwworm fly (SWF) invasion model. The extent and distribution of female SWF 2 years after incursions on 1 January in Sydney, Cairns, Darwin and Fremantle are shown for (a) an average year and (b) a wet year. The estimated range in an endemic situation (unhindered growth for 10 years) is shown for summer (c) and winter (d). Although there was limited spread after 2 years around the Sydney and Fremantle invasions compared with the more northerly incursions, the endemic pattern revealed contiguity of spread and a large population north of Sydney in the summer months. Reproduced with permission from R. Glanville, DPI Queensland.

18.

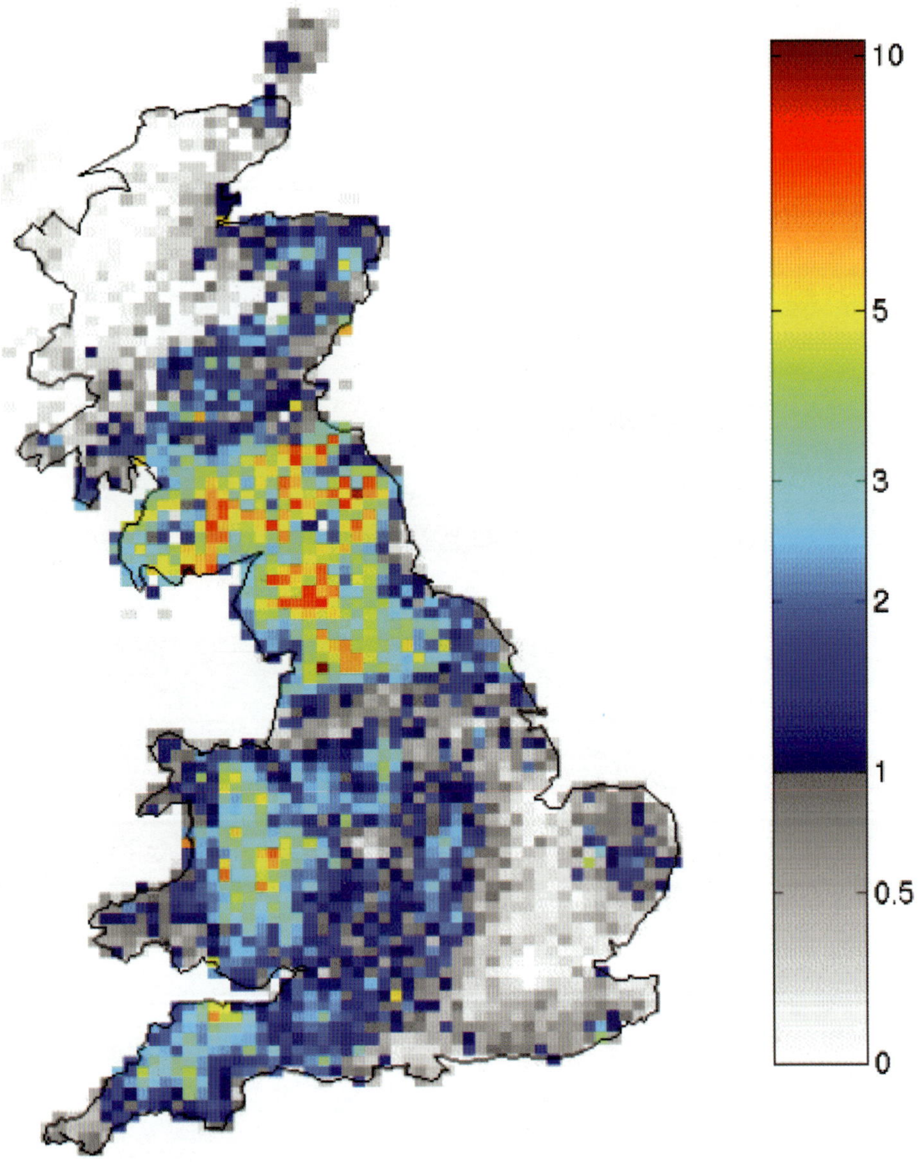

Plate 18. R0 map produced from the estimated number of secondary foot-and-mouth disease (FMD) infections arising from each of the 144,000 farms in the UK. The results are aggregated into 10 x 10 km squares. The colour coding highlights those areas with R0 > 1, where the number of cases would increase in the absence of intervention. Reproduced with permission from Keeling *et al.* (2001). Supplementary material: http://www.sciencemag.org/cgi/content/full/1065973/DC1/1

19.

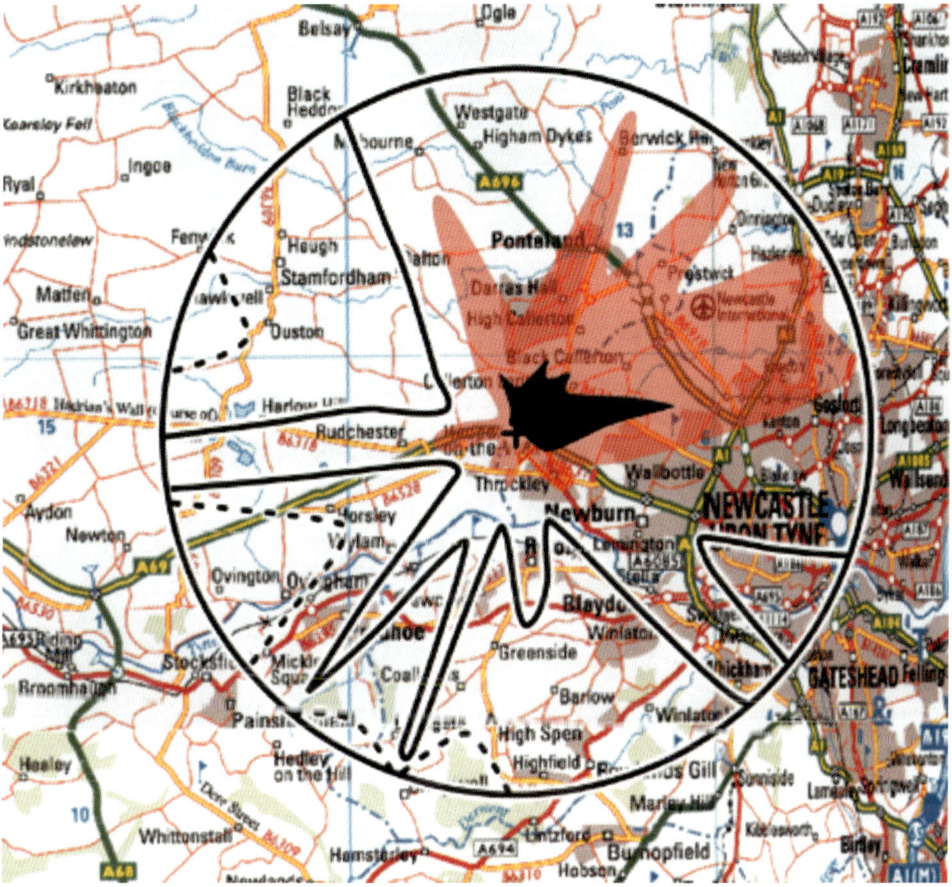

Plate 19. Plume map of foot-and-mouth disease (FMD) virus generated off the presumed index case farm at Heddon-on-the-Wall, near Newcastle, for the UK 2001 FMD epidemic. Map supplied courtesy of Veterinary Laboratories Agency, Weybridge.

20.

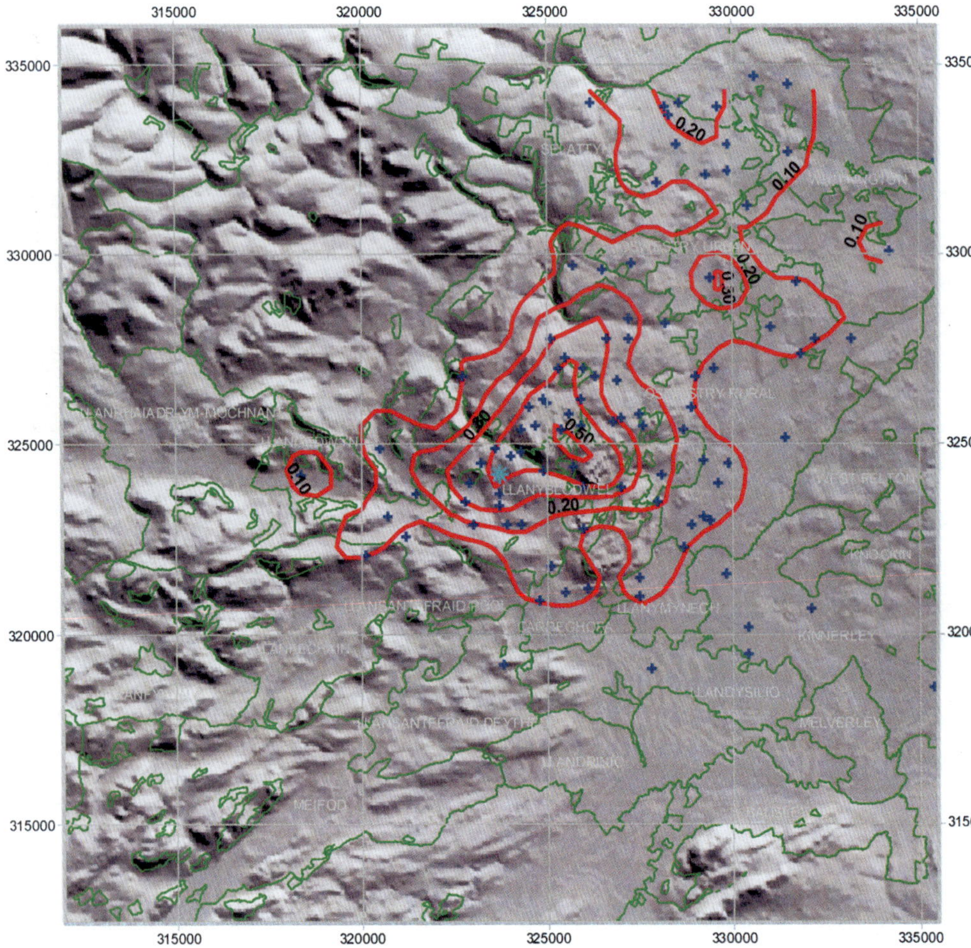

Plate 20. Map showing farms infected within the first 3 weeks of the UK 1967/68 foot-and-mouth disease epidemic in Shropshire, UK. Asterisks indicate the source farm and crosses indicate secondary farms. Estimated mean infection probability isolines (0.1 increments) are shown. The background shows parishes and a shaded relief model. From Sanson *et al.* (2000). Background map reproduced with permission of Ordnance Survey (Crown Copyright NC/00/724).

21.

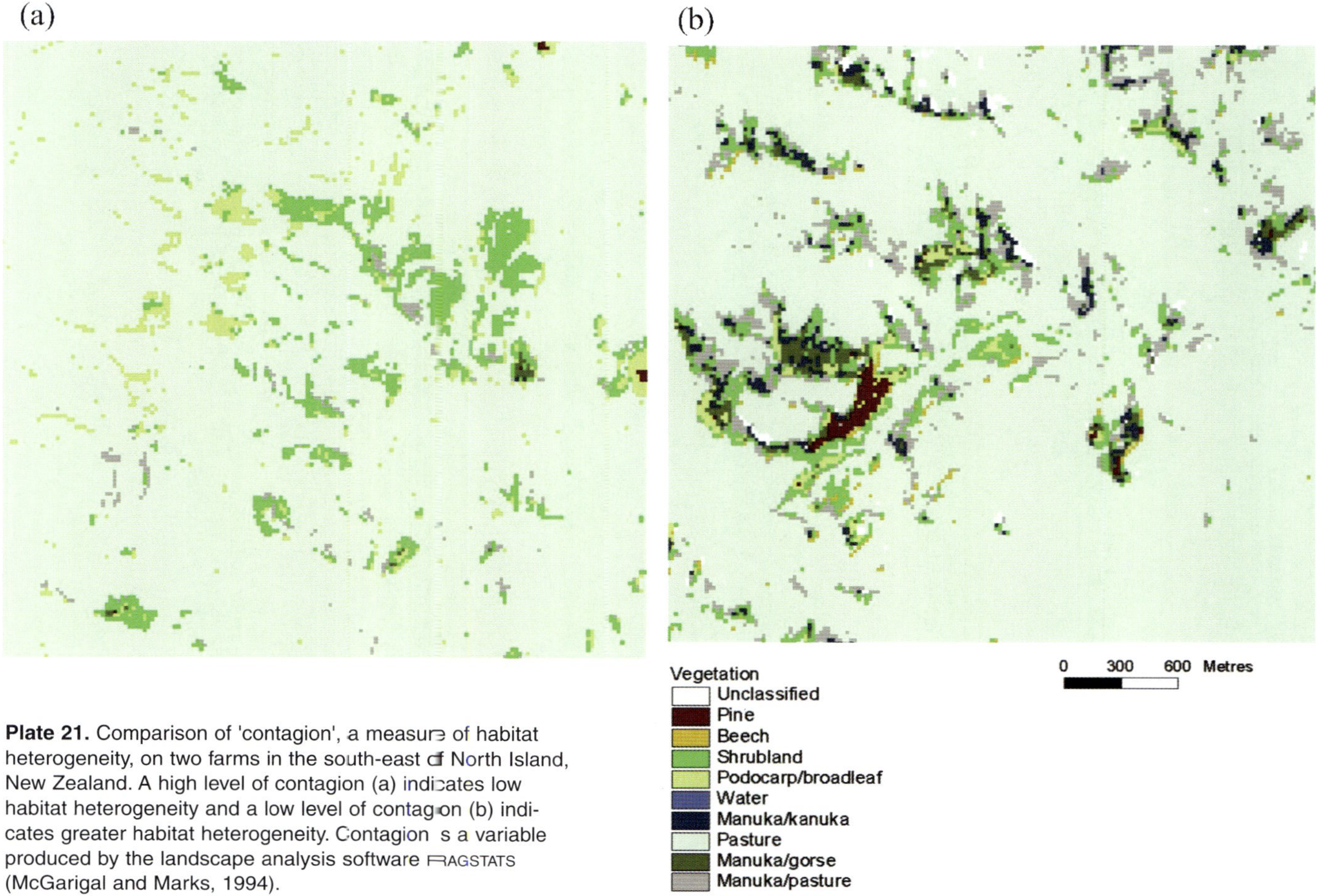

Plate 21. Comparison of 'contagion', a measure of habitat heterogeneity, on two farms in the south-east of North Island, New Zealand. A high level of contagion (a) indicates low habitat heterogeneity and a low level of contagion (b) indicates greater habitat heterogeneity. Contagion is a variable produced by the landscape analysis software FRAGSTATS (McGarigal and Marks, 1994).

22.

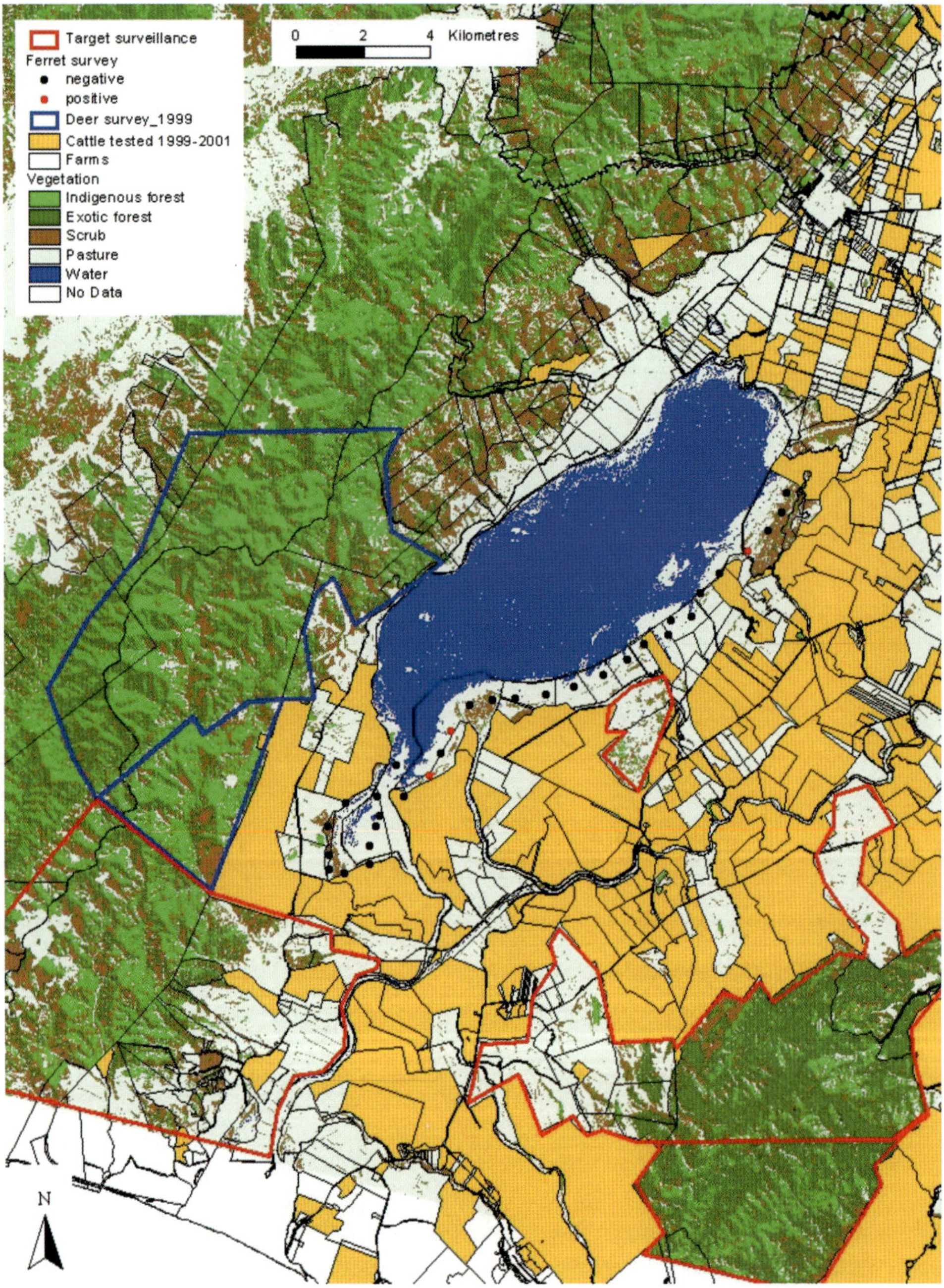

Plate 22. A map combining three sources of information on TB status of the underlying possum population: farms on which cattle have been TB-tested (coloured orange), a survey of ferrets (red dots, TB-positive; black dots, TB-negative) and the hypothetical area covered by a hunter-based survey of TB in feral deer (outlined in blue). The areas where the TB status of possums is uncertain and which can be targeted for future surveillance activities are outlined in red.

Geographical Information Science and Spatial Analysis in Animal Health

5

Dirk U. Pfeiffer

5.1 Introduction

Animal disease data are collected as part of surveillance or research activities. Each data item normally has a spatial as well as an animal and a temporal dimension. Classic epidemiological analysis focused mainly on the animal dimension, whereas time and space were usually explored using fairly basic methods. Most national disease surveillance systems still only have a limited capacity to work with georeferenced information. However, recent outbreaks of classical swine fever and foot-and-mouth disease in the UK have demonstrated that geographical information systems (GIS) have now become an indispensable tool, particularly when dealing with emergency responses to exotic disease outbreaks. While surveillance systems lag behind in the adoption of spatial data analysis (SDA), its use for the purpose of specific epidemiological investigations has already become widespread.

Transmission of an infectious agent requires direct or indirect contact between the source of infection and the susceptible animal, which means that spatial proximity has to be considered as a key factor when determining the risk of infection for individual animals or herds. GIS has the advantage over a standard database management system that it has a concept of spatial neighbourhood, so that it is possible to determine spatial proximity between individual herds and animals. As a consequence, incorporating GIS into a national disease surveillance information system will allow the development of refined control strategies with higher spatial resolution. In dealing with difficult disease control problems, it will also be possible to use spatial risk assessment methods to characterize farms according to the risk of being or becoming infected and the exposure that they may represent for other herds, given their spatial proximity.

While GIS technology has the potential to become a significant component of modern animal disease surveillance, it makes substantial demands in terms of data quality, cost, training and development. The effectiveness of a disease surveillance system will depend on the quality and quantity of data collected. But it is not sufficient merely to generate large amounts of data; in addition, the data have to be analysed and interpreted in order to be of benefit for the disease control effort. It is much easier to meet these demands as part of specific epidemiological investigations.

5.2 Background

GIS emerged from the introduction of computer-assisted cartography in the late 1970s via a multiplicity of initially separate development efforts in different fields including cartography, geology, geography, soil science, surveying, urban and rural planning, utility networks and remote sensing to become an essential data management tool in today's information society (Burrough and McDonnell, 1998; see also Chapter 1). SDA has developed in parallel, but largely independently. As a result, modern GIS software still has fairly limited SDA functionality.

SDA has been used for many years, particularly in ecology and geology, and a number of textbooks have been published over the last 10 years, such as Haining (1990), Cressie (1993), Bailey and Gatrell (1995) and Griffith and Layne (1999). Other textbooks have covered specific areas within SDA, such as the analysis of point patterns (Diggle, 2003) or geostatistics (Isaaks and Srivastava, 1989). Applications of SDA in medical epidemiology have appeared in the scientific literature for many years, but comprehensive textbooks and edited collections have only been published relatively recently; for example, Elliott *et al.* (1993), Gatrell and Löytönen (1998), Lawson *et al.* (1999), Elliott *et al.* (2000), Lawson and Williams (2001) and Lawson (2001b). In general, textbooks emphasize either GIS or SDA. One of the few exceptions is the book by Bonham-Carter (1994), although its coverage of SDA is fairly specialized for geological applications. Thomas (2002) states that the statistical methods used to exploit the resources that have become available through the explosion in the availability of georeferenced data on health and exposures are still in their infancy. This seems a somewhat strong statement, given the range of textbooks recently published and the range of methods now available.

Potential uses of GIS in animal disease control have been described by Sanson *et al.* (1991), McGinn *et al.* (1996) and Pfeiffer and Hugh-Jones

(2002). Veterinary applications of cluster detection methods have been reviewed by Ward and Carpenter (2000a,b) and Carpenter (2001). Pfeiffer (2000) presented an overview of spatial analysis applications in veterinary epidemiology. Apart from the review by Sanson and colleagues, all others were published from 2000 onwards, which clearly demonstrates that the interest in the spatial analysis of veterinary problems has only emerged fairly recently (see also Chapter 2).

5.3 Characteristics of spatial data

GIS have specific requirements with respect to data collection, the most important being the addition of a georeference to each record in the database. Geographical information science defines the simplest data model as a basic data entity that is further specified by geographical location and attributes. Making effective use of GIS requires an understanding of these two components.

5.3.1 Geographical location

Geographical phenomena can be viewed as discrete entities or continuous fields (Burrough and McDonnell, 1998) in which locations of diseased animals or infected farms represent examples of the former and elevation or rainfall examples of the latter. They can be represented using raster or vector format. In the case of raster data, a grid is superimposed on an area so that the resolution of the data depends on the size of the grid cells. This format is suited for representing continuous fields. Vector data allow a more exact definition of discrete entities, using points, lines or polygons. Ideally, farms or herds should be represented as polygons reflecting the property boundaries of individual farms. Usually, this is considered to be too costly and complicated, particularly if a farm includes several non-contiguous land parcels, and it is therefore more easily represented as a single point location (see Chapter 2). One then has to decide whether to use the geographical coordinates of the farmhouse or those of the centroid calculated from the main farm area. The disadvantages of condensing a farm's area into a single point location include the need to base any neighbourhood calculations on distance rather than true property boundary adjacency, and the need to assume a circular shape for any farm property. Point location data can be easily collected using a handheld global positioning system (GPS) while on the farm, or by reading it directly from a map. Durr and Froggatt (2002) analysed the impact of using different methods for representing farm properties and concluded that the use of single point locations is currently the most cost-effective method. But the aim has to be to develop methods for integrating the true boundaries of multi-land-parcel properties into the spatial analysis, since this will allow more accurate representations of the spatial relationships.

Most surveillance data are currently presented as tabulated summary statistics generated at a defined administrative level of aggregation, such as the district or province level. These data can be easily presented using a GIS, since the boundaries of these administrative units are available in digital formats for most countries in the world. It is important to match the level of administrative aggregation with the spatial resolution at which epidemiological inferences are to be drawn. For example, if one were to make broad assessments with respect to the occurrence of cattle tuberculosis in Great Britain at a national scale, aggregation at the county level can be acceptable. Alternatively, if clusters resulting from point sources of infection are to be identified, it will be necessary to work with data aggregated at a much higher resolution or, ideally, with point locations.

Epidemiological interpretation of disease surveillance data requires access to denominator information and the spatial distribution of this information. Ideally, this will mean that the actual locations of all livestock holdings around the country, or at least summary estimates at some administrative level of aggregation, for example county or parish in Great Britain, are available. It is also important to recognize that changing the level of data aggregation may result in very different observed spatial patterns. This process has been called the 'modifiable areal unit problem', and it is similar to the ecological fallacy.

5.3.2 Attribute data

In addition to geographical location, a spatial entity such as a farm may have a range of attributes, such as the number of animals of each species or, for example, the herd's infection status with respect to cattle tuberculosis. Some of this information will already be available in national animal disease information systems, but it is not necessarily georeferenced. An increasing number of countries are also now collecting information on animal movements, and this will introduce a dynamic component to spatial data because individual animals may be associated with several geographical locations during their lifetime. In the case of raster data, continuous fields, such as average rainfall and elevation, are the attributes of individual raster cells. Raster data can now be obtained relatively cost-effectively through satellite remote sensing.

5.3.3 Spatial effects

The spatial dimension of animal disease data can be the objective of an epidemiological analysis or a nuisance effect that has to be taken into account when investigating animal or herd characteristics. Spatial processes are the result of a mixture of first- and second-order effects. The first-order effect represents large-scale variation in the mean value of a spatial process; that is, a global trend. Disease risk, for example, may increase from the south to the north of a region. Second-order effects, on the other hand, describe the local dependence of a spatial process; for example, local clustering. This could be expressed as clusters of disease around livestock markets. Statistical analysis of spatial data becomes particularly complicated if both these effects are present simultaneously. Most methods currently available will only allow modelling of one or the other, and may produce biased results in the presence of both effects. Stationarity or homogeneity of a second-order effect implies that the model describing the spatial dependence will be independent from absolute location. A second-order effect is considered isotropic if it depends only on the distance between locations and not on the direction between them. This will be a problem if wind direction affects the spatial spread of a disease. Bailey and Gatrell (1995) provide an excellent discussion of first- and second-order effects.

5.4 Methods for spatial analysis of animal diseases

In the past, one of the constraints on making effective use of GIS for research on animal diseases and particularly the surveillance of diseases has been that spatial analytical methods were not easily accessible to applied epidemiologists. The last 10 years have seen some important changes in this regard. These changes began with the evolution of user-friendly and powerful GIS software packages, and this was followed more recently by the emergence of spatial analysis frameworks and more user-friendly analysis tools. But it should be noted that there is still a notable difference between the accessibility of GIS and that of spatial analysis methods.

The objectives of SDA are the description of spatial patterns, the identification of disease clusters and the explanation or prediction of disease risk. The individual methods used depend on whether the data are available as individual case locations or aggregated data. Most currently available statistical methods will represent polygon data using the centroid point location together with any associated attributes, if available. A framework for the spatial analysis of epidemiological data adapted from Bailey and Gatrell (1995) includes the following groups of analytical methods: data visualization, exploratory analysis and modelling. The first two groups include methods that focus purely on examining the spatial dimension of the data. With visualization, this involves mainly presentation and, to a limited extent, analysis, but the primary objective is a descriptive analysis of the spatial data. Exploratory analysis will introduce statistical hypothesis-testing, but still remains within the spatial domain. Modelling involves the combination of different spatial and non-spatial data sources for explanatory or predictive purposes. There is some overlap between the groups, particularly between visualization and exploration, since meaningful visual presentation may require extensive data manipulation.

5.4.1 Data visualization

The most commonly applied spatial analysis technique in research and surveillance of animal diseases is data visualization. This involves generating maps to present the spatial and temporal patterns of disease occurrence, which are then used to develop hypotheses about possible cause–effect relationships. The visualization of area data is considered first, before I turn to point data.

If the data are available in an aggregated format, such as the number of foxes identified as infected with *Echinococcus multilocularis* in each of the administrative regions within the state of Lower Saxony in Germany, they can be presented as a choropleth map (Berke, 2001). While this type of map is easy to interpret, it can introduce bias because the size of the regions and the locations of their boundaries are typically a reflection of administrative requirements rather than of the spatial distribution of epidemiological factors. As the objective of these map presentations is to identify locations with unusually high or low disease levels, different types of epidemiological parameters can be calculated to take account of potential confounding factors, such as the spatial heterogeneity of the underlying population at risk. This means that, in the case of foxes identified as infected with *E. multilocularis* in Lower Saxony, one needs to take into account the number of foxes examined from each administrative region (Fig. 5.1).

The standardized mortality or morbidity ratio (SMR) has been used extensively for the description of spatial patterns of disease distribution in medical epidemiology. It uses indirect standardization to re-express the data as the ratio between the observed number of cases and the number that would have been expected in a standard population. The disease risk or rate calculated after aggregating the data from all regions included in the analysis can be used to calculate the expected number of cases for each local area (Lawson and Williams, 2001). It differs from a prevalence or incidence map in that it emphasizes deviation from the average risk of infection across the total area included in the analysis. It

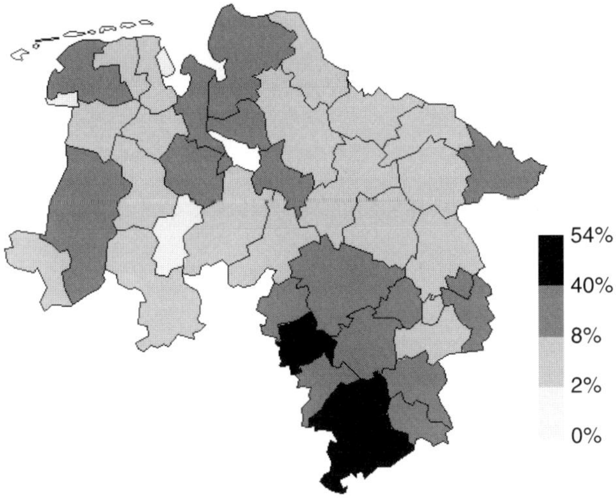

Fig. 5.1. Choropleth map of raw mean annual prevalences of *Echinococcus multilocularis* infections among red foxes in 43 administrative districts of Lower Saxony, 1991–1997. Reprinted from Berke (2001), Fig. 2, page 124, with permission from Elsevier.

is important to recognize that the presentation of risk maps does not provide an indication of the statistical confidence limits of the data presented. As this is largely a function of sample size, it is appropriate to accompany these maps with presentations of the variability of estimates, such as standard errors of confidence limits. The unit of analysis for the SMR calculations has to be very clearly defined; it could be, for example, herds or animals. The standard SMR approach is particularly problematic with small area units and/or rare diseases. High SMR values for areas with small populations will result in a map being dominated by the least reliable information. Adoption of empirical or fully Bayesian estimation methods will correct this problem by taking advantage of knowledge about the disease risk in the rest of the map. In this case, a posterior distribution of relative risk is estimated from a weighted combination of observed data, such as the local risk, and prior information, such as the neighbourhood risk (Clayton and Bernardinelli, 1992; Wakefield *et al.*, 2000a). Empirical Bayesian methods will estimate the posterior distribution on the basis of applying maximum likelihood procedures to existing data, whereas fully Bayesian methods will generate the posterior using a sampling process.

The relative weights given to the local data and the prior information will depend on the sample size in the local area. If the local population size is large, the local data will receive a stronger weighting in the calculation process than the neighbourhood data. If it is relatively

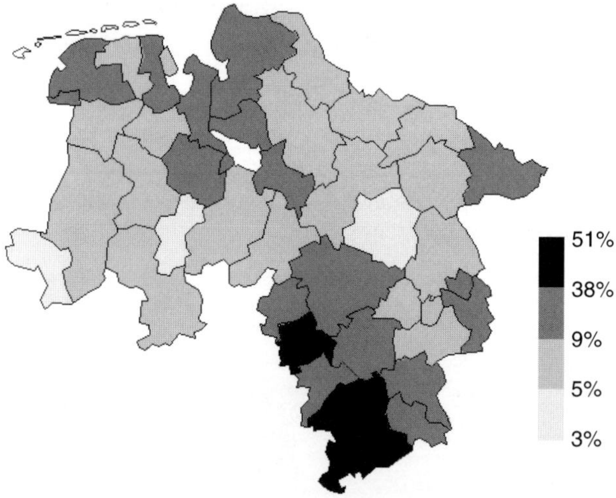

Fig. 5.2. Choropleth map of empirical Bayesian estimated mean annual prevalences of *Echinococcus multilocularis* infections among red foxes in 43 administrative districts of Lower Saxony, 1991–1997. Reprinted from Berke (2001), Fig. 3, page 125, with permission from Elsevier.

small, its weighting will be small, and the derived estimate will be shrunk towards the mean of the neighbouring areas. The geographical extent of the neighbourhood can be defined as anything between the total map area and the immediate neighbourhood. As a result of the smoothing, the estimated relative risk will be more stable and have higher specificity. Bernardinelli and Montomoli (1992) emphasize that the confidence intervals obtained using the empirical Bayes approach will be too narrow, since they are based on point estimates of the prior. Fully Bayesian estimation uses the probability distributions of these parameters, and will therefore reflect the underlying uncertainty more accurately. These methods will be discussed in more detail in Section 5.4.3. Figure 5.2 shows the empirical Bayesian estimates of the mean annual prevalence of *E. multilocularis* infected red foxes in Lower Saxony (Berke, 2001). Unfortunately, this map cannot be compared with Fig. 5.1 since the legend is scaled differently. Inspection of the data presented in the paper (Berke, 2001) shows that the empirical Bayesian estimates predict the presence of infection in two areas where none had been found on the basis of sample sizes below ten foxes. As a result, the epidemiologically sensible conclusion was reached that *E. multilocularis* infection was endemic in red foxes in Lower Saxony. The estimates generated for regions in the boundary areas close to the edge of the map have to be interpreted with caution since observations in these locations are subject to a spatial censoring effect. These so-called edge effects can be compensated for during the estimation process through weighting systems or the inclusion of external guard areas (Lawson *et al.*, 1999b).

The visual analysis of point data includes the simple map display of the point locations and the use of smoothing methods to generate surface representations of point density. In general, the first method should only be used if the number of points is small and the points are not too densely clustered. If the point density is too high, such that it is not possible to obtain an impression of the density pattern visually, interpretation of the map can be facilitated either by generating estimates aggregated at an administrative level or by applying smoothing methods. Spatial smoothing can be achieved through estimation of localized averages by using a spatial filter or by applying a mathematical function such as kernel smoothing. Spatial filters are used in image enhancement to remove random noise, but are also available as a standard neighbourhood function in GIS (Bonham-Carter, 1994). With epidemiological spatial data, they can be applied to point as well as aggregated data. Talbot *et al.* (2000) describe the use of filters with fixed geographical size as well as with constant population size to generate smoothed map representations of disease ratios. They demonstrate that a filter with constant population size retains adequate spatial resolution in high-density areas while at the same time producing stable rate estimates in low-density areas. Kernel density estimation uses a bivariate probability density function to determine the intensity of a spatial point process (Bailey and Gatrell, 1995). The appearance of the smoothed density surface is dependent on the type of probability density function chosen, the bandwidth and the size of the grid cells for which the individual estimates are generated. The bandwidth defines the distance from the centre of the kernel over which points will be included in the calculations, and the larger it is the smoother the surface will be. The appropriate choice of bandwidth and grid cell size should reflect the spatial scale of the biological process to be represented as well as the geographical scale that is relevant to decision making, and, of course, the actual density of points. It is also possible to use mathematical calculations to choose the bandwidth. Diggle (1981) recommends the use of the smoothing value $h = 0.68n^{-0.2}$ (n being the number of observations) scaled to the size of the study area (multiplying by the square root of the size of the study area). It is also possible to use adaptive bandwidth selection methods which vary the local bandwidth during the estimation process so that a minimum number of observations is included (Bailey and Gatrell, 1995).

The ratio of two density surfaces (one representing cases and the second a set of controls or a population at risk) is a very useful tool (see, e.g. Kelsall and Diggle, 1995, and Chapters 3 and 4). There is some debate as to whether the numerator and denominator kernel density surfaces used in this ratio calculation should be generated using the same or different bandwidths (Bithell, 1990; Bailey and Gatrell, 1995; Diggle, 2000). In any case, the bandwidths chosen for producing the individual density surfaces are not necessarily appropriate for the generation of the ratio surface. Stevenson *et al.* (2000) conducted a descriptive spatial analysis of the occurrence of BSE in the UK. They used kernel density estimation based on a Gaussian kernel and a fixed bandwidth of 30 km estimated using the normal optimal method described by Bowman and Azzalini (1997). Figure 5.3 shows a time series of kernel ratio maps expressing the incidence of confirmed BSE cases per 100 adult cattle per square kilometre between 1987 and 1997. While the maps provide a useful impression of the temporal dynamics of the incidence of BSE during that period, they do not allow an interpretation of the uncertainty associated with the estimates. This information would be particularly useful for areas with relatively small population sizes where high risks were calculated, such as in Scotland. Increasing the grid cell size and/or bandwidth would have increased the certainty about the estimates, but at the expense of reduced spatial differentiation in the main areas of interest, such as in the south-west of England and Wales. Monte Carlo methods could have been used to quantify the statistical precision of the ratio estimates (Kelsall and Diggle, 1995).

5.4.2 Exploratory analysis

While visualization can be used to present spatial information and to develop preliminary hypotheses with respect to unusual occurrences of disease, exploratory analysis has the specific objective of using a statistical hypothesis-testing framework for the identification of spatial clusters of disease. The term 'clusters' refers to locations at which disease occurrence is higher or lower than would have been expected if disease were randomly distributed in space. Such investigations have to take into account the spatial distribution of the population at risk, which is often clustered itself. The statistical methods can be grouped into global and local statistics depending on whether they generate a single statistic for the whole area or statistics for individual locations within that area. In addition, there is a category of focused tests that examine whether disease risk is increased around known locations. Cluster detection can also incorporate space–time clustering. Significance testing with these methods involves the use of Monte Carlo simulation

Fig. 5.3. (Opposite.) Kernel-smoothed map representations of the incidence of BSE in Great Britain. Abbreviations refer to Ministry of Agriculture administrative regions (SW, Southwest; SE, Southeast; EA, Eastern; MW, Mid and West; WA, Wales; SC, Scotland). From Stevenson *et al.* (2000); reproduced with permission.

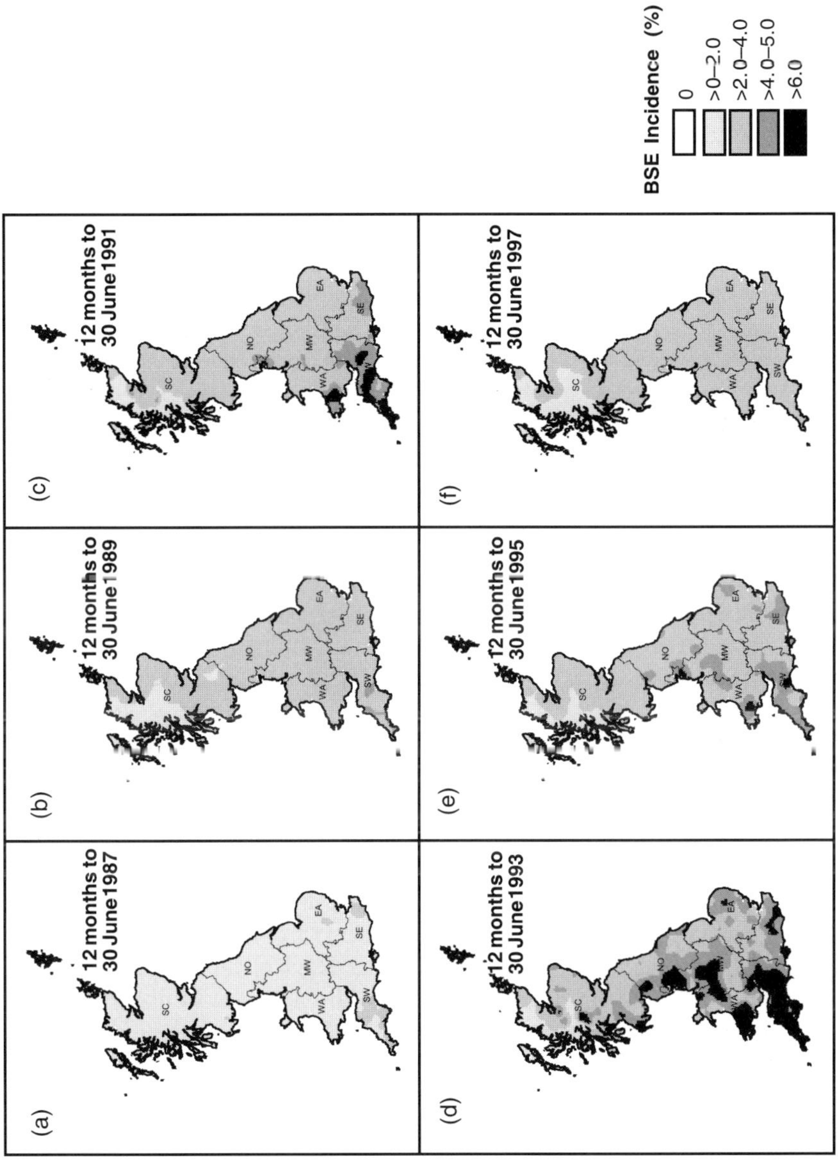
(a)
12 months to 30 June 1987
(b)
12 months to 30 June 1989
(c)
12 months to 30 June 1991
(d)
12 months to 30 June 1993
(e)
12 months to 30 June 1995
(f)
12 months to 30 June 1997
SC
NO
MW
EA
WA
SW
SE
BSE Incidence (%)
0
>0–2.0
>2.0–4.0
>4.0–5.0
>6.0

or permutation methods. It is important to bear in mind that these methods are potentially affected by type I error (i.e. they may erroneously detect clusters where there are none). They should therefore be used as screening methods, and any apparent clusters will require further epidemiological investigation. Alexander and Cuzick (1992) emphasize the need for extreme caution when interpreting single clusters resulting from *post hoc* investigation. Application of different methods to the same data or the repeated testing of the same region over many time periods will increase the risk of false-positive clusters (type I error) (Wartenberg and Greenberg, 1990). Kulldorff (1998) and Wakefield *et al.* (2000b) provide more comprehensive reviews of spatial clustering methods than that presented below.

Spatial monitoring or surveillance involves the assessment of temporal case occurrence data in a spatial context. The aim is to alert decision makers if there are unusual patterns in space and time. Statistical process control methods can be used to determine when a sequence of disease events exceeds its 'control' limits. Lawson (2001) concludes that there is considerable scope for the development of new methods in the general area of time–space surveillance data.

As mentioned for visual analysis, the definition of the spatial extent of the areas used to generate aggregated data may introduce bias when attempts are made to investigate the epidemiology of a disease process. For example, the resulting maps may hide any existing clusters that occur at a scale that is smaller than the size of the area over which the data were aggregated. The data are typically measured on an ordinal or continuous scale, such as the number of diseased animals or the prevalence of infection per unit area. If the data can be treated as continuous, the presence of spatial autocorrelation can be assessed visually using a variogram or Moran's I statistic (see Chapter 1). Variograms express the variation among pairs of data points within a given distance. These are presented as graphs with distance (spatial lag) on the x-axis and variation on the y-axis. Variogram estimation assumes stationarity of the spatial process, i.e. the spatial dependence described is independent of location (Bailey and Gatrell, 1995). A variogram curve with a flat shape suggests the absence of spatial dependence. A curve with an exponential shape, expressing increasing variability between pairs of locations with distance, reflects the presence of spatial dependence. Moran's I is calculated as the correlation between values of the same variable in different locations. Ward and Carpenter (2000b) applied Moran's I to assess the clustering of fly strike in sheep. However, they acknowledge its weakness in that, in its unmodified implementation, it does not take account of spatial heterogeneity in the underlying population at risk. Tango (1999) concludes that there are only four tests for assessing the tendency to cluster that are free from statistical inappropriateness, among them a global statistic by Besag and Newell (1991) and a local statistic by Kulldorff and Nagarwalla (1995). Besag and Newell's test is suitable for detecting clusters of rare diseases in a large area comprising many small administrative units. It requires that the number of cases forming a cluster is set before the analysis, which is rarely possible. The spatial scan statistic by Kulldorff and Nagarwalla (1995) does not have this requirement. It is based on the construction of circles of varying size around the centroid of each area and comparison of the risk of being a case between the areas inside and outside the circle.

If geographical coordinates are available to precisely indicate the locations of herds or animals that are affected or unaffected, the *K*-function can be used as a global spatial statistic to describe the second-order effect which has led to a particular spatial pattern of cases and controls (Bailey and Gatrell, 1995). It is based on the distances between all pairs of points. These are modelled separately for cases and controls, so that the resulting *K*-functions express the expected number of cases (or controls) within a certain distance from a random point. The function resulting from differencing the individual *K*-functions for cases and controls indicates the extra clustering of either the cases or the controls. This difference function can be evaluated statistically using Monte Carlo methods. The *K*-function has the restricting assumption that the underlying spatial process is stationary and isotropic. While it may be that it is stationary (i.e. the spatial relationship is independent from location), it also has to be independent of direction. It is also extremely sensitive to edge effects (Cressie, 1993). O'Brien *et al.* (2000) investigated the spatial relationship in the occurrence of specific types of cancers in humans and dogs in Michigan by comparison of the shape of the *K*-functions. They did not take the heterogeneity of the underlying population at risk into account since their focus was on an inter-species comparison. Therefore, as acknowledged by the authors, their finding of a lack of independence between the spatial case distributions could have been the result of similar population distributions. They also found that clustering occurred at distances of <2000 m, and discuss several potential reasons for this finding. The *K*-function can be extended to assess the presence of space–time interaction (Diggle *et al.*, 1995). French *et al.* (1999) used the method to investigate the space–time pattern of sheep scab in Great Britain between 1973 and 1992. They focused on outbreak data, i.e. they did not take into account the spatial distribution of the population at risk. The analysis indicated that there was strong evidence of space–time interaction among outbreaks occurring within 12 km and 5 months of each other. Figure 5.4 shows the results of an investigation of the spatial dependence of a Newcastle disease outbreak in Northern Ireland (Abernethy *et al.*, 2000). The difference function presented in Fig. 5.4c indicates that extra clustering of cases occurred at distances of up to about 8 km. With all three examples presented above, it is not possible to assess if the assumptions of stationarity and isotropy were met.

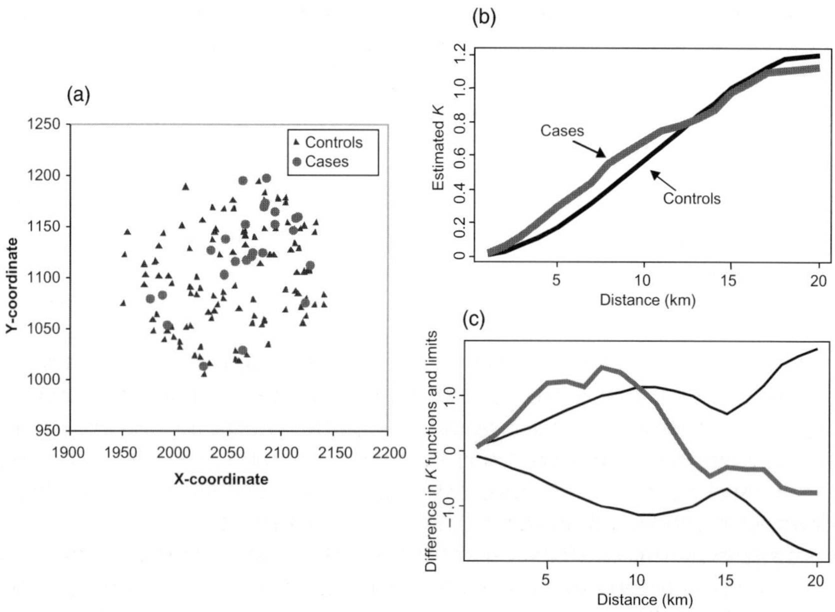

Fig. 5.4. *K*-function analysis of the spatial dependence of a Newcastle disease outbreak in Northern Ireland. (a) Locations of infected (case) and non-infected (control) poultry flocks. (b) *K*-functions for cases and controls. (c) Difference function (thick line), including Monte Carlo simulation envelope (thin lines).

The Cuzick and Edwards test can be applied to obtain a global spatial cluster statistic from point locations of disease cases and random controls (Cuzick and Edwards, 1990). It assesses whether, within the predefined neighbourhood of *K* neighbours of a case, there are more likely to be more other cases than controls. The method does not suffer from assumptions as restrictive as those for the *K*-function, and it inherently takes the spatial heterogeneity of the population at risk into account. But it is critical to decide on an appropriate number of nearest neighbours, and it is important to be aware that even using Bonferroni-type adjustments it is not possible to fully adjust for the effect of multiple testing (Wakefield *et al.*, 2000b). Ward and Armstrong (1999) used the technique to assess spatial clustering of louse infestation in Queensland sheep flocks on the basis of postal questionnaire data. They found no indication of the presence of clustering when they included all data. When they conducted the analysis separately for each of the four regions in Queensland that were included in the survey, they found clustering of louse infestation in the South region ($P=0.02$). While the algorithm applied to each of the five analyses used the Simes method (Simes, 1986) to reduce the chance of a type I error occurring, re-running it for each region will also have represented multiple testing. A similar approach was used by Doherr *et al.* (1999), who repeated the Cuzick and Edwards test for the same area, reporting both Bonferroni- and Simes-adjusted *P*-values, but for each of 19 months. In both cases, the results may have been affected by type I error.

Apart from aggregated spatial data, as described above, Kulldorff's spatial scan test can also be used to obtain a local statistic for point location data. Kulldorff's spatial scan statistic has good characteristics for the identification of circular, compact clusters. It has low power for other cluster shapes and multiple small clusters in different locations (Lawson and Kulldorff, 1999). Wakefield *et al.* (2000b) point out that the choice of population size to be included in cluster detection with the spatial scan statistic is somewhat arbitrary. Kulldorff recommends including a maximum of 50% of the total population. Values much below this may be sensible if the focus of the investigation is on identifying clusters occurring at a relatively small spatial scale. Also, if the data to be tested include a very large number of locations (e.g. all herds from a country), setting a lower limit will speed up the calculations substantially.

Stevenson *et al.* (2000) used the spatial scan statistic to identify three spatial clusters of high incidence of BSE-infected cattle herds in the UK until June 1997. They attributed this pattern to localized differences in management and feeding practices. Ward and Carpenter (2000b) applied the spatial scan statistic as well as Cuzick and Edwards' test to investigate spatial clustering of flystrike in sheep flocks in south-east Queensland. The most probable clusters were detected using the spatial scan statistic, but the global statistic produced by the Cuzick and Edwards test for up to ten neighbours was not significant. The authors did not discuss possible reasons for this discrepancy.

Space–time clustering indicates that disease cases occur close to each other in time as well as space. The appropriate methods can be grouped into those aimed at the detection of cluster locations and those for the description of the space–time interaction. Kulldorff's spatial scan statistic can be easily extended to allow detection of clusters with both a temporal and a spatial dimension (Kulldorff *et al.*, 1998). It will take account of the population at risk and can also control for confounding factors. This method will detect clusters that might be missed as a result of averaging out if one applies a spatial clustering method to data collected over a period of time. The spatial scan statistic will identify clusters that are stable in space. Space–time interaction is investigated using only the point locations of cases, and its presence is considered to be evidence of a contagious process. Such a process can be dynamic in space. The Knox test (Knox, 1964), one of the most commonly used methods, requires prior definition of a threshold time and space distance at which clustering is hypothesized to occur. While this decision can sometimes be made on the basis of the epidemiological characteristics of an infectious process, e.g. its incubation period and potential for aerosol transmission, it is often difficult to justify. Fuchs and Deutz (2002) suggest the use of indicator variograms (allowing for modelling of binomial variables) to determine the spatial distance criterion for Knox's test. The approach requires knowledge of the appropriate time criterion and assumes an isotropic stationary spatial process. Mantel regression (Mantel, 1967), on the other hand, uses the actual data values and assesses the correlation between the distances in space and time between all pairs of data points, and weighting can be applied through the use of value transformation. Jacquez (1996) developed a method which requires the analyst to define a threshold number of *k* nearest neighbours. It is possible to calculate a statistic for different *k* values. All three methods therefore introduce a level of arbitrariness through the need to define either a threshold value or a data transformation. They are not affected by heterogeneity of the population in space and generalized changes in population size over time, except if the latter occur at different rates in different areas (Kulldorff, 1998). Kulldorff and Hjalmars (1999) emphasize that *P*-values derived from the space–time interaction methods should be interpreted very cautiously. It is important to recognize that cases which occur within the same area and at specific times are not a reflection of space–time interaction.

Norström *et al.* (2000) investigated the presence of space–time clustering during an outbreak of acute respiratory disease in Norwegian cattle. They identified space–time interaction using both the Knox and the Jacquez test, which suggested the presence of airborne infection, particularly since the Knox test was significant at a threshold value of 500 m. The use of Kulldorff's space–time statistic revealed the location of a most likely as well as three secondary space–time clusters within the study area (Fig. 5.5). The findings were interpreted as suggesting that bovine respiratory syncytial virus had caused the outbreak. Fuchs *et al.* (2000) assessed the space–time clustering of scabies in chamois in Austria using Mantel regression and Knox's test. Ward and Carpenter (2000a) used blowfly capture data to demonstrate the use of space–time clustering methods. They recommend the use of several methods to increase the statistical power of the analysis. As mentioned above, this approach will increase type I error.

5.4.3 Modelling

Visualization and exploration are both used as mechanisms for generating causal hypotheses. Epidemiological modelling of spatial data, on the other hand, aims to explain or predict the occurrence of disease. Various static or dynamic relationships defined by the underlying models are used to derive new output maps from a set of input maps. The methods used for this purpose can be grouped into data-driven and

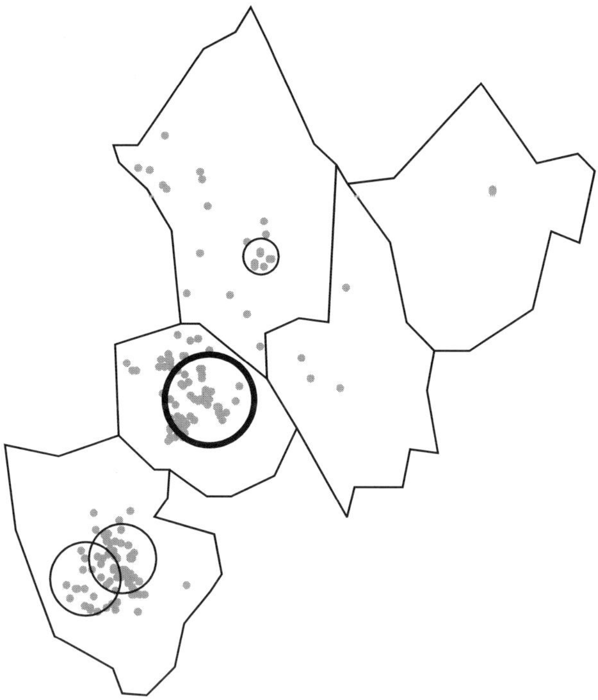

Fig. 5.5. Map of locations of cattle farms affected by acute respiratory disease in south-east regions of Norway during the winter and spring of 1995 showing clusters of disease identified using the space–time scan statistic. The most probable cluster is indicated by a thick circle; secondary clusters are indicated by thin circles. Reproduced from Norström *et al.* (2000), Fig. 4, page 115, with permission from Elsevier.

knowledge-driven models (Bonham-Carter, 1994). It has to be emphasized that the model output should only be used to guide decision making if the decision makers are conscious of the underlying assumptions, uncertainty and variability of the predictions. It is also important to investigate the potential effects of error propagation since, during the modelling process, the errors inherent in individual maps will be combined to generate new errors in the output maps, which will potentially be affected by unpredictable bias (Burrough and McDonnell, 1998). This can, for example, be done by introducing random error into the input data and assessing the sensitivity of the model output to this effect. Combining data collected at different spatial resolutions can be particularly dangerous since it may lead to the identification of spurious associations.

Data-driven models are generated from existing georeferenced data sets about disease occurrence as well as potential risk factors. Statistical methods such as regression analysis, weights of evidence or neural network techniques are then used to provide the weightings, combining the inputs to generate output maps (Bonham-Carter, 1994). A critical assumption of ordinary regression analysis is that the observations used to generate the model are statistically independent of one other. Spatial data that are subject to second-order effects may therefore require the use of analytical methods that take account of the local dependence. The presence of such effects can be investigated, for example, using cluster detection methods or variograms of the model residuals. The dependent variable in epidemiological regression models typically consists of either point locations of cases and non-cases or aggregated area data representing the number of cases in an area, given a certain size population at risk. Statistical regression methods suitable for incorporating spatial dependence with these types of dependent variables include generalized linear mixed models (GLMM) and Bayesian estimation methods. The GLMM is an extension of the generalized linear model that allows for fixed as well as random effects. The random effects can be structured or unstructured, the former representing spatial and the latter non-spatial overdispersion (Lawson, 2001b). Information about spatial dependence is provided to the modelling algorithm in the format of a spatial contiguity or weights matrix based on neighbourhood or distance criteria (Cressie, 1993). Wakefield *et al.* (2000a) provide a discussion of different approaches to modelling variability in the data. They emphasize that the appropriate form of representing spatial dependence should be selected on the basis of sensitivity analysis and the aim of the analysis, so that, for example, distance-based models are more appropriate than neighbourhood models for aerosol exposure. Besag *et al.* (1991) first proposed a Bayesian model for expressing heterogeneity in the data, which is now often applied in spatial regression analysis. It includes a trend component, a non-spatial component and a spatial component. Unfortunately, these complex models resulted in computational difficulties because of the need for integration over the random effects. Until the emergence of Markov chain Monte Carlo (MCMC) techniques, approximate inference methods, such as penalized or marginal maximum likelihood, had to be used as discussed in Clayton and Bernardinelli (1992). With MCMC, samples are drawn from approximate distributions to provide starting values for a Markov chain of simulated values that should converge to a stationary distribution representing the posterior distribution. This approach became computationally tractable through the development of the Metropolis–Hastings algorithm (a method for drawing samples from Bayesian posterior distributions) and particularly its special case, the Gibbs sampler (Gelman *et al.*, 1995). Lawson *et al.* (2000) compared several methods for modelling mapped disease risk, including approximate inference and fully Bayesian methods. As a preliminary conclusion, they reported that none of the approaches performed consistently well, but that the fully Bayesian approach, which included a structured and unstructured random effect, achieved the best goodness of fit. While the development of MCMC has been a great leap forward for spatial disease modelling, it is important to recognize that this approach is also not without its problems, and misleading results can be produced; for example, through the specification of inappropriate priors or inadequate investigation of convergence. Given all this, the current trend in spatial risk modelling clearly indicates that MCMC estimation of Bayesian models may become the standard statistical modelling approach for spatial data (Wakefield *et al.*, 2000a; Lawson, 2001). However, it is important to remember that the use of such more complex procedures can be avoided by choosing a spatial resolution for the unit of analysis that is less than the scale at which the local dependence occurs. An alternative approach to the regression approaches presented above is 'kriging', which is based on mathematical modelling of the local spatial dependence using information obtained from a variogram (Isaaks and Srivastava, 1989; Cressie, 1993). It can be applied to multiple data variables measured at different scales, but special care has to be taken when dealing with non-stationarity or a directional spatial process.

An increasing number of applications of spatial risk modelling to animal disease problems have been published over the last 10 years. Baylis *et al.* (2001) modelled the disease vector distribution to identify areas of bluetongue infection risk in the Mediterranean. Their discriminant analysis model predicts three abundance categories of *Culicoides imicola* on the basis of a combination of various remotely sensed climate variables. The accuracy of these predictions depends highly on the spatially and temporally representative collection of the data used to indicate the presence or absence of biting midges. McKenzie *et al.* (2002) used remotely sensed information to predict the risk of *Mycobacterium bovis* infection in wildlife as part of a decision support system for tuberculosis control (see Chapter 10, this volume). The logistic regression model predicts the presence of hotspots of tuberculosis infection on the basis of information about vegetation and slope. The output is used to design tailored disease control programmes. Duchateau *et al.* (1997) generated a risk map of theileriosis outbreaks in Zimbabwe. They applied principal components analysis to climate variables to control for the multicollinearity between the variables, so that selected components could be included in the logistic regression analysis. None of the models described above considered spatial dependence. 'Cokriging' was used by Estrada-Peña (1999) to predict habitat suitability for *Boophilus microplus* ticks in South America by linking tick presence/absence data for selected locations with remotely sensed temperature and vegetation information. The resulting model, which takes account of spatial dependence, had 91% sensitivity and 88% specificity. Pfeiffer *et al.* (1997) refined the model presented by Duchateau *et al.*

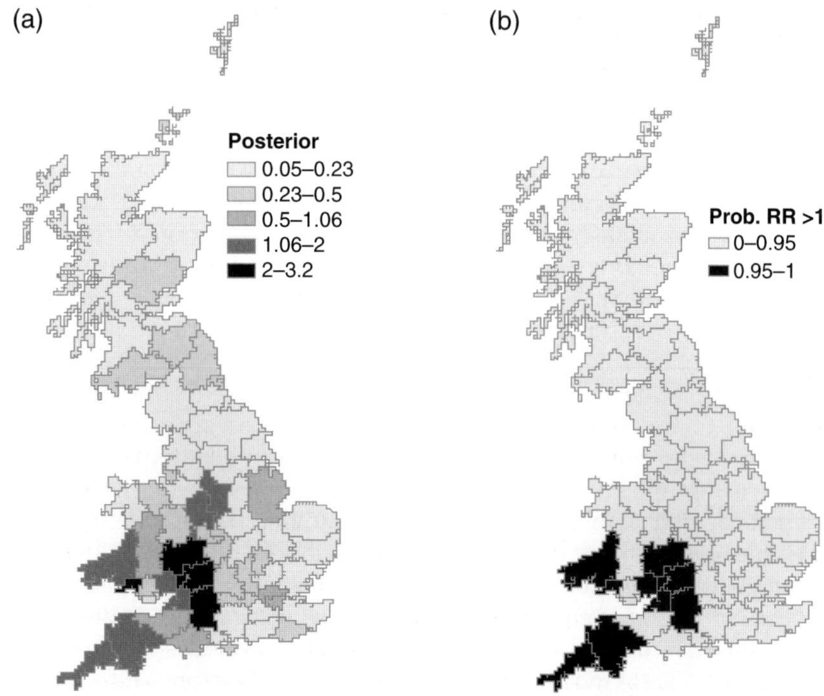

Fig. 5.6. Choropleth maps of Bayesian relative risk estimates for tuberculin herd test results for cattle in 1999 aggregated by county in Great Britain. (a) Bayesian estimates of relative risk (RR) of tuberculin test reactor herds. (b) Statistically significant Bayesian relative risks. Data are from DEFRA.

(1997) to take account of spatial dependence by using generalized linear mixed logistic regression. The underlying model includes environmental and land-use risk factors, as well as a random effect to take account of the local dependence between neighbouring observations. The resulting risk map could be used to guide decision-making with respect to the geographical locations that are the most suitable for vaccination (Colour Plate 10a). The predictive accuracy of the model is summarized using the ROC (receiver operating characteristic) curve shown in Colour Plate 10b, which also allows the decision makers to choose desirable sensitivity and specificity levels of the predicted model probability cut-offs.

An example of the MCMC approach is the relative risk map for cattle herds testing positive for tuberculosis in Great Britain in 1999 shown in Fig. 5.6a. Fully Bayesian modelling was used to generate estimates for each county on the basis of a convolution prior, as described in Besag *et al.* (1991). The map shown in Fig. 5.6b identifies three groupings of counties which had a statistically significantly elevated risk of tuberculosis-infected herds in comparison with the rest of the country.

If no empirical data are available, the existing quantitative and qualitative knowledge that is available from the literature or experts can be used to provide the weightings for linking different types of spatial inputs to produce output maps. The information can be quantitatively evaluated using multicriteria decision-making models (MCDM), which can then be incorporated into expert systems. MCDM has already been used with spatial data to evaluate land suitability (Pereira and Duckstein, 1993). It is based on the definition of a range of criteria, which are then used to generate the decision rules to satisfy given objectives. A very useful feature of this method is that it is possible to incorporate decision rule uncertainty through the use of fuzzy logic or Dempster–Shafer theory (Bonham-Carter, 1994). Luo and Caselton (1997) emphasize that, for the purpose of combining decision rules, Dempster–Shafer theory has the advantage over Bayesian methods in that it allows more accurate capture of information from both weak data and weak subjective data sources. The maps presented in Colour Plate 11 were generated using Dempster–Shafer theory. The underlying model incorporates factors which were included in the logistic regression model that produced the map shown in Colour Plate 10a. The knowledge base consists of decision rules that were defined for each factor depending on whether it provided evidence for separate hypotheses about the presence or absence of *Theileria parva*. Each factor was re-expressed using a fuzzy probability scale from 0 to 1 to indicate the certainty with which it supported either of the two hypotheses. For example, the detection of *T. parva* in the field was considered to support with absolute certainty the presence of the vector in the respective location, whereas the observed absence of *T. parva* was interpreted as a less than certain indication of vector absence, since it might have been affected, for example, by under-reporting bias. The map presented in Colour Plate 11a shows the spatial pattern of the degree of belief in the presence of *T. parva*. Colour Plate 11b indicates the degree of uncertainty about the quantity shown in the belief map. The higher the value, the more certainty can be gained about the prediction in the belief maps by obtaining better local information. This suggests that the predictions made for the southern part of the country are very uncertain. Obviously, this model depends strongly on the decision rules derived from existing knowledge that have been used to generate the maps.

5.5 Conclusions

Modern animal disease surveillance information systems need to embrace GIS as a standard component, and at least make use of its visualization and exploration capabilities. These methods are reasonably well understood and are already widely available. Improvements are required with respect to the data quality of spatial information as well as the diagnostic methods to assess it. Decision support systems require the integration of many different data sources to generate disease intelligence information. Modelling of spatial data can fulfil this function, for example, through the production of risk maps or expert system rules that can directly guide the decision-making process. The methodology of statistical spatial modelling is still an area of intensive research, but it currently appears that MCMC modelling will be able to provide the appropriate estimation methods.

References

Abernethy, D.A., Pfeiffer, D.U., Denny, G.O., Torrens, T.D., McCullough, S.J. and Graham, D.A. (2000) Evaluating airborne spread in a Newcastle epidemic in Northern Ireland. In: Salmon, M.D., Morley, P.S. and Ruch-Gallie, R. (eds) *Proceedings of the 9th Symposium of the International Society for Veterinary Epidemiology & Economics, Breckenridge, Colorado, August 6–11, 2000*, pp. 1115–1117.

Alexander, F.E. and Cuzick, J. (1992) Methods for the assessment of disease clusters. In: Elliott, P., Cuzick, J., English, D. and Stern, R. (eds) *Geographical and Environmental Epidemiology: Methods for Small-area Studies*. Oxford University Press, Oxford, UK, pp. 238–250.

Anyamba, A., Linthicum, K.J., Mahoney, R., Tucker, C.J. and Kelley, P.W. (2002) Mapping potential risk of rift valley fever outbreaks in African savannas using vegetation index time series data. *Photogrammetric Engineering and Remote Sensing* 68, 137–145.

Bailey, T.C. and Gatrell, A.C. (1995) *Interactive Spatial Data Analysis*. Longman, Harlow, UK.

Baylis, M., Mellor, P.S., Wittmann, E.J. and Rogers, D.J. (2001) Prediction of areas around the Mediterranean at risk of bluetongue by modelling the distribution of its vector using satellite imaging. *Veterinary Record* 149, 639–643.

Berke, O. (2001) Choropleth mapping of regional count data of *Echinococcus multilocularis* among red foxes in Lower Saxony, Germany. *Preventive Veterinary Medicine* 52, 119–131.

Bernardinelli, L. and Montomoli, C. (1992) Empirical bayes versus fully bayesian analysis of geographical variation in disease risk. *Statistics in Medicine* 11, 983–1007.

Besag, J. and Newell, J. (1991) The detection of clusters in rare diseases. *Journal of the Royal Statistical Society, Series A* 154, 143–155.

Besag, J., York, J. and Molliè, A. (1991) Bayesian image restoration, with applications in spatial statistics (with discussion). *Annals of the Institute of Statistics and Mathematics* 43, 1–59.

Bithell, J.F. (1990) An application of density estimation to geographical epidemiology. *Statistics in Medicine* 9, 691–701.

Bonham-Carter, G.F. (1994) *Geographic Information Systems for Geoscientists: Modelling with GIS*. Elsevier Science, Oxford, UK.

Bowman, A.W. and Azzalini, A. (1997). *Applied Smoothing Techniques for Data Analysis: The Kernel Approach with S-Plus Illustrations.* Oxford University Press, Oxford, UK.

Burrough, P.A. and McDonnell, R.A. (1998) *Principles of Geographical Information Systems.* Oxford University Press, Oxford, UK.

Carpenter, T.E. (2001) Methods to investigate spatial and temporal clustering in veterinary epidemiology. *Preventive Veterinary Medicine* 48, 303–320.

Clayton, D. and Bernardinelli, L. (1992) Bayesian methods for mapping disease risk. In: Elliott, P., Cuzick, J., English, D. and Stern, R. (eds) *Geographical and Environmental Epidemiology: Methods for Small Area Studies.* Oxford University Press, Oxford, UK, pp. 205–220.

Clements, A.C.A., Pfeiffer, D.U., Otte, M.J., Morteo, K. and Chen, L. (2002) A global livestock production and health atlas (GLiPHA) for interactive presentation, integration and analysis of livestock data. *Preventive Veterinary Medicine* 56, 19–32.

Cressie, N.A.C. (1993) *Statistics for Spatial Data.* John Wiley & Sons, New York.

Cuzick, J. and Edwards, R. (1990) Spatial clustering for inhomogenous populations. *Journal of the Royal Statistical Society, Series B* 52, 73–104.

Diggle, P.J. (1981) Some graphical methods in the analysis of spatial point patterns. In: Barnett, V. (ed.) *Interpreting Multivariate Data.* John Wiley & Sons, Chichester, UK, pp. 55–73.

Diggle, P.J. (2000) Overview of statistical methods for disease mapping and its relationship to cluster detection. In: Elliott, P., Wakefield, J.C., Best, N.G. and Briggs, D.J. (eds) *Spatial Epidemiology: Methods and Applications.* Oxford University Press, Oxford, UK, pp. 87–103.

Diggle, P.J. (2003) *Statistical Analysis of Spatial Point Patterns*, 2nd edn. Edward Arnold, London.

Diggle, P.J., Chetwynd, A.G., Haggkvist, R. and Morris, S.E. (1995) Second-order analysis of space–time clustering. *Statistical Methods in Medical Research* 4, 124–136.

Doherr, M.G., Carpenter, T.E., Wilson, W.D. and Gardner, I.A. (1999) Evaluation of temporal and spatial clustering of horses with *Corynebacterium pseudotuberculosis* infection. *American Journal of Veterinary Research* 60, 284–291.

Duchateau, L., Kruska, R.L. and Perry, B.D. (1997) Reducing a spatial database to its effective dimensionality for logistic-regression analysis of incidence of livestock disease. *Preventive Veterinary Medicine* 32, 207–218.

Durr, P.A. and Froggatt, A.E.A. (2002) How best to geo-reference farms? A case study from Cornwall, England. *Preventive Veterinary Medicine* 56, 51–62.

Elliott, P., Cuzick, J., English, D. and Stern, R. (1993) *Geographical and Environmental Epidemiology: Methods for Small-area Studies.* Oxford University Press, Oxford, UK.

Elliott, P., Wakefield, J.C., Best, N.G. and Briggs, D.J. (2000) *Spatial Epidemiology: Methods and Applications.* Oxford University Press, Oxford, UK.

Estrada-Peña, A. (1999) Geostatistics and remote sensing using NOAA-AVHRR satellite imagery as predictive tools in tick distribution and habitat suitability estimations for *Boophilus microplus* (Acari: Ixodidae) in South America. *Veterinary Parasitology* 81, 73–82.

French, N.P., Berriatua, E., Wall, R., Smith, K. and Morgan, K.L. (1999) Sheep scab outbreaks in Great Britain between 1973 and 1992: spatial and temporal patterns. *Veterinary Parasitology* 83, 187–200.

Fuchs, K. and Deutz, A. (2002) Use of variograms to detect critical spatial distances for the Knox's test. *Preventive Veterinary Medicine* 54, 37–45.

Fuchs, K., Deutz, A. and Gressmann, G. (2000) Detection of space-time clusters and epidemiological examinations of scabies in chamois. *Veterinary Parasitology* 92, 63–73.

Gelman, A.B., Carlin, J.S., Stern, H.S. and Rubin, D.B. (1995) *Bayesian Data Analysis*. Chapman and Hall/CRC, Boca Raton, Florida.

Griffith, D.A. and Layne, L.J. (1999) *A Casebook for Spatial Statistical Data Analysis*. Oxford University Press, Oxford, UK.

Haining, R. (1990) *Spatial Data Analysis in the Social and Environmental Sciences*. Cambridge University Press, Cambridge, UK.

Isaaks, E.H. and Srivastava, R.M. (1989) *Applied Geostatistics*. Oxford University Press, New York.

Jacquez, G.M. (1996) A *k* nearest neighbour test for space–time interaction. *Statistics in Medicine* 15, 1935–1949.

Keeling, M.J., Woolhouse, M.E.J., Shaw, D.J., Matthews, L., Chase-Topping, M., Haydon, D.T., Cornell, S.J., Kappey, J., Wilesmith, J. and Grenfell, B.T. (2001) Dynamics of the 2001 UK foot and mouth epidemic: stochastic dispersal in heterogeneous landscape. *Science* 294, 813–817.

Kelsall, J.E. and Diggle, P.J. (1995) Non-parametric estimation of spatial variation in relative risk. *Statistics in Medicine* 14, 2335–2342.

Knox, E.G. (1964) The detection of space–time interactions. *Applied Statistics* 13, 25–29.

Kulldorff, M. (1998) Statistical methods for spatial epidemiology: tests for randomness. In: Gatrell, A. and Löytönen, M. (eds) *GIS and Health*. Taylor and Francis, London, pp. 49–62.

Kulldorff, M. and Hjalmars, U. (1999) The Knox method and other tests for space–time interaction. *Biometrics* 55, 544–552.

Kulldorff, M. and Nagarwalla, N. (1995) Spatial disease clusters: detection and inference. *Statistics in Medicine* 14, 799–810.

Kulldorff, M., Athas, W.F., Feuer, E.J., Miller, B.A. and Key, C.R. (1998) Evaluating cluster alarms: a space–time scan statistic and brain cancer in Los Alamos, New Mexico. *American Journal of Public Health* 88, 1377–1380.

Lawson, A.B. (2001a) Disease map reconstruction. *Statistics in Medicine* 20, 2183–2204.

Lawson, A.B. (2001b) *Statistical Methods in Spatial Epidemiology*. John Wiley & Sons, Chichester, UK.

Lawson, A.B. and Kulldorff, M. (1999) A review of cluster detection methods. In: Lawson, A., Biggeri, A., Böhning, D., Lessaffre, E., Viel, J.-F. and Bertollini, R. (eds) *Disease Mapping and Risk Assessment for Public Health*. John Wiley & Sons, Chichester, UK, pp. 99–110.

Lawson, A.B. and Williams, F.L.R. (2001) *An Introductory Guide to Disease Mapping*. John Wiley & Sons, Chichester, UK.

Lawson, A., Biggeri, A., Böhning, D., Lesaffre, E., Viel, J.F. and Bertollini, R. (1999a) *Disease Mapping and Risk Assessment for Public Health*. John Wiley & Sons, Chichester, UK.

Lawson, A.B., Biggeri, A. and Dreassi, E. (1999b) Edge effects in disease mapping.

In: Lawson, A., Biggeri, A., Böhning, D., Lessaffre, E., Viel, J.-F. and Bertollini, R. (eds) *Disease Mapping and Risk Assessment for Public Health*. John Wiley & Sons, Chichester, UK, pp. 83–98.

Lawson, A.B., Biggeri, A.B., Boehning, D., Lesaffre, E., Viel, J.F., Clark, A., Schlattmann, P. and Divino, F. (2000) Disease mapping models: an empirical evaluation. *Statistics in Medicine* 19, 2217–2241.

Luo, W.B. and Caselton, B. (1997) Using Dempster–Shafer theory to represent climate change uncertainties. *Journal of Environmental Management* 49, 73–93.

Mantel, N. (1967) The detection of disease clustering and a generalized regression approach. *Cancer Research* 27, 209–220.

McGinn, T.J., Cowen, P. and Wray, D.W. (1996) Geographic information systems for animal health management and disease control. *Journal of the American Veterinary Medical Association* 209, 1917–1921.

McKenzie, J.S., Morris, R.S., Pfeiffer, D.U. and Dymond, J.R. (2002) Application of remote sensing to enhance the control of wildlife-associated *Mycobacterium bovis* infection. *Photogrammetric Engineering and Remote Sensing* 68, 153–159.

Morris, R.S., Wilesmith, J.W., Stern, M.W., Sanson, R.L. and Stevenson, M.A. (2001) Predictive spatial modelling of alternative control strategies for the foot-and-mouth disease epidemic in Great Britain, 2001. *Veterinary Record* 149, 137–144.

Myers, M.F., Rogers, D.J., Cox, J., Flahault, A. and Hay, S.I. (2000) Forecasting disease risk for increased epidemic preparedness in public health. In: Hay, S.I., Randolph, S.E. and Rogers, D.J. (eds) *Remote Sensing and Geographical Information Systems in Epidemiology*. Academic Press, London, pp. 309–330.

Norström, M., Pfeiffer, D.U. and Jarp, J. (2000) A space–time cluster investigation of an outbreak of acute respiratory disease in Norwegian cattle herds. *Preventive Veterinary Medicine* 47, 107–119.

O'Brien, D.J., Kaneene, J.B., Getis, A., Lloyd, J.W., Rip, M.R. and Leader, R.W. (1999) Spatial and temporal distribution of selected canine cancers in Michigan, USA, 1964–1994. *Preventive Veterinary Medicine* 42, 1–15.

O'Brien, D.J., Kaneene, J.B., Getis, A., Lloyd, J.W., Swanson, G.M. and Leader, R.W. (2000) Spatial and temporal comparison of selected cancers in dogs and humans, Michigan, USA, 1964–1994. *Preventive Veterinary Medicine* 47, 187–204.

Pereira, J.M.C. and Duckstein, L. (1993) A multiple criteria decision-making approach to GIS-based land suitability evaluation. *International Journal of Geographical Information Systems* 7, 407–424.

Pfeiffer, D.U. (2000) Spatial analysis – a new challenge for veterinary epidemiologists. In: Thrusfield, M.V. and Goodall, E.A. (eds) *Proceedings of the Annual Meeting of Society for Veterinary Epidemiology & Preventive Medicine, Edinburgh 29th–31st March, 2000*. Society for Veterinary Epidemiology and Preventive Medicine, Edinburgh, pp. 86–106.

Pfeiffer, D.U. and Hugh-Jones, M. (2002) Geographical information systems as a tool in epidemiological assessment and wildlife disease management. *Revue Scientifique et Technique – Office International des Épizooties* 21, 91–102.

Pfeiffer, D.U. and Morris, R.S. (1994) Comparison of four multivariate techniques for causal analysis of epidemiological field studies. In: Rowlands, G.J., Kyule, M.N.

and Perry, B.D. (eds) *Proceedings of the 7th International Symposium on Veterinary Epidemiology & Economics, Nairobi, 15–19 August 1994*, pp. 165–170.

Pfeiffer, D.U., Duchateau, L., Kruska, R.L., Ushewokunze-Obatolu, U. and Perry, B.D. (1997) A spatially predictive logistic regression model for the occurrence of theileriosis outbreaks in Zimbabwe. In: *Proceedings of the VIII International Symposium on Veterinary Epidemiology & Economics, Paris, 8–11 July, 1997*, pp. 12.12.1–12.12.3.

Sanson, R.L., Pfeiffer, D.U. and Morris, R.S. (1991) Geographic information systems: their application in animal disease control. *Revue Scientifique et Technique de l'Office International des Epizooties* 10, 179–195.

Sheather, S.J. and Jones, M.C. (1992) The performance of six popular bandwidth selection methods on some real data sets. *Computational Statistics* 7, 225–250.

Simes, R.J. (1986) An improved Bonferroni procedure for multiple tests of significance. *Biometrika* 73, 751–754.

Stevenson, M.A., Wilesmith, J.W., Ryan, J.B.M., Morris, R.S., Lawson, A.B., Pfeiffer, D.U. and Lin, D. (2000) Descriptive spatial analysis of the epidemic of bovine spongiform encephalopathy in Great Britain to June 1997. *Veterinary Record* 147, 379–384.

Talbot, T.O., Kulldorff, M., Forand, S.P. and Haley, V.B. (2000) Evaluation of spatial filters to create smoothed maps of health data. *Statistics in Medicine* 19, 2399–2408.

Tango, T. (1999) Comparison of general tests for spatial clustering. In: Lawson, A., Biggeri, A., Böhning, D., Lessaffre, E., Viel, J.-F. and Bertollini, R. (eds) *Disease Mapping and Risk Assessment for Public Health.* John Wiley & Sons, Chichester, UK, pp. 111–117.

Thomas, D.C. (2002) Some contributions of statistics to environmental epidemiology. In: Raftery, A.E., Tanner, M.A. and Wells, M.T. (eds) *Statistics in the 21st Century.* Chapman and Hall/CRC, Boca Raton, Florida.

Wakefield, J.C., Best, N.G. and Waller, L. (2000a) Bayesian approaches to disease mapping. In: Elliott, P., Wakefield, J.C., Best, N.G. and Briggs, D.J. (eds) *Spatial Epidemiology: Methods and Applications.* Oxford University Press, Oxford, UK, pp. 104–127.

Wakefield, J.C., Kelsall, J.E. and Morris, S.E. (2000b) Clustering, cluster detection and spatial variation in risk. In: Elliott, P., Wakefield, J.C., Best, N.G. and Briggs, D.J. (eds) *Spatial Epidemiology: Methods and Applications.* Oxford University Press, Oxford, UK, pp. 128–152.

Ward, M.P. and Armstrong, R.T.F. (1999) Prevalence and clustering of louse infestation in Queensland sheep flocks. *Preventive Veterinary Medicine* 82, 243–250.

Ward, M.P. and Carpenter, T.E. (2000a) Analysis of time–space clustering in veterinary epidemiology. *Preventive Veterinary Medicine* 43, 225–237.

Ward, M.P. and Carpenter, T.E. (2000b) Techniques for analysis of disease clustering in space and in time in veterinary epidemiology. *Preventive Veterinary Medicine* 45, 257–284.

Wartenberg, D. and Greenberg, M. (1990) Detecting disease clusters: the importance of statistical power. *American Journal of Epidemiology* 132, Supplement 1, S156–S166.

6 The Use of GIS in Veterinary Parasitology

Guy Hendrickx, Jan Biesemans and Reginald de Deken

6.1 Introduction

During the past few decades the publication of papers of veterinary and human health interest related to the use of geographical information systems (GIS) and/or remote sensing (RS) has followed an exponential trend (Fig. 6.1a). Some key events have marked the curve. Prior to the review published by Hugh-Jones (1989) in *Parasitology Today* on the applications of remote sensing to the identification of habitats of parasites and disease vectors, only a few papers were published. Of these, one-third were related to parasitology and were aimed mainly at the identification of mosquito habitats (malaria and Rift Valley fever). A second major event was the publication in 1991 of an issue of *Preventive Veterinary Medicine* devoted to the applications of remote sensing to epidemiology and parasitology. This clearly raised interest in these new technologies; the average number of publications increased from three papers every 2 years to 17 per year in the first half of the 1990s. In the second half of the 1990s, numbers further increased exponentially, and currently more than 60 papers are recorded per year, 60% of which are related to parasitology and vector-borne diseases. A further breakdown by subject is given in Fig. 6.1b. Papers on four major disease vectors predominate (69% of published papers). These vectors are: (i) mosquitoes (29%), with topics including malaria, Rift Valley fever, Lacrosse encephalitis, dengue, West Nile fever and eastern equine encephalitis; (ii) tsetse (16%) and (mainly) animal trypanosomiasis; (iii) ticks (13%) as vectors of Lyme disease and tick-borne encephalitis in Europe and northern America as well as some African tick-borne diseases; and (iv) snail intermediary hosts (11%) of

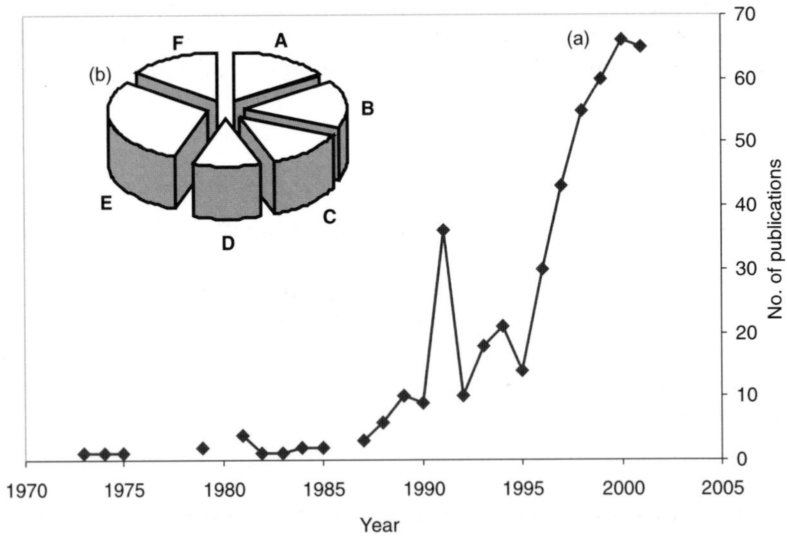

Fig. 6.1. Time distribution of (a) GIS/RS parasitology-related papers and (b) GIS/RS-related parasitology papers on different topics. A, review papers; B, tsetse and trypanosomiasis; C, ticks and tick-borne diseases; D, intermediary snail hosts, schistosomiasis and fasciolosis; E, mosquitoes, malaria, etc.; F, other topics. Data are from CABHealth and VetCD.

schistosomes and liver fluke. Currently *Culicoides* midges, major players on the arboviruses and emerging diseases scene, are a topical subject.

The applications of GIS and RS in epidemiology and parasitology have been reviewed by several authors (44 recorded papers). The most recent in-depth summary of one decade of research was by Hay *et al.* (2000), who reviewed all relevant topics in great detail, providing the scientific community with the latest landmarks in this field.

The use of GIS and RS is now generally accepted by the scientific community as a major tool contributing to the understanding of epidemiological processes *sensu lato*: disease, vector, host, environment. Nevertheless, whilst most people are now aware of the potential of these techniques, many still hesitate to use them for research or decision making. This chapter reviews recent advances towards the more widespread routine use of GIS/RS and of space–time information systems (STIS) in parasitology.

First we will review past trends. To do this we will focus on three case studies. The first is an insect-borne disease: tsetse-transmitted animal trypanosomiasis, with particular reference to West Africa. Secondly, we consider an intermediary host disease, *Fasciola hepatica* in the southern USA and East Africa. Thirdly, we examine a tick-borne disease, East Coast fever in East and southern Africa.

In the second part of the chapter we consider current and future trends, starting with a discussion about the implications of using GIS at an operational level and the need to fully integrate all aspects of time and space to achieve this goal. In this part, a review of literature published since 2000 on topics relevant to GIS and parasitology is given.

6.2 Tsetse-transmitted trypanosomiasis

Arguably, area-wide knowledge of the different factors affecting the interactions between vectors, parasites and hosts is required in order to understand the spatial epidemiology of the disease and to provide a strong basis for rational trypanosomiasis management. Thus, a first step towards understanding those interactions at a macro scale will include the systematic mapping of:

- The distribution and abundance of the different tsetse species (vectors).
- The occurrence (prevalence) and expression (anaemia) of trypanosomes (parasites).
- The distribution and relative importance of cattle breeds and cattle management systems (hosts).

6.2.1 Area-wide mapping

Since the early workers established, 100 years ago, the link between nagana, caused by trypanosomes, and the tsetse vector, considerable efforts have been made to map the distributions of the different tsetse species. This wealth of information, gathered by often anonymous field workers at country level, has regularly been compiled to produce distribution maps on a subregional or continental scale (Nash, 1948; Ford, 1963; Ford and Katondo, 1973).

The maps produced by Ford and Katondo (1973) are still considered to be an international standard. They include nine sheets of 1:5,000,000 maps describing the distributions of the different tsetse species of each group (palpalis, morsitans, fusca) and for each subregion (western, eastern and southern Africa). They have been locally updated by several authors (Katondo, 1984; Moloo, 1985; Gouteux, 1990). A detailed review of past and present tsetse distributions in southern Africa is given by Van den Bossche and Vale (2000) for Malawi, Mozambique, eastern Zambia and Zimbabwe.

Whilst historical tsetse distribution patterns are often well documented on a country scale, the problem of mapping tsetse abundance has been addressed less frequently. Most efforts towards that goal are limited to the monitoring of tsetse populations in areas earmarked for vector eradication before, during and after suppression campaigns; for example, the pastoral zone of Sidéradougou (3000 km^2) of Burkina Faso (Cuisance *et al.*, 1984b). In northern Côte d'Ivoire (134,000 km^2) tsetse surveys carried out between 1978 and 1981 to help define a rational control strategy for the whole area yielded detailed tsetse distribution and abundance maps of all species present (Clair and Lamarque, 1984). In The Gambia (10,000 km^2) an abundance map of *Glossina morsitans submorsitans* was produced (Rawlings *et al.*, 1993). More recently, in Togo (56,000 km^2) a set of national distribution maps at a grid resolution of 0.125° for all species present (*G. m. submorsitans, G. longipalpis, G. tachinoides, G. palpalis palpalis, G. fusca and G. medicorum*) and abundance maps for both riverine species (*G. tachinoides* and *G. p. palpalis*) was produced in the 1990s (Hendrickx *et al.*, 1999a).

Whilst tsetse survey results are well documented, there are few known records of the systematic mapping of trypanosome distribution and prevalence rates. Most studies report results in tabular form according to administrative units (e.g. Awan *et al.*, 1988; Agu *et al.*, 1989). Other examples include some spatial aspects, such as reported by Corten *et al.* (1988) in south-west Zambia, where surveys revealed that the extent of the trypanosomiasis problem covered a wider area than expected from historical fly distribution data alone.

The recorded fly abundance was expected to reflect disease risk (Clair and Lamarque, 1984; Cuisance *et al.*, 1984a). Therefore, trypanosomiasis surveys were often not conducted. In parts of the northern Côte d'Ivoire area, Camus (1981a) conducted prevalence surveys in 191 herds of the 1200 herds monitored by the Société pour le Développement de la Production Animale. Sixteen cattle were sampled from each herd. Herds were classified as either positive or negative. Results were summarized in a table and some spatial variation of disease prevalence was shown. No link was made with tsetse maps. An analysis of contemporary zootechnical data showed a significant difference between positive and negative herds. In the Gambia example (Rawlings *et al.*, 1993), a series of integrated trypanosomiasis control measures was proposed, adapted to the different levels of *G. m. submorsitans* abundance. In a later study, Snow *et al.* (1997) showed positive correlations between the recorded tsetse abundance figures and disease prevalence in cattle, small ruminants and equids.

Only a few studies were aimed at area-wide trypanosomiasis mapping. In Togo, in addition to the entomological surveys mentioned above, herds were systematically sampled at the same spatial resolution. After transformation, results yielded detailed countrywide raster maps of parasite distributions and prevalence as well as of herd anaemia (Hendrickx *et al.*, 1999b). This work was later extended to western Burkina Faso along the Mouhoun river system. Data on disease prevalence and the prevalence of anaemic cattle were combined to map epidemiological patterns, and this showed clearly the changing risk levels according to the importance of drainage systems (Hendrickx and Tamboura, 2000).

In southern Africa, point measurement maps were produced, summarizing trypanosomiasis surveys conducted in the 1990s in Malawi (159 sampling sites), Mozambique (274 sampling sites), Zambia (128 sampling sites) and Zimbabwe (62 sampling sites) (Van den Bossche and Vale, 2000).

In western and central Africa, the International Livestock Centre for Africa (1979) produced cattle breed maps for different countries with details for the larger administrative regions. Maps combined with pie charts depict the presence of dominant cattle breeds. In addition, information is provided on breed performance and husbandry systems. No maps are given of the latter.

In northern Côte d'Ivoire, Camus *et al.* (1981b) studied, as part of the same investigation into trypanosomiasis prevalence mentioned above, breed distributions and the effect of increasing zebu pressure on sedentary taurine herds after the droughts of the 1970s. Cattle were classified as either Baoulé (West African Shorthorn taurine), N'dama (West African Longhorn taurine), zebu or taurine × zebu crosses. Data were gathered from the SODEPRA (Société de Développement des Productions Animales) extension workers. Schematic maps are given of distributions of sedentary cattle of individual breeds for reproductive females and males. Densities are shown as dots representing 500 and 5000 head respectively.

In The Gambia, the ITC (International Trypanotolerance Centre) team involved in the examples given above have developed a low-cost rapid appraisal method whereby results of field surveys are combined with two socioeconomic questionnaires, including topics on farming systems and village economics and livestock and tsetse (Snow *et al.*, 1995).

Finally, during the Togo study mentioned above an exhaustive countrywide cattle survey yielded distribution and breed maps for cattle (Hendrickx *et al.*, 1999b). Cattle breeds were characterized as either trypanosusceptible (zebu), trypanotolerant (West African Shorthorn Somba) or crossbreds (Colour Plate 12). Results obtained using a phenotypic key were validated using microsatellite technology (to measure zebu introgression) on a subsample.

6.2.2 Remote sensing to assist disease mapping

The influence of climatic variables on the distribution and abundance of tsetse has long been recognized, at both the local (Nash, 1937) and the regional (Nash, 1948) level, through years of field study. Nowadays, the increased availability of satellite imaging allows us to draw up much improved vector distribution maps (Hay *et al.*, 1997). Satellite images offer several advantages over field surveys: the data are free from any human bias, make remote places accessible, are continuously produced and show real-time information.

Rogers and Randolph (1993) pioneered the application of NOAA (National Oceanic and Atmospheric Administration, USA)-derived NDVI (normalized difference vegetation indices, a measure of the amount of vegetation activity) data plus ground-measured temperature and elevation data to predict the distribution of *G. morsitans* and *G. pallidipes* in Kenya and Tanzania. Taking the historical fly distribution (Ford and Katondo, 1973) as a reference, satellite-derived predictor variables were selected and an accuracy of 84 and 79% correct predictions was obtained when predicting the presence of *G. morsitans* and *G. pallidipes* respectively.

For West Africa, Rogers *et al.* (1996) carried out a similar exercise and produced distribution limits of eight tsetse species encountered in Burkina Faso and Côte d'Ivoire at 0.167° resolution. The satellite data in this study comprised Fourier-processed NDVI, channel 4 (linked to ground temperature) and CCD (cold cloud duration, linked to rainfall) values. As before, historical records served as the reference for fly distribution. Selecting the ten best predictor variables, the percentage of correct predictions of the abundance of *G. tachinoides*, *G. palpalis*, *G. m. submorsitans* and *G. longipalpis* was 74, 87, 67 and 71%, respectively.

In Togo, Hendrickx *et al.* (1995) and Rogers *et al.* (1994) introduced discriminant analysis of satellite data to identify tsetse habitat in an attempt to minimize the use of ground-collected data and to optimize the application of satellite imaging. Hendrickx *et al.* (2001b) used non-linear discriminant analysis models in combination with Fourier-processed AVHRR–NOAA (AVHRR = Advanced Very High Resolution Radiometer) predictor data to produce spatial predictions of fly distribution for *G. m. submorsitans, G. longipalpis, G. tachinoides, G. p. palpalis, G. fusca* and *G. medicorum*. The results yielded presence/absence accuracies greater than 90%. Low-, medium- and high-abundance models were also produced for both riverine species, *G. tachinoides* (70% correct) and *G. p. palpalis* (56% correct). Three other aspects linked to vector prediction were also studied: (i) the effects on accuracy of using a spatial subsample to predict the remainder of the country; (ii) the effects on accuracy of the number of predictor variables included in the models; and (iii) the accuracy of using training sets to predict the presence of flies in non-adjacent areas. Not surprisingly, decreasing the size of the training set systematically reduced the accuracy of the predictions. The effect of the number of predictor variables was less straightforward. It was shown that accuracy increased to a maximum with an increasing number of predictor variables for sampled grids included in the training set. However, for grids not included in the training set predictions were always maximized with fewer predictor variables compared with results obtained in grids included in the training set. This highlighted the risk of overfitting models to restricted subsamples. Finally, it was clearly shown that one should be cautious when using training sets to predict the presence of flies in non-adjacent areas. The huge discrepancies observed between the prediction of fly presence in Togo using data from Côte d'Ivoire and Burkina Faso and the observed Togo maps clearly suggested that, whilst training set quality may certainly play a role, multivariate conditions at the grid level were (are) far too different between these two areas to produce results that are accurate enough. This work was later extended to western Burkina Faso in ecoclimatically drier areas complementary to the prevailing conditions in Togo. The aim was to map fly ecology patterns along the Mouhoun river system (Colour Plate 13) as a contribution to the understanding of riverine fly fragmentation patterns at their distribution limits.

The Togo approach developed for georeferenced trypanosomiasis management was extended to Burkina Faso. Results included maps of epidemiological patterns and fly ecology patterns for the Mouhoun river in western Burkina Faso (Hendrickx and Tamboura, 2000).

In southern Africa, Robinson *et al.* (1997a,b) analysed the historical distribution of *G. m. centralis*, *G. m. morsitans* and *G. pallidipes* in the common fly belt of Malawi, Mozambique, Zambia and Zimbabwe (Ford and Katondo, 1973) using NDVI, ground-measured temperatures, rainfall and elevation. Multivariate techniques included were linear discriminant analysis, maximum likelihood classification and principal component analysis. For each species, the best predictor variables were selected and the discriminant functions were applied to produce 84–92% correct predictions. Interestingly, the analysis successfully identified the geographical limits of both subspecies of *G. morsitans* present.

As for field surveys, remote sensing has been used mainly to assist in mapping the vectors whose distribution and abundance depend on ecovariables. The sole example of predicting trypanosome distribution and prevalence rates is the above-mentioned Togo study. Using techniques similar to those described for the spatial prediction of tsetse flies, models were produced for the prevalence of *Trypanosoma congolense* and *T. vivax* (Hendrickx *et al.*, 2000). In addition, prediction maps were also produced for average herd packed cell volume (PCV, a measure of anaemia, the most important symptom of trypanosomiasis). For trypanosomiasis, the highest prediction accuracy was obtained (83 and 89% for the two species of *Trypanosoma* respectively) when, in addition to remote sensing, a set of anthropogenic predictor variables was used. Not surprisingly, since many other causes may affect anaemia, the accuracy of PCV predictions was significantly lower than the accuracy of prediction of trypanosomiasis.

6.2.3 Integrated spatial data analysis and management in a GIS environment

To date, different approaches have been explored to use GIS towards a better understanding of the epidemiology and impact of tsetse-transmitted trypanosomiasis in order to assist rational disease management. Such studies have been conducted at the continental, subregional, national and local levels.

At the continental scale, Reid and Ellis (1995) performed GIS simulations using data on tsetse distributions, human population, cattle densities and protected or conservation areas with the aim of identifying the possible environmental implications of eventual trypanosomiasis control. Maps were generated depicting the areas where trypanosomiasis control may, from an ecological perspective, be encouraged, i.e. areas of agricultural intensification, banned, i.e. areas of high ecological integrity, or recommended with caution, i.e. areas of agricultural extensification. In a further study Reid *et al.* (2000) modelled, also at the continental level, the effect of an expanding human population and associated agriculture on the distribution of tsetse fly species. The spatial model included a combination of fine-resolution human population data, field data and the distribution of different types of tsetse. Results suggest that many of the 23 species of tsetse fly will begin to disappear by the year 2040, and that the area of land infested and the number of people in contact with flies will also decline. However, an area of Africa larger than Western Europe will remain infested by tsetse and under threat of trypanosomiasis for the foreseeable future.

At the subcontinental scale, Wint *et al.* (1997) conducted a series of studies in eastern, western and southern Africa. The rationale here was to select areas where trypanosomiasis control would yield high agricultural benefits, by integrating data on tsetse fly distributions, the pattern of human habitation, cropping areas and cattle densities. Tentative farming systems were defined on the basis of ecozone-related, geographic clusters of typical combinations of farmer densities, the proportion of land brought into the cultivation cycle and cattle numbers. These different farming systems were next matched with the tsetse distributions, to allow the likely outcome of any tsetse control, expressed in terms of expected changes in the amount of cropping and livestock to be predicted. In the case of missing field data, multivariate analysis models and NOAA satellite data were used to compensate for these shortfalls. The results are believed to aid the prioritization of areas particularly in the eastern and western parts of Africa. The results obtained have been embedded in the Food and Agriculture Organization (FAO) Programme Against African Trypanosomiasis (PAAT) information system (http:// www.fao.org/paat/html/home.htm).

At the regional scale, data layers from the PAAT information system have been used, together with other data, to assist in the area-wide planning of tsetse control in West Africa (Hendrickx *et al.*, 2004). On the basis of the results of a livestock production systems analysis and a series of hypotheses concerning riverine fly ecology, different approaches for integrated vector control have been suggested and pathways for future research proposed.

In southern Africa (Malawi, Mozambique, Zambia, Zimbabwe) Doran and Van den Bosche (2000) developed a strategy to identify priority areas for control on the basis of detailed knowledge of socioeconomic, institutional, technical and environmental (SITE) variables. To be fully operational, this decision-making process must be seen as a dynamic process in which potential and existing control activities need to be filtered by each SITE criterion on an ongoing basis. Whilst it is not yet applied in practice, this system is the only one that includes a strong time factor.

At a national level, Robinson (1998) integrated data from eastern Zambia on tsetse distribution, agricultural land use intensity, net stocking rates and arable potential in order to identify areas where tsetse control may be appropriate for relieving direct disease pressure and areas where control could potentially relieve land pressure. This approach was refined in a second paper (Robinson *et al.*, 2002).

In Togo, Hendrickx *et al.* (1999b) developed a GIS-based decision support system using the various data layers on vectors, parasites and hosts described elsewhere in this chapter. Different decision tree models were developed that were adapted to the prevailing mapped livestock production systems. The system was used to plan a national extension campaign focused on disease management and the involvement of private veterinary practitioners and auxiliaries ('barefoot vets'). This also included some areas earmarked for vector control. In these selected priority areas an additional study was conducted to model soil fragility, a crucial factor in the development of sustainable mixed farming.

Finally, a series of fine-scale studies were conducted at the local level using high-resolution satellite imaging. De Wispelaere (1994) integrated SPOT (Satellite Pour l'Observation de la Terre)-derived data on vegetation and land use to discern *G. m. submorsitans* habitat on the Adamawa plateau in Cameroon. Kitron *et al.* (1996) used Landsat imagery in the remote Lambwe Valley (Kenya) to predict favourable fly habitat. De La Rocque (2001b) combined high-resolution satellite imaging with entomological, disease prevalence, hydrography, landscape patterns, land-use and animal husbandry data in an attempt to identify major discriminating factors of tsetse presence and trypanosomiasis risk at a resolution of 30 metres in Sidéradougou, Burkina Faso. Currently targeted vector control activities focus on epidemiological hotspots (personal communication, S. De La Rocque). In addition, the combined experience of the Togo and Burkina Faso projects (see also above) serves as a basis to further study fly fragmentation and dispersion patterns on the Mouhoun river in western Burkina Faso.

In the Didessa Valley (Ethiopia) Erkelens *et al.* (2000) used a series of environmental variables and Landsat TM (Thematic Mapper) imagery to map priority areas for tsetse control on the basis of a cost–benefit approach addressing the following questions: (i) where does trypanosomiasis have a negative effect on (agricultural) development? (ii) In which areas will control measures have the highest impact/economic benefit? Currently, different ongoing projects in the area are further refining this approach.

6.3 Snails and liver flukes

6.3.1 Hard-copy maps

Prior to the 1990s, few attempts were made to map fasciolosis. Interestingly, most of these early studies did not focus on habitat mapping of the intermediary hosts but rather on observed disease data; that is, they looked at the problem from a veterinary perspective.

In this pre-GIS period, Ollerenshaw (1966) published crude choropleth maps for England and Wales at the county level showing predicted and observed disease in sheep. Forecasts were made using climatic conditions occurring in the previous 6 months excluding winter, a method derived from a pioneering model developed in Anglesey, Wales (Ollerenshaw and Rowlands, 1959). On the basis of a visual comparison between the expected incidence and the observed cases it was concluded that a 'reasonable correlation' could be shown. Some years later, Boray (1969) published a sketch map of south-east Australia that divided the area into five endemic areas of fluke, defined by temperature–rainfall regimes. The approach used was very crude and was mainly based on the extrapolation of disease prevalence results from a limited number of tracer studies.

In 1980 Watt published choropleth maps of Victoria, Australia, showing the prevalence of condemned bovine livers (slaughterhouse data) at the shire level. High-prevalence areas were visually correlated with high-rainfall and irrigation areas (see Chapter 1). The last significant study of this pre-GIS era involved small-area mapping of the intermediary hosts. Maps produced by Wright and Swire (1984) show a broad visual association between snail habitat and gley soil classes. The distribution of snails is shown to be patchy within given wet soil classes and the associated wetland plants.

6.3.2 Digital spatial data

On the basis of previous work, which concluded that a developed climate forecast model did not account for local variations in observed prevalence of fasciolosis, Zukowski *et al.* (1991) used a raster GIS to overlay snail habitats traced on to an aerial photograph and digitized US Geological Survey (USGS) soil maps of the coastal area of Louisiana, USA. As a first step, snail habitat was associated with certain soil types on a primary study farm. These results were confirmed when the association was extended to another 12 maps. In a further study, Zukowski *et al.* (1993) found a good association between the proportion of high-risk soil types and snail habitats; this relationship was less clear for disease risk.

Malone *et al.* (1992) used a more complex GIS approach to produce a composite risk index for 25 farms in the Red River Basin, Louisiana. The risk index included data from digitized USGS soil data updated using multispectral scanner (MSS) images, slopes, and length of pasture/water course per hectare. A significant regression was found between the weighted risk index and measured egg counts per farm, a measure of disease in live animals. The importance of GIS in quantifying local risk at farm level was further stressed by Malone and Zukowski (1992).

In Africa, a series of studies attempted to relate the distribution and abundance of *Fasciola* to NDVIs derived from low-resolution meteorological satellite data. In East Africa, Malone *et al.* (1998) used a set of digital agroecological data layers from the FAO and a climate forecast computer model that had been developed previously for crop productivity models to construct forecast index maps, i.e. abundance estimates, for *F. hepatica* and *F. gigantica* for different crop production system zones. The calculated risk forecast for both species combined was shown to be significantly correlated with average monthly NDVI values, and less so with available disease prevalence data. This approach was also applied separately to Ethiopia (Yilma and Malone, 1998) using the NDVI rather than a forecast index. The spatial association between the predicted and observed distributions of *Fasciola* was mainly based on visual map interpretation.

More recently, Fuentes *et al.* (2001) made an attempt to predict human fasciolosis in the northern Altiplano of Bolivia. Best results were obtained when fasciolosis was predicted using 1.1 km NDVI data. Nevertheless, whilst the model correctly predicted abundance ranges in known fasciolosis hotspots, it failed to identify the absence of disease in areas where the intermediary snail host was known to be absent. Little detail was given about the statistical techniques used. Finally, Cringoli *et al.* (2002) report the mapping of *F. hepatica* and *Dicrocoelium dendriticum* in the southern Appennines of Italy, using faecal samples from cattle and sheep. The GIS analysis of point distribution maps revealed a homogeneous distribution for *D. dendriticum* and a focal distribution for *F. hepatica*.

No attempt was made to use these training data to forecast the spatial distribution of liver flukes in the area.

6.4 Tick-transmitted East Coast fever

6.4.1 The pre-GIS era

Early studies focused mainly on the relationship between the distributions of cattle and East Coast fever. Robson *et al.* (1961) showed that in Tanzania, East Coast fever was confined to areas of tsetse absence and cattle presence. In north-west Tanzania, Yeoman (1966a) produced maps of cattle density and East Coast fever outbreaks in the study area. It was possible to draw a line separating endemic (ticks always present) and epidemic (ticks only present in favourable years) areas and map the spatial development of the epidemic over a 4-year period. The relationship between endemicity/epidemicity and rainfall isolines was also studied (Yeoman, 1966b). No direct relationship was found between the number of ticks on cattle and the annual variation in rainfall.

6.4.2 The ecoclimatic index, CLIMEX and the prediction of tick distributions

In the 1980s the idea of ecoclimatic matching for predicting the potential distribution and relative abundance of species by matching climates inside and outside sampled areas was first applied to animal disease vectors. Sutherst and Maywald (1985) calculated an ecoclimatic index (EI) for *Rhipicephalus appendiculatus* for selected sites worldwide on the basis of the distribution of the tick in Kenya. A reasonable correlation was obtained between the observed and predicated distributions. The absence of this tick in West Africa despite predicted climatic suitability was noted. Implementation of ecoclimatic matching was through a specifically developed software package, CLIMEX (http://www.ento.csiro.au/climex/climex.htm)

In the early 1990s, the International Livestock Research Institute (ILRI) initiated the use of CLIMEX to forecast tick distributions. Norval and Perry (1990) determined CLIMEX values for the period 1972–1986 at a single weather station in south-east Zimbabwe. Though this paper did not involve a spatial study as such, the authors explained the spread and subsequent disappearance of ticks by a run of favourable years as determined by EI values. A first spatial data set was depicted by Lessard *et al.* (1990), who used the ARCINFO software to map the disease (theileriosis), the vector (*R. appendiculatus*) and the hosts (cattle and buffalo) for Africa, with a special focus on East and southern Africa. Interpolated climatic data at a resolution of 625 km^2 were used to train CLIMEX predictions for all pixels. A vegetation map based on average monthly NDVI values was also included. In this paper the authors discuss biological processes only briefly. The discussion was taken further by Perry *et al.* (1990), who mapped CLIMEX dry and heat stresses and discussed tick distribution in relation to such climatic stresses in East and southern Africa, and by Norval *et al.* (1991), who identified similar EI and NDVI values between the Kenyan and Ethiopian highlands. The absence of ticks in south-west Ethiopia despite favourable conditions was related to the presence of tsetse (the tsetse corridor). These different results (Colour Plate 14) were summarized by Perry *et al.* (1991a), who also reproduced some of the earlier CLIMEX map outputs in greater detail, showing the sensitivity and specificity of CLIMEX EI for *R. appendiculatus* according to grid cell. The authors showed a visual correlation between NDVI values greater than or equal to a value of 0.150 and tick presence.

In southern Africa, historical data on East Coast fever outbreaks (at administrative region resolution) which occurred between 1901 and 1960 were visually related by the use of a CLIMEX-generated map of climatic suitability for *R. apendiculatus* (Lawrence, 1991). This built on the results published by Mayward and Sutherst in 1987. It was concluded that the CLIMEX favourability map overestimated tick suitability areas.

6.4.3 Remote sensing, an added value for mapping tick distribution patterns

The growing availability of remote sensing products since the late 1980s and early 1990s has opened new avenues for understanding and predicting area-wide tick distributions.

Early exploratory studies covering Zimbabwe explored the relationship between mean monthly NDVI and ecoclimatic zones. NDVI was related to rainfall and it was shown that commercial grazing lands averaged a higher NDVI value than adjacent communal areas (Kruska and Perry, 1991). On the basis of an extensive georeferenced data set that included ecoclimatic data, cattle distributions, boundaries between commercial and communal land, EI for ticks and East Coast fever outbreaks, Perry *et al.* (1991b) and Kruska and Perry (1992) reported (no analysis given) a visual relationship between ticks, disease outbreaks, EI and agro-ecoclimatic zones. The boundaries between commercial and communal lands were obtained from Landsat MSS images, and Thiessen polygons were used to convert cattle numbers at dip-tanks into area distribution values.

By relating seasonally variable tick mortality rates to remotely sensed vegetation data for Burundi, Uganda, Tanzania, Zimbabwe and South Africa, a major breakthrough in the understanding of area-wide tick distributions and abundance was achieved (Randolph, 1993). By showing that meteorological satellite sensor data (i.e. NDVI) seem to be a reliable marker for tick performance, taking regional heterogeneities into consideration, a sound biological justification was provided for using this type of variable in a purely statistical GIS framework to define the environmental characteristics of sites where ticks do occur and others where they do not (Randolph, 2000). Using discriminant analysis and NDVI, temperature and altitude as predictor variables, the spatial distribution of *R. appendiculatus* was modelled for Zimbabwe, Kenya and Tanzania (Rogers and Randolph, 1993) (Colour Plate 14).

6.4.4 Towards mapping disease risk

Whilst the relationship between spatial tick distribution patterns and remotely sensed and ground-measured ecoclimatic data has been shown, this relationship is less clear for the disease. As was shown for trypanosomiasis (Hendrickx *et al.*, 1999b), anthropogenic factors, such as husbandry systems, grazing management, vector control and treatment against the disease, are mostly not related to ecoclimatic spatial settings and therefore blur the picture.

Most efforts towards mapping East Coast fever were conducted by ILRI teams to aid in decision support in the planning of 'infect-and-treat' immunization campaigns. The aim was to infect young cattle with a live strain of *Theileria parva*, the causative agent of East Coast fever, and to administer at the same time a curative drug treatment. This approach provides protection for up to 3 years (Perry and Young, 1995). Since, in most cases, studies with this goal involve several visits to the same farms over a period of time, the collection of samples for laboratory analysis and the implementation of socioeconomic questionnaires, these studies usually cover limited areas. Results are therefore difficult to extrapolate.

Delehanty (1993) used a GIS to map agroecological and socioeconomic variables of livestock farmers in the Uasin Gishu district in west Kenya. The aim was to identify areas where immunization may be most applicable. In his discussion, the author mainly addresses the difficulty of extrapolating from data-rich to data-poor areas. In the Coast Province of Kenya, Deem *et al.* (1993) showed an East Coast fever gradient in three out of four coastal agroecozones. In a later study, Gitau *et al.* (2000) analysed epidemiological patterns in a series of contrasting agroecological and grazing strata in the Muranga district in highland Kenya. It was concluded, as in the previous studies, that the link between East Coast fever and agroecozone may be a key to understanding the spatial patterns of East Coast fever outbreaks.

Duchateau *et al.* (1997) developed a spatial logistic regression model to predict the presence and absence of East Coast fever using the georeferenced data set of Kruska and Perry (1992). Results included maps of outbreak probabilities for Kenya and residual distribution patterns. Much attention was given to reducing the size, whilst retaining the maximum amount of information, of the spatial predictor variable database, which included ground-measured climatic data, remotely sensed NDVI and land cover data. This was achieved using principal components analysis and subsequent varimax rotation of the principal components that were obtained. The same data set was revisited by Pfeiffer *et al.* (1997) using three spatial regression models. The spatial models selected the same variables as in the previous study.

Recently, ILRI has put effort into collating the results of different longitudinal and cross-sectional epidemiological studies conducted in the framework of their East Coast fever immunization activities and covering a series of different settings (from both the agroecozone and the animal husbandry point of view) in coastal and highland Kenya. Currently, efforts are under way to improve these results (personal communication, B.D. Perry).

6.5 About GIS, semantics and teamwork

The acronym 'GIS' can be interpreted in two ways (see Chapter 3). First, as geographical information *systems*, which encapsulates the different commercial software packages; secondly, as geographical information *science*, which recognizes the fact that almost every process in nature displays some pattern in the space domain. While the first interpretation involves only the systems that are used to store data and to perform some elementary operations on the data, the latter includes the multidisciplinary techniques for the description of the spatial patterns of natural processes.

As GIScience evolves, one could argue that GISystems will never meet the full requirements of every end-user: a geologist may need a totally different tool-set from that of a parasitologist. Although the tool-sets become larger as new versions of GIS software systems emerge, GIS system developers recognize that it is impossible to fulfil everyone's needs and are therefore developing and commercializing application programming interfaces (APIs) to enable the end-user to develop her or his own specific tools without having to deal with data file formats or elementary GIS operations (e.g. point-in-polygon operations, buffering, overlays). However, because IT standards develop rapidly and because the traditional educational background of the majority of environmental scientists is not focused on IT-related problem-solving, this may strengthen the general feeling that GIS is nice, but ...

In addition, most GIS-related research focuses on 'where?' and

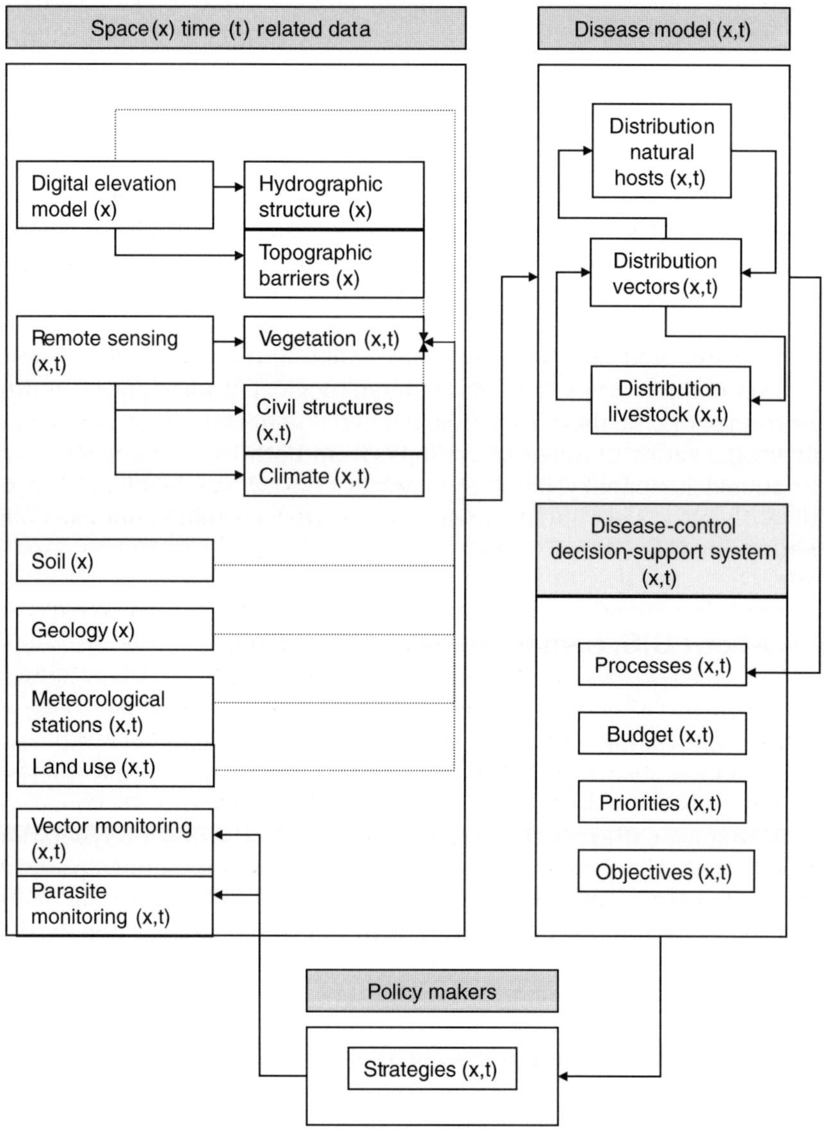

Fig. 6.2. Structural framework of an STIS decision-support system.

'what?', and often completely ignores 'when?'. Because this time domain is equally important in most environmental processes, it has been suggested that 'GIS' should be replaced by 'STIS', standing for space–time information science/systems (Kyriakidis and Journel, 2001). STIS aims to model processes in order to support our decisions and is now emerging in many university departments (Fig. 6.2). Also, STIS recognizes that all data feature some degree of error/uncertainty and that our knowledge is imprecise or not exhaustive and tries to incorporate this uncertainty throughout any analysis (Heuvelink, 1998; Biesemans *et al.*, 2000). Although knowledge of the confidence level of the model results is vital in making decisions, uncertainty propagation is often (if not almost always) neglected.

The list of techniques encapsulated by this new concept of STIS is massive and reaches far beyond the capabilities of currently available GIS software packages. It is therefore an advantage to form multidisciplinary groups to tackle the problems involved. This idea of 'scientific clustering' is nowadays embraced by many governmental organizations, which assign research funds only if such clusters are formed.

STIS reasoning offers a series of advantages. First, it is an important step towards the integrated management of our natural resources. Secondly, it increases awareness of the techniques used in other scientific research fields. Thirdly, STIS reasoning stimulates the integration of uncertainty analysis in expert systems; therefore, in the decision-making process uncertainty and/or error should no longer be considered to be bad.

But there are not only advantages in STIS reasoning. The major disadvantages are that the level of complexity is rising and it is a demanding task to keep pace with technological developments. Further, there is a lack of standards, which does not favour the portability of STIS/GIS data and the software modules that operate on this type of data.

Obviously, one can pinpoint many subjects in which STIS science and technology can be improved. However, it is clear that the disadvantages are best regarded as topics for further research and development rather than fundamental concerns. It may be that the only real disadvantage or pitfall in STIS reasoning is that some might link complexity with accuracy. Complex models may be 'better' than simple models, but this should certainly not be used as a rule of thumb. It all depends on the manner of implementation, and thus the manner of reasoning. If one takes this attitude, it is clear that STIS reasoning is a major step forward: it initiates and consolidates a more holistic approach in the decision-support cycle.

6.6 STIS: from theory to practice

Whilst it is clear that the proposed expansion of the GIS concept to STIS opens new avenues for collaborative research, we may ask what products we may expect and how far the parasitologist is from the routine use of these tools.

6.6.1 Mapping

Mapping is a crucial step towards understanding the spatial epidemiology of parasitic diseases. Vector and host distributions are directly related to ecoclimatic conditions. Therefore, populations can be described in great detail using a variety of ground-measured and remotely sensed environmental and geographical correlates. Apart from simple presence/absence modelling, the mapping of spatial patterns may also address population density and time-dependent seasonal fluctuations or longer-term trends. The latter includes the likely impact of climate change.

The collection of field data on parasites, vectors or (intermediary) hosts, including the identification of gathered samples, is notoriously time-consuming and expensive. Different approaches have been developed to allow the extrapolation of point field survey data to continuous probability maps of presence/absence or abundance. Although in some studies the distribution of sampling points may be dense enough to produce usable point density maps without need for further interpolation or extrapolation, as in the study on liver flukes in southern Italy (Cringoli *et al.*, 2002), in most cases it is not.

One way round this problem is to establish correlations between distribution data and landscape categories. These techniques were already in use prior to the RS/GIS era; for example, the mapping of ixodid ticks, including *Ixodes persulcatus*, in Siberia and the Soviet Far East by Korenberg (1973) and Korenberg and Lebedeva (1976). On the basis of historical and field-collected transect data, tick populations were related to landscape types at a local and regional scale. Ten main types and 26 regional subtypes of habitat were identified in Asiatic Russia. Further subdivisions were characterized by the relative proportions of the different tick species found in each area. The aim of these maps was to link discrete tick populations with foci of tick-borne encephalitis and rickettsiosis and to conduct epidemiological forecasting, also based on seasonal activity patterns.

Such techniques have since been refined and now include the use of high-resolution satellite imagery (Landsat, SPOT) to fingerprint landscape types using various supervised and unsupervised classification techniques. The most recent examples include the mapping of *Culiseta melurna*, the vector of eastern equine encephalomyelitis in Massachusetts, USA (Moncayo *et al.*, 2000) and a study of the transmission and intermediary hosts of alveolar echinococcosis in Tibet (Danson *et al.*, 2002).

Whilst the cost of high-resolution satellite data, as used in the studies listed above, limits their use to relatively small areas, other techniques, relying on data from meteorological satellites, have been developed for area-wide mapping. Using this approach, distribution maps at a resolution of between 8 and 1 km are now routinely produced. Point measurements of the variable to map (e.g. a vector) are related to gridded environmental predictor variables. Various statistical techniques are then used, including regression models and discriminant analysis, to calculate the probability of presence in non-sampled grids, thus creating a continuous distribution map based on scattered point observations.

This approach has been adapted to a wide range of (vectors of) diseases and geographical settings relevant to the veterinary parasitologist. Recent examples include the mapping of fasciolosis in Bolivia (Fuentes *et al.*, 2001), the mapping of tsetse in South Africa (Hendrickx *et al.*, 2002) and the mapping of *Culicoides* midges in the Mediterranean basin (Baylis *et al.*, 2001; Wittmann *et al.*, 2001).

In addition to mapping the distribution of parasites, vectors and intermediary hosts, similar approaches have also been used to map the distribution of livestock. Currently, distribution data at a grid resolution of 5 km are available for Europe, Asia and Africa on the World Wide Web (Wint *et al.*, 2001). Data on North, Central and South America have been processed and will soon be available to the user community, as will be regular updates and improvements of existing maps.

Whilst it is not the purpose of this chapter to discuss statistical methods (see elsewhere in this book), it is important to discuss briefly some issues related to training data, i.e. observed or historical data used to feed spatial prediction models. Ideally, the sampling procedure should follow the following steps: (i) define homogeneous ecoclimatic strata in the area under consideration; (ii) randomly select grids to sample within each stratum; and (iii) sample the variable to be modelled according to the same standard procedure in each selected grid.

Ecoclimatic strata may be defined by clustering the available ground-measured and remotely sensed environmental correlates using standard statistical software. A dendrogram should be used to determine the number of relevant clusters to include. Whilst this is relatively straightforward, deciding how many grids to sample is far less so. If the total area is large enough and the sampled grids are carefully selected, as few as 1% of the grids under consideration may be sufficient (Lark, 1994). Often the final number sampled will be a compromise between statistical relevance and the funding, infrastructure and manpower available.

Some additional tools are available to upgrade observed training data before predicting continuous spatial distribution patterns. Recently geostatistics have been used to achieve this goal (Hendrickx *et al.*, 2002). For example, we have modelled the distribution of *G. austeni* in KwaZulu Natal, using a geostatistics (indicator kriging) approach (Colour Plate 15) and multivariate logistic regression. In the latter, a model was fitted using the presence/absence of *G. austeni* and a set of environmental covariates including NOAA–AVHRR Local Area Coverage satellite images at 1.1 km resolution (Colour Plate 15).

6.6.2 Spatial epidemiology and the time dimension

The previous section dealt with the development of individual data layers; here some recent developments towards understanding the spatial epidemiology of vector-borne and/or parasitic diseases are highlighted, with emphasis on studies including a time dimension.

In a series of studies conducted in China (Yang *et al.*, 2000, 2002) the impact of flooding on the habitat and distribution of the intermediary snail host of schistosomiasis has been studied in great detail. Ground validation indicated that such an ecology-based approach, taking into consideration specific environmental conditions associated with the extent of annual floods, correctly predicted potential snail habitats and contributed to the understanding of seasonal habitat differences, a key factor in integrated disease control. In an additional study, Seto *et al.* (2002) identified two key factors hampering the development of predictive models of the spatial distribution of schistosomiasis: (i) different subspecies of *Oncomelania hupensis*, the intermediary snail host, are adapted to distinct habitats ranging from mountainous to floodplain habitats; and (ii) environmental changes resulting from the construction of the Three Gorges Dam and global warming threaten to increase snail habitats. The understanding of these factors is a prerequisite for accurate risk mapping and the identification of priority areas for schistosomiasis control.

In Burkina Faso, historical tsetse distribution records and high-resolution satellite imaging (SPOT) time series analysis made it possible to link changes in the distribution and density of two riparian tsetse species, *G. palpalis* and *G. tachinoides*, and increased human activity as depicted by land use changes and cattle densities. Results identified anthropogenic and environmental factors affecting riparian tsetse populations either positively or negatively (De La Rocque *et al.*, 2001a). Such indicators are essential in predicting the human impact on riparian tsetse populations in the region; little is known about this, but such knowledge is a key to current area-wide tsetse suppression plans.

The study of historical outbreaks of Rift Valley fever in Kenya between 1950 and 1998 revealed that outbreaks followed periods of abnormally high rainfall in otherwise dry habitats (Linthicum *et al.*, 1999). More than three-quarters of these events have been linked to the warm phase of the El Niño southern oscillation phenomenon. During these abnormal rainfall periods, dry dambos (distinct mosquito habitats) are flooded, resulting in the hatching of transovarially infected mosquito eggs – the start of a new epidemic. The mapping of ecological conditions using satellite recordings of vegetation shows increased greenness up to 5 months before outbreaks, indicating the forecasting potential of this type of approach.

An analysis of the seasonal variation in abundance of larvae and nymphs of ticks in seven European countries showed that, at sites within foci of Western type tick-borne encephalitis, larvae consistently started feeding and questing several months earlier in the year compared with sites where the disease did not occur, when nymphs are also active (Randolph *et al.*, 2000). Such synchronization between live stages is necessary for outbreaks to occur (Randolph *et al.*, 1999). Using satellite-derived time series of land surface temperature, it was shown that this behavioural pattern was associated with a higher than average rate of autumnal cooling relative to the peak midsummer land surface temperature. It was concluded that this link between satellite signals and biological processes is a key to predictive risk mapping (Randolph *et al.*, 2000). Such information is crucial in the testing of different 'what if?' temperature scenarios linked to anticipated global climate change patterns to predict the spread or decline of this disease (Randolph and Rogers, 2000).

Other teams have also used multivariable GIS models to study the spatial epidemiology of tick-borne disease outbreaks. In the north-central USA (Guerra *et al.*, 2002) results showed that the presence and abundance of *Ixodes scapularis* varied, even when the host population was adequate. Using different modelling techniques, risk maps were produced indicating suitable habitats and areas of high probability where ticks are likely to become established should they be introduced, thus highlighting both the explanatory and predictive capability of such models. This is an important feature, given the upsurge of these emerging diseases. In Italy a multivariable GIS model was developed to link the probability of tick (*I. ricinus*) occurrence with the probability of occurrence of infected tick nymphs at 50/50 metre resolution (Rizzoli *et al.*, 2002).

6.6.3 Decision-support systems

Spatial decision-support systems take spatial analysis one step further: from understanding epidemiological patterns to planning integrated control schemes.

As seen in Section 6.4.4 of this chapter, a leading field in this domain is African tsetse-transmitted trypanosomiasis, where decision-support tools have been developed at various scales. Data feeding these systems originated from: (i) extensive pluridisciplinary field surveys on vectors, hosts, parasites and socioeconomics; (ii) a wide range of contemporary ecogeographical environmental correlates; and (iii) access to various historical databases. Decisions are made by ranking identified sets of key variables. The different approaches used in these models have been reviewed in Section 6.2.2 of this chapter. Nevertheless, it is important to note here that, except for the Sidéradougou study, in which historical data on land use and tsetse distribution changes are part of the decision-making procedure, and for SITE criteria (see Van den Bossche and Vale, 2000), in which continuous data influx is considered a condition *sine qua non* for success, none of the systems that have been developed include a time component dealing with seasonal variation and medium-term forecasting.

No other examples are known to us of multidisciplinary information systems intended to aid in planning the integrated control of animal parasitic diseases over a large area. Most other existing information systems focus on vector-transmitted 'emerging' infectious diseases (West Nile fever, bluetongue, Rift Valley fever) or human parasitic diseases (malaria, schistosomiasis).

In Mpumalanga province, South Africa, a GIS-based information system was implemented for use in planning malaria control (Booman *et al.*, 2000). The system functioned in three steps: (i) data collection – a simplified reporting system to allow improved malaria reporting at the village and town levels; (ii) data analysis – the definition of high-risk areas and the stratification of malaria risk within these areas; and (iii) disease control – the planning and implementation of more efficient disease control. In the Republic of Korea (Claborn *et al.*, 2002) a GIS-based information system was used to compare the costs of malaria chemoprophylaxis with the costs of larvicidal treatment of potential mosquito breeding areas around two US military camps.

In China, mathematical models are being developed to describe the transmission of schistosomiasis using georeferenced field data and remote sensing inputs (Spear *et al.*, 2002). Though still at an experimental stage, it is expected that such models will produce sufficiently precise predictions to discriminate among competing control options.

The advent of diseases that may have an impact on public health has boosted the funding of research towards web-based forecasting systems. It is clear that other fields, such as veterinary parasitology, will greatly benefit from these developments.

A leading example in this field is the NASA-based website on the spread of West Nile virus in the USA (see http://www.gsfc.nasa.gov/topstory/20020828phap.html and http://www.gsfc.nasa.gov/topstory/20020204westnile.html). Data on virus occurrence in migratory birds, human cases of disease, the monitoring of mosquito populations, and satellite-derived forecasts are combined to produce updated risk maps. 'The idea is to let the satellite capture where the disease is spreading from year to year and make some predictions about where the disease is going. Computer models can determine which areas have the right combinations of temperatures and moisture levels most suitable for mosquitoes and transmission. Then, efforts and resources can target those high-risk areas. The goal of the programme is to extend the benefits of NASA's investments in Earth system science, technology and data toward public-health decision making and practice.'

In Australia, the National Arbovirus Monitoring Program operates a web-based information system, http://www.namp.com.au, which maps risk areas for bluetongue, Akabane virus and ephemeral fever virus. The aims are to: (i) facilitate international trade in Australian livestock (export certification); (ii) act as an early warning system for bluetongue; and (iii) assist producers and exporters in risk management. Risk models are based on seroconversion data from a network of sentinel animals and data on *Culicoides* midges from insect traps located near these animals. Efforts are also under way to develop disease-forecasting systems (Cameron, 2000). Results obtained with such information systems are of particular interest in Europe and the Mediterranean Basin, where bluetongue is currently emerging following the invasion of *Culicoides imicola*, a major vector of the disease (Wittmann *et al.*, 2001).

6.7 Discussion

Current trends show that systems based on spatial data analysis and the use of remote sensing are now applied to a wide variety of diseases and geographical areas. This is particularly the case with respect to the use of meteorological satellite data to predict spatial distribution patterns of parasites, vectors, intermediary hosts and hosts, not only in the tropics but also at subtropical and temperate latitudes (Green and Hay, 2002).

Developed methods are now robust enough to be included more routinely in spatial epidemiology studies and for decision support. Though meteorological satellite data are freely downloadable from the Internet (e.g. NOAA–AVHRR data; see http://www.saa.noaa.gov) data processing to transform raw data into usable formats remains a bottleneck. We have recently developed software (Avia-GIS NOAA Tools 1.0: see http://www.avia-gis.com) that allows the user to process downloaded data and to produce composite images in different formats compatible with commercial GIS software. Apart from the parasitologist's knowledge of epidemiological processes and creativity, the sole remaining limit now is hard disk space and computing memory: typically, gigabytes of meteorological data are needed to produce time series covering several years of information.

An increasing number of studies also consider time in addition to spatial analysis. Examples that have been cited include the analysis of historical trends, the impact of recurrent natural phenomena such as floods and El Niño, and the seasonal variation of vector populations. Nevertheless, many obstacles still have to be overcome before operational parasitic disease forecasting systems can be produced. It is anticipated that the current efforts deployed to monitor and forecast emerging diseases, e.g. West Nile virus in the USA and arboviruses in Australia, will further boost the development of such systems.

Another opportunity to develop such tools arises from the increasing (and not unrelated) interest in monitoring global changes. These include not only climate changes but also changes related to globalization: increases in mobility and trade, population shifts towards densely populated areas, increasing numbers of livestock in close contact with human populations, and changes in consumption patterns. All these factors have a major impact on the epidemiology of animal diseases and can be measured and monitored in space and time.

It is suggested that parasitic and vector-borne diseases are more likely to be affected by global climate change (Harvell *et al.*, 2002). Human-induced climate change is having measurable effects on ecosystems, communities and populations and therefore will most likely affect free-living stages and vectors or intermediary hosts. Greater overwintering success of free-living stages and effects on stages in hypobiosis will have a direct impact on parasite populations, resulting in increased disease severity and changing epidemiological patterns. Shifts in the geographic range and abundance of vectors and intermediary hosts may occur: known vectors of disease may invade new territory and existing (potential) vector populations may now reach the critical size that will allow disease transmission. An increase in temperature will also affect parasite development and transmission rates, resulting in the spread of disease as a result of the increased vectorial capacity of endemic vectors. But in some cases the opposite may also be true: changing habitats and climatic conditions may cause vector extinction or disrupt fragile epidemiological pathways. In any case, one will have to remain cautious and avoid oversimplification when interpreting results, as was recently shown by a study on the lack of a relationship between the spread of malaria and meteorological trends in the East African highlands (Hay *et al.*, 2002).

Both the variety of subjects and the increasing use of the time dimension in spatial analysis suggest that GIS and RS are now widely used and accepted. Most of the tools and ingredients are now available to further promote the emergence of STIS reasoning in veterinary parasitology, provided scientists from different disciplines are prepared to share data and experience. More than ever, such technologies and collaborative networks are needed to help understand and cope with a changing world.

References

Agu, W.E., Kalejaiye, J.O. and Olatunde, A.O. (1989) Prevalence of bovine trypanosomiasis in Kaduna and Plateau states of Nigeria. *Bulletin of Animal Health and Production in Africa* 37, 161–166.

Awan, M.A.Q., Maiga, S. and Bouare, S. (1988) Bovine trypanosomiasis in the Niger valley of the republic of Mali. Occurence and seasonal variation. *Bulletin of Animal Health and Production in Africa* 36, 330–333.

Baylis, M., Mellor, P.S., Wittmann, E.J. and Rogers, D.J. (2001) Prediction of areas around the Mediterranean at risk of bluetongue by modelling the distribution of its vector using satellite imaging. *Veterinary Record* 149, 639–643.

Biesemans, J., Van Meirvenne, M. and Gabriels, D. (2000) Extending the RUSLE with the Monte Carlo error propagation technique to predict longtime off-site sediment accumulation. *Journal of Soil and Water Conservation* 35, 35–43.

Booman, M., Durrheim, D.N., LaGrange, K., Martin, C., Mabuza, A.M., Zitha, A., Mbokazi, F.M., Fraser, C. and Sharp, B.L. (2000) Using a geographical information system to plan a malaria control programme in South Africa. *Bulletin of the World Health Organization* 78, 1438–1444.

Boray, J.C. (1969) Experimental fascioliasis in Australia. *Advances in Parasitology* 7, 95–210.

Cameron, A.R. (2000) Modelling the risk of arbovirus transmission in time and space. *Arbovirus Research in Australia* 8, 56–58.

Camus, E. (1981a) Epidémiologie et incidence clinique de la trypanosomose bovine dans le nord de la Côte d'Ivoire. *Revue d'Elevage et de Médecine Vétérinaire des Pays Tropicaux* 34, 289–295.

Camus, E. (1981b) Evaluation économique des pertes provoquées par la trypanosomose sur quatre types génétiques bovins dans le nord de la Côte-d'Ivoire. *Revue d'Elevage et de Médecine Vétérinaire des Pays Tropicaux* 34, 297–300.

Camus, E., Landais, E. and Poivey, J.P. (1981) Structure génétique du cheptel bovin sédentaire du Nord de la Côte-d'Ivoire. Perspectives d'avenir en fonction de la diffusion croissante de sang zébu. *Revue d'Elevage et de Médecine Vétérinaire des Pays Tropicaux* 34, 187–198.

Claborn, D.M., Masuoka, P.M., Klein, T.A., Hooper, T., Lee, A. and Andre, R.G. (2002) A cost comparison of two malaria control methods in Kyunggi Province, Republic of Korea, using remote sensing and geographic information systems. *American Journal of Tropical Medicine and Hygiene* 66, 680–685.

Clair, M. and Lamarque, G. (1984) Répartition des glossines dans le nord de la Côte d'Ivoire. *Revue d'Elevage et de Médecine Vétérinaire des Pays Tropicaux* 37, 60–83.

Corten, J., Ter Huurne, A., Moorhouse, P.D.S. and De Rooij, R.C. (1988) Prevalence of trypanosomiasis in cattle in South-West Zambia. *Tropical Animal Health and Production* 20, 78–84.

Cringoli, G., Rinaldi, L., Veneziano, V., Capelli, G. and Malone, J.B. (2002) A cross-sectional coprological survey of liver flukes in cattle and sheep from an area of the southern Italian Apennines. *Veterinary Parasitology* 108, 137–143.

Cuisance, D., Politzar, H., Tamboura, I., Mérot, P. and Lamarque, G. (1984a) Répartition des glossines dans la zone pastorale d'accueil de Sidéradougou, Burkina Faso. *Revue d'Elevage et de Médecine Vétérinaire des Pays Tropicaux* 37, 99–113.

Cuisance, D., Politzar, H., Merot, P. and Tamboura, I. (1984b) Les lâchés de mâles irradiés dans la campagne de lutte intégrée contre les glossines dans la zone pastorale de Sidéradougou, Burkina Faso. *Revue d'Elevage et de Médecine Vétérinaire des Pays Tropicaux* 47, 69–75.

Danson, F.M., Craig, P.S., Man, W., Shi, D.Z., Pleydell, D.R.J. and Giradoux, P. (2002)

Satellite remote sensing and geographical information systems for risk modelling of alveolar echinococcus. In: *Proceedings of the NATO Advanced Research Workshop on Cestode Zoonosis: Echinococcus and Cysticercosis: an Emergent and Global Problem, Poznan, Poland, 10–13 September, 2000*, pp. 237–248.

De La Rocque, S., Augusseau, X., Guillobez, S., Michel, J.F., De Wispeleare, G., Bauer, B. and Cuisance, D. (2001a) The changing distribution of two riverine tsetse flies over 15 years in an increasingly cultivated area of Burkina Faso. *Bulletin of Entomological Research* 91, 157–166.

De La Rocque, S., Michel, J.F., De Wispeleare, G. and Cuisance, D. (2001b) De nouveaux outils pour l'étude des trypanosimoses en zone soudanienne: modélisation de paysages épidémiologiquement dangereaux par télédétection et systèmes d'information géographique. *Parasite* 8, 171–195.

De Wispeleare, G. (1994) Contribution of satellite remote sensing to the mapping of land use and of potential *Glossina* biotopes. Case study of the Adamawa plateaux in Cameroon. In: *A Systematic Approach to Tsetse and Trypanosomiasis Control. Proceedings of the FAO Panels of Experts, Rome, 1–3 December 1993*. FAO, Rome, pp. 74–89.

Deem, S.L., Perry, B.D., Katende, J.M., McDermott, J.J., Mahan, S.M., Maloo, S.H., Morzaria, S.P., Morzaria, A.J., Musoke, A.J. and Rowlands, G.J. (1993) Variations in prevalence rates of tick-borne diseases in zebu cattle by agroecological zone: implications for East Coast fever immunization. *Preventive Veterinary Medicine* 16, 171–187.

Delehanty, J. (1993) Spatial projection of socioeconomic data using geographic information systems: results from a Kenya study in the strategic implementation of a livestock disease control intervention. In: Dvorak, D.A. (ed.) *Social Science Research for Agricultural Technology Development: Spatial and Temporal Dimensions*. CAB International, Wallingford, UK, pp. 37–50.

Doran, M. and van den Bossche, P. (2000) *SITE Analysis. An Approach to Strategy Formulation for Tsetse and Trypanosomiasis Control. Bovine Trypanosomiasis in Southern Africa – Volume 1.* Regional Tsetse and Trypanosomiasis Control Programme for Southern Africa, Harare, Zimbabwe.

Duchateau, L., Kruska, R.L. and Perry, B.D. (1997) Reducing a spatial database to its effective dimensionality for logistic-regression analysis of incidence of livestock disease. *Preventive Veterinary Medicine* 32, 207–218.

Erkelens, A.M., Dwinger, R.H., Bedane, B., Slingenbergh, J.H.W. and Wint, W. (2000) Selection of priority areas for tsetse control in Africa: a decision tool using GIS in Didissa Valley, Ethiopia, as a pilot study. In: Dwinger, R. (ed.) *Animal Trypanosomiasis: Diagnosis and Epidemiology*. Backhuys Publishers, Leiden, The Netherlands, pp. 213–236.

Ford, J. (1963) The distribution of the vectors of African pathogenic trypanosomes. *Bulletin of the World Health Organization* 28, 653–669.

Ford, J. and Katondo, K.M. (1973) *The Distribution of Tsetse Flies (Glossina) in Africa*. Interafrican Bureau of Animal Resource, Nairobi.

Fuentes, M.V., Malone, J.B. and Mas-Coma, S. (2001) Validation of a mapping and prediction model for human fasciolosis transmission in Andean very high altitude endemic areas using remote sensing data. *Acta Tropica* 79, 87–95.

Gitau, G.K., McDermott, J.J., Katende, J.M., O'Callaghan, C.J., Brown, R.N. and Perry, B.D. (2000) Differences in the epidemiology of theileriosis on smallholder dairy farms in contrasting agro-ecological and grazing strata of highland Kenya. *Epidemiology and Infection* 124, 325–335.

Gouteux, J.P. (1990) Current considerations on the distribution of *Glossina* in West and Central Africa. *Acta Tropica* 47, 185–187.

Green, R.M. and Hay, S.I. (2002) The potential of Pathfinder AVHRR data for providing surrogate climatic variables across Africa and Europe for epidemiological applications. *Remote Sensing of Environment* 79, 166–175.

Guerra, M.A., Walker, E.D., Jones, C., Paskewitz, S., Cortinas, M.R., Stancil, A., Beck, L., Bobo, M. and Kitron, U. (2002) Predicting the suitability of Lyme disease: habitat suitability for *Ixodes scapularis* in the north central United States. *Emerging Infectious Diseases* 8, 289–297.

Harvell, C.D., Mitchell, C.E., Ward, J.S., Altizer, S., Dobsob, A., Ostfeld, R.S. and Samuel, M.D. (2002) Climate warming and disease risks for terrestrial and marine biota. *Science* 296, 2158–2162.

Hay, S.I., Packer, M.J. and Rogers, D.J. (1997) The impact of remote sensing on the study and control of invertebrate intermediate hosts and vectors for disease. *International Journal of Remote Sensing* 18, 2899–2930.

Hay, S.I., Randolph, S.E. and Rogers, D.J. (eds) (2000) *Remote Sensing and Geographical Information Systems in Epidemiology*. Academic Press, London.

Hay, S.I., Cox, J., Rogers, D.J., Randolph, S.E., Stern, D.I., Shanks, G.D., Myers, M.F. and Snow, R.W. (2002) Climate change and the resurgence of malaria in the East African highlands. *Nature* 415, 905–909.

Hendrickx, G. and Tamboura, I. (2000) Epidémiologie spatiale de la trypanosomose animale au Burkina Faso: le cas de la boucle du Mouhoun. In: *Colloque International sur les Techniques de l'Information Spatiale et de l'Epidémiologie, Bobo Dioulasso, Burkina Faso, 7 to 9 March, 2000*. (CD-ROM.)

Hendrickx, G., Rogers, D.J., Napala, A. and Slingenbergh J.H.W. (1995) Predicting the distribution of riverine tsetse and the prevalence of bovine trypanosomiasis in Togo using ground-based and satellite data. In: *International Scientific Council for Trypanosomiasis Research and Control (ISCTRC), Twenty-Second Meeting, Kampala, Uganda, 1993*. Organisation of African Unity – Scientific and Technical Research Commission (OUA-STRC), Nairobi, pp. 218–232.

Hendrickx, G., Napala, A., Dao, B., Batawui, D., de Deken, R., Vermeilen, A. and Slingenbergh, J.H.W. (1999a) A systematic approach to area-wide tsetse distribution and abundance maps. *Bulletin of Entomological Research* 89, 231–244.

Hendrickx, G., Napala, A., Dao, B., Batawui, K., Bastiaensen, P., de Deken, R., Vermeilen, A., Vercruysse, J. and Slingenbergh, J.H.W. (1999b) The area-wide epidemiology of bovine trypanosomiasis and its impact on mixed farming in subhumid West Africa; a case study in Togo. *Veterinary Parasitology* 84, 13–31.

Hendrickx, G., Napala, A., Slingenbergh, J.H.W., De Deken, R., Vercruysse, J. and Rogers, D.J. (2000) The spatial pattern of trypanosomiasis prevalence predicted with the aid of satellite imagery. *Parasitology* 120, 121–134.

Hendrickx, G., de La Rocque, S., Reid, R. and Wint, W. (2001a) Spatial trypanosomiasis management: from data-layers to decision making. *Trends in Parasitology* 17, 35–41.

Hendrickx, G., Napala, A., Slingenbergh, J.H.W., De Deken, R. and Rogers, D.J. (2001b) A contribution towards simplifying area-wide tsetse surveys using

medium resolution meteorological satellite data. *Bulletin of Entomological Research* 91, 333–346.
Hendrickx, G., Biesemans, J. and Van Camp, N. (2002) Tsetse presence–absence prediction model for *Glossina austeni* and *Glossina brevipalpis* in KwaZulu Natal. Unpublished technical report for the International Atomic Energy Agency. Avia-GIS, Zoersel, Belgium. http://www.avia-gis.com
Hendrickx, G., de La Rocque, S. and Mattioli, R. (2004) *Systems dynamics and fly distribution patterns: towards longterm tsetse and trypanosomiasis management in West Africa.* Program Against African Trypanosomiasis Technical and Scientific Series (in press).
Heuvelink, G.B.M. (1998) *Error Propagation in Environmental Modelling with GIS.* Taylor and Francis, London.
Hugh-Jones, M. (1989) Applications of remote sensing to the identification of the habitats of parasites and disease vectors. *Parasitology Today* 5, 244–251.
International Livestock Centre for Africa (1979) *Trypanotolerant Livestock in West and Central Africa* (2 volumes). ILCA, Addis Ababa.
Katondo, K.M. (1984) Revision of second edition of tsetse distribution maps: an interim report. *Insect Science and its Applications* 5, 381–388.
Kitron, U., Otieno, L.H., Hungerford, L.L., Odulaja, A., Brigham, W.U., Okello, O.O., Joselyn, M., Mohamed-Ahmed, M.M. and Cook, E. (1996) Spatial analysis of the distribution of tsetse flies in the Lambwe Valley, Kenya, using Landsat TM satellite imagery and GIS. *Journal of Animal Ecology* 65, 371–380.
Korenberg, E.I. (1973) An experiment in detailed large-scale mapping of the distribution of the taiga tick. [In Russian.] *Parazitologiya* 7, 238–243.
Korenberg, E.I. and Lebedeva, N.N. (1976) Regionalisation of the range of the taiga tick (*Ixodes persulcatus*). [In Russian.] *Zoologicheskii Zhurnal* 55, 1468–1475.
Kruska, R.L. and Perry, B.D. (1991) Evaluation of grazing lands of Zimbabwe using the AVHRR normalised difference vegetation index. *Preventive Veterinary Medicine* 11, 361–363.
Kruska, R.L. and Perry, B.D. (1992) Development of spatial databases for analysis of tick-borne diseases of cattle in Zimbabwe. In: Unpublished paper presented at the SADDC Regional Workshop on GIS for Natural Resource Management, Harare, April 1992, pp. 1–11.
Kyriakidis, P.C. and Journel, A.G. (2001) Stochastic modeling of atmospheric pollution: a spatial time series framework. Part I: Methodology. *Atmospheric Environment* 35, 2331–2337.
Lark, R.M. (1994) Sample size and class variability in the choice of a method of discriminant analysis. *International Journal of Remote Sensing* 15, 1551–1555.
Laveissière, C.D., Eouzan, J.P., Grebaut, P. and Lemasson, J.J. (1990) The control of riverine tsetse. *Insect Science and its Applications* 11, 427–441.
Lawrence, J.A. (1991) Retrospective observations on the geographical relationship between *Rhipicephalus appendiculatus* and East Coast fever in southern Africa. *Veterinary Record* 128, 180–183.
Lessard, P., L'Eplattenier, R., Norval, R.A.I., Kundert, K., Dolan, T.T., Croze, H., Walker, J.B., Irvin, A.D. and Perry, B.D. (1990) Geographical information systems for studying the epidemiology of cattle diseases caused by *Theileria parva*. *Veterinary Record* 126, 255–262.
Linthicum, K.J., Anyamba, A., Tucker, C.J., Kelley, P.W., Myers, M.F. and Peters,

C.J. (1999) Climate and satellite indicators to forecast Rift Valley fever epidemics in Kenya. *Science* 285, 397–400.

Malone, J.B. and Zukowski, S.H. (1992) Geographic models and control of cattle liver flukes in southern USA. *Parasitology Today* 8, 266–270.

Malone, J.B., Fehler, D.P., Loyacano, A.F. and Zukowski, S.H. (1992) Use of LANDSAT MSS imagery and soil type in a geographic information system to assess site-specific risk of fascioliasis on Red River Basin farms in Louisiana. *Annals of the New York Academy of Sciences* 653, 389–397.

Malone, J.B., Gommes, R., Hansen, J., Yilma, J.M., Slingenberg, J., Snijders, F., Nachtergaele, F. and Ataman, E. (1998) A geographic information system on the potential distribution and abundance of *Fasciola hepatica* and *F. gigantica* in east Africa based on Food and Agriculture Organization databases. *Veterinary Parasitology* 78, 87–101.

Moloo, S.K. (1985) Distribution of *Glossina* species in Africa. *Acta Tropica* 42, 275–281.

Moncayo, A.C., Edman, J.D. and Finn, J.T. (2000) Application of geographic information technology in determining risk of eastern equine encephalomyelitis virus transmission. *Journal of the American Mosquito Control Association* 16, 28–35.

Nash, T.A.M. (1937) Climate, the vital factor in the ecology of *Glossina*. *Bulletin of Entomological Research* 28, 75–127.

Nash, T.A.M. (1948) *Tsetse Flies in British West Africa.* His Majesty's Stationery Office, London.

Norval, R.A.I. and Perry, B.D. (1990) Introduction, spread and subsequent disappearance of the brown ear-tick, *Rhipicephalus appendiculatus*, from the southern lowveld of Zimbabwe. *Experimental and Applied Acarology* 9, 103–111.

Norval, R.A.I., Perry, B.D., Gebreab, F. and Lessard, P. (1991) East Coast fever: a problem of the future for the horn of Africa? *Preventive Veterinary Medicine* 10, 163–172.

Ollerenshaw, C.B. (1966) The approach to forecasting the incidence of fascioliasis over England and Wales 1958–1962. *Agricultural Meteorology* 3, 35–53.

Ollerenshaw, C.B. and Rowlands, W.T. (1959) A method of forecasting the incidence of fascioliasis in Anglesey. *Veterinary Record* 71, 591–598.

Perry, B.D. and Young, A.S. (1995) The past and future roles of epidemiology and economics in the control of tick-borne diseases of livestock in Africa: the case of theileriosis. *Preventive Veterinary Medicine* 25, 107–120.

Perry, B.D., Lessard, P., Norval, R.A.I., Kundert, K. and Kruska, R. (1990) Climate, vegetation and the distribution of *Rhipecephalus appendiculatus* in Africa. *Parasitology Today* 6, 100–104.

Perry, B.D., Kruska, R., Lessard, P., Norval, R.A.I. and Kundert, K. (1991a) Estimating the distribution and abundance of *Rhipicephalus appendiculatus* in Africa. *Preventive Veterinary Medicine* 11, 261–268.

Perry, B.D., Norval, R.A.I., Kruska, R.L., Ushewokunze-Obatolu, U. and Booth, T.H. (1991b) Predicting the epidemiology of tick-borne diseases of cattle in Zimbabwe using geographic information systems. In: Martin, S.W. (ed.) *Proceedings of the 6th International Symposium on Veterinary Epidemiology and Economics, Ottawa, October 12–16, 1991*, pp. 214–216.

Pfeiffer, D.U., Duchateau, L., Kruska, R.L., Ushewokunze-Obatolu, U. and Perry,

B.D. (1997) A spatially predictive logistic regression model for the occurrence of theileriosis outbreaks in Zimbabwe. In: *Proceedings of the VIII International Symposium on Veterinary Epidemiology and Economics, Paris, 8–11 July, 1997*, pp. 12.12.1–12.12.3.

Randolph, S.E. (1993) Climate, satellite imagery and the seasonal abundance of the tick *Rhipicephalus appendiculatus* in southern Africa: a new perspective. *Medical and Veterinary Entomology* 7, 243–258.

Randolph, S.E. (2000) Ticks and tick-borne disease systems in space and from space. In: Hay, S.I., Randolph, S.E. and Rogers, D.J. (eds) *Remote Sensing and Geographical Information Systems in Epidemiology*. Academic Press, London, pp. 217–243.

Randolph, S.E. and Rogers, D.J. (2000) Fragile transmission cycles of tick-borne encephalitis virus may be disrupted by predicted climate change. *Proceedings of the Royal Society of London, Series B* 267, 1741–1744.

Randolph, S.E., Miklisova, D., Lysy, J., Rogers, D.J. and Labuda, M. (1999) Incidence from coincidence: patterns of tick infestations on rodents facilitate transmission of tick-borne encephalitis virus. *Parasitology* 118, 177–186.

Randolph, S.E., Green, R.M., Peacey, M.F. and Rogers, D.J. (2000) Seasonal synchony: the key to tick-borne encephalitis foci identified by satellite data. *Parasitology* 121, 15–23.

Rawlings, P., Ceesay, M.L., Wacher, T.J. and Snow, W.F. (1993) The distribution of the tsetse flies *Glossina morsitans submorsitans* and *G. palpalis gambiensis* (Diptera: Glossinidae) in The Gambia and the application of survey results to tsetse and trypanosomiasis control. *Bulletin of Entomological Research* 83, 625–632.

Reid, R.S. and Ellis, J.E. (1995) The environmental implications of controlling tsetse-transmitted trypanosomiasis. Final report to the Rockefeller Foundation. ILRI, Nairobi.

Reid, R.S., Kruska, R.L., Deichmann, U., Thornton, P.K. and Leak, S.G.A. (2000) Human population growth and the extinction of the tsetse fly. *Agriculture Ecosystems and Environment* 77, 227–236.

Rizzoli, A., Merier, S., Furanello, C. and Genchi, C. (2002) Geographical information systems and bootstrap aggregation (bagging) of tree-based classifiers for Lyme disease risk prediction in Trentino, Italian Alps. *Journal of Medical Entomology* 39, 485–492.

Robinson, T.P. (1998) Geographic information systems and the selection of priority areas for control of tsetse-transmitted trypanosomiasis in Africa. *Parasitology Today* 14, 457–461.

Robinson, T., Rogers, D. and Williams, B. (1997a) Mapping tsetse habitat suitability in the common fly belt of Southern Africa using multivariate analysis of climate and remotely sensed vegetation data. *Medical and Veterinary Entomology* 11, 235–245.

Robinson, T., Rogers, D. and Williams, B. (1997b) Univariate analysis of tsetse habitat in the common fly belt of southern Africa using climate and remotely sensed vegetation data. *Medical and Veterinary Entomology* 11, 223–234.

Robinson, T.P., Harris, R.S., Hopkins, J.S. and Williams, B.G. (2002) An example of decision support for trypanosomiasis control using a geographical information system in eastern Zambia. *International Journal of Geographical Information Science* 16, 345–360.

Robson, J., Yeoman, G.H. and Ross, J.P.J. (1961) *Rhipicephalus appendiculatus* and East Coast fever in Tanganyika. *East African Medical Journal* 38, 206–214.

Rogers, D.J. and Randolph, S.E. (1993) Distribution of tse-tse and ticks in Africa: past, present and future. *Parasitology Today* 9, 266–271.

Rogers, D.J., Hendrickx, G., Slingenbergh, J.H.W. and Uilenberg, G. (1994) Tsetse flies and their control. *Revue Scientifique et Technique Office International des Epizooties* 13, 1075–1124.

Rogers, D.J., Hay, S.I. and Packer, M.J. (1996) Predicting the distribution of tsetse flies in West Africa using temporal Fourier processed meteorological satellite data. *Annals of Tropical Medicine and Parasitology* 90, 225–241.

Seto, E., Xu, B., Liang, S., Gong, P., Wu, W., Davis, G., Qiu, D.C., Gu, X.G. and Spear, R. (2002) The use of remote sensing for predictive modeling of schistosomiasis in China. *Photogrammetric Engineering and Remote Sensing* 68, 167–174.

Snow, W.F., Rawlings, P. and Norton, G.A. (1995) A framework for the rapid field appraisal of tsetse and trypanosomiasis problems. In: *International Scientific Council for Trypanosomiasis Research and Control (ISCTRC), Twenty-Second Meeting, Kampala, Uganda, 1993.* Organisation of African Unity – Scientific and Technical Research Commission (OUA-STRC), Nairobi, pp. 218–232.

Snow, W.F., Wacher, T.J. and Rawlings, P. (1997) Observations on the prevalence of trypanosomiasis in small ruminants, equines and cattle, in relation to tsetse challenge, in The Gambia. *Veterinary Parasitology* 66, 1–11.

Spear, R.C., Hubbard, A., Liang, S. and Seto, E. (2002) Disease transmission models for public health decision making: towards an approach for designing intervention strategies for *Schistosomiasis japonica*. *Environmental Health Perspectives* 110, 907–915.

Sutherst, R.W. and Maywald, G.F. (1985) A computerised system for matching climates to ecology. *Agriculture, Ecosystems and Environment* 13, 281–299.

Van den Bossche, P. and Vale, G.A. (2000) *Tsetse and Trypanosomiasis in Southern Africa. Bovine Trypanosomiasis in Southern Africa, Volume 2.* Regional Tsetse and Trypanosomiasis Control Program for Southern Africa, Harare.

Watt, G.E.L. (1980) An approach to determining the prevalence of liver fluke in a large region. In: Geering, W.A., Roe, R.T. and Chapman, L.A. (eds) *Proceedings of the 2nd International Symposium on Veterinary Epidemiology and Economics, Canberra, Australia, 7–11 May, 1979,* pp. 152–155.

Wint, W., Rogers, D.J. and Robinson, T. (1997) Ecozones, farming systems and priority areas for tsetse control in East, West and Southern Africa. Unpublished consultant's report to the FAO. http://ergodd.zoo.ox.ac.uk/download

Wint, W., Slingenbergh, J., Hendrickx, G. and Bourn, D. (2001) Livestock geography: new perspectives on global resources. http://ergodd.zoo.ox.ac.uk/livatl2/index.htm

Wittmann, E.J., Mellor, P.S. and Baylis, M. (2001) Using climate data to map the potential distribution of *Culicoides imicola* (Diptera: Ceratopogonidae) in Europe. *Revue Scientifique et Technique Office International des Epizooties* 20, 731–740.

Wright, P.S. and Swire, P.W. (1984) Soil type and the distribution of *Lymnaea truncatula. Veterinary Record* 114, 294–295.

Yang, G.J., Zhou, X.N., Wang, T.P., Lin, D.D., Hu, F., Hong, Q.B. and Sun, L.P. (2002) Establishment and analysis of GIS databases on schistosomiasis in three provinces in the lower reaches of the Yangtze River. *Chinese Journal of Schistosomiasis Control* 14, 21–24.

Yang, H.M., Peng, H., Hu, H.B., Xie, Z.Y., Qiu, L., Huang, J.Z., Sun, L.P., Hong, Q.B. and Zhou, X.N. (2000) Prediction by remote sensing of snail habitats in the marshland along the Yangtze River affected by flood in 1998. *Chinese Journal of Schistosomiasis Control* 12, 337–339.

Yeoman, G.H. (1966a) Field vector studies of epizootic East Coast fever. I. A quantitative relationship between *R. appendiculatus* and the epizooticity of East Coast fever. *Bulletin of Epizootic Diseases of Africa* 14, 5–27.

Yeoman, G.H. (1966b) Field vector studies of epizootic East Coast fever. II. Seasonal studies of *R. appendiculatus* on bovine and non-bovine hosts in East Coast fever enzootic, epizootic and free areas. *Bulletin of Epizootic Diseases of Africa* 14, 113–140.

Yilma, J.M. and Malone, J.B. (1998) A geographic information system forecast model for strategic control of fasciolosis in Ethiopia. *Veterinary Parasitology* 78, 103–127.

Zukowski, S.H., Hill, J.M., Jones, F.W. and Malone, J.B. (1991) Development and validation of a soil-based geographical information system model of habitat of *Fossaria bulimoides*, a snail intermediate host of *Fasciola hepatica*. *Preventive Veterinary Medicine* 11, 221–227.

Zukowski, S.H., Wilkerson, G.W. and Malone, J.B. Jr (1993) Fasciolosis in cattle in Louisiana. II. Development of a system to use soil maps in a geographic information system to estimate disease risk on Louisiana coastal marsh rangeland. *Veterinary Parasitology* 47, 51–65.

7 The Use of GIS in Modelling the Spatial and Temporal Spread of Animal Diseases

Nigel P. French and Piran C.L. White

7.1 Introduction

There have been considerable advances in the mathematical and computational tools available to modellers in recent years, especially within spatial modelling (Keeling, 1999a). However, the pace of theoretical developments has exceeded that of the practical implementations, so that the perceived gap between modelling theory and empirical evidence or application has widened (Tompkins and Wilson, 1998). Since one of the major roles of modelling in animal disease is to inform control policy, this is of considerable concern from a management perspective. The greater use of GIS in modelling provides one means by which this problem can be addressed and the theoretical advances can be brought to bear on the realities of disease management.

This chapter describes basic approaches to modelling the spatial and temporal spread of animal disease and considers the role of GIS in the development and application of simulation models. The review is limited to simulation models in which model parameters are used within a spatial and temporal framework to generate data in the form of predicted patterns of disease. The work does not include 'statistical' models in which data are used solely to provide empirical summaries and parameter estimates; the use of GIS for providing summaries of information relevant to disease management has been reviewed recently by Pfeiffer and Hugh-Jones (2002). Following the summary of different modelling approaches, three case studies (rabies and tuberculosis in wildlife, myiasis in livestock and foot-and-mouth disease (FMD) in livestock) are considered in more detail to illustrate the application of different forms of modelling and the use of GIS. The final example of FMD enables four contrasting approaches to modelling to be compared directly.

7.2 The use of spatial simulation models

Epidemiological models have contributed greatly to increases in our understanding and management of infectious diseases in animal populations (Barlow, 1995, 1996). The most common approach has been to use deterministic, non-spatial models. These models operate in continuous time and are deterministic in the sense that their predictions are determined by the initial values of parameters included in the model. Thus, for each unique combination of parameter values there is just one solution. These models can be useful in providing estimates of disease spread over a wide area, or the reduction in host population density required to eliminate an infection. They have been useful in informing policy for a number of wildlife species (Anderson *et al.*, 1981; Anderson and Trewhella, 1985; Barlow, 1991a,b). However, they have no explicit definition of space, and assume that the distribution of hosts, the pattern of contact between them and the landscape in which they live are all homogeneous. As a result, they are not well suited to situations where there are marked heterogeneities in the disease–host system, such as restricted interactions between individuals or states, and finite populations.

Heterogeneities can cause or be caused by the distribution or behaviour of individual hosts. For diseases of livestock, heterogeneities will arise at a broad scale as a result of transfer of animals between farms, at a medium scale as a result of fragmentation of farm units, occurring for either administrative or landscape reasons, and at a fine scale as a result of patterns of grazing behaviour. For diseases of wildlife, heterogeneities may arise at a broad scale as a result of patterns of suitable habitat and dispersal behaviour, at medium scales as a result of territoriality of the hosts, and at finer spatial scales as a result of patterns of foraging within home ranges. For disease–host systems where there are marked heterogeneities or where control strategies are required for specific locations, spatial simulation models have been increasingly applied. Within these models, the host population and the landscape it occupies are spatially compartmentalized, thereby enhancing the realism of the model structure and the applicability of the results to policy.

Simulation models have been used to describe the spatial and temporal spread of a number of animal disease-related outcomes. These include:

- *Parasite abundance.* The use of models in this way has been most frequent for vectors of disease such as ticks and tsetse flies and other ectoparasites, such as myiasis flies.

- *Patterns of disease (endemic and epidemic).* Both endemic and epidemic diseases in a range of host species, including farm animals (e.g. FMD, myiasis) and wildlife (e.g. parapox, morbillivirus), have been modelled, as have zoonotic diseases (e.g. bovine tuberculosis, rabies).
- *The impact of control measures.* Interventions and their impact on disease frequency (incidence and prevalence) have been modelled using scenario analysis.
- *The economic impact of disease.* Models have been used to assess the cost of disease incursions and provide data for cost–benefit analyses of interventions.

7.3 The importance of the spatial dimension and the contribution of GIS

Models incorporating both spatial and temporal dimensions can be used to explore the dynamics of disease spread with reference to the role of spatial heterogeneity in parasite abundance, host populations and contact structures. They can also consider spatial separation as a determinant of disease transmission. However, relatively few animal disease models reported in the literature have considered the spatial dimension and even fewer have used GIS at any stage of the modelling process.

There are several ways in which GIS can be used in disease modelling. A GIS can serve as a database for the storage and retrieval of spatially referenced information, which may be used by a model. It can be used as a means of enhancing the displays of model input or output. It can also potentially be an integral component of the model, deriving information from other sources, feeding it into the model, and storing the output. Where GIS technology has played a role in model development to date, it has been used mainly to provide input variables and display model output, although there are some examples of the use of GIS to provide a more interactive means of assessing the impact of control measures.

There are a number of examples of simulation studies that have used existing GIS-linked databases to provide raw and summarized data. For example, raw data may be provided on the distribution of animal hosts and the location of farms, or summarized data such as the number of animals per unit area. Satellite imagery, combined with predictive modelling, has also been used to provide predicted distributions of wildlife hosts. Other kinds of information of potential value as spatially dependent input variables include climate and vegetation data. For example, variation in temperature is likely to be important when considering local variation in populations whose dynamics are driven by temperature. The pattern of local or regional control strategies may also be an important consideration and, particularly for zoonotic diseases, the distribution of human hosts.

GIS may be very useful, although not essential, for displaying the output from simulation studies. In many situations the information generated by the model can be represented as a simple map, with a polygon indicating land margins; hence there is no advantage in linking the model to a GIS. However, a GIS is of greater value if further detailed interrogation of the output is required, particularly if the output is to be compared with other spatially related variables. Current software may also be used to display time series data as repeated fixed images for interrogation and analysis, or converted into moving images for animated displays.

7.4 Spatial disease modelling

7.4.1 Classification of spatial models with reference to the role of GIS

If we consider the classical spectrum between strategic and tactical models (May, 1974), there is arguably a greater role for GIS in the more specific, tactical models, in which the emphasis is on detail rather than generality. Spatial disease models can be classified by the degree of abstraction of spatial processes into spatially abstract, spatially explicit and spatially specific models.

Spatially abstract models are those with summarized, abstract representations of space in which spatial arrangement is considered but where absolute distances, or locations, are not required. Examples include lattice models, such as the *Mycobacterium bovis* models of White *et al.* (1997), White and Harris (1995a,b) and Smith *et al.* (1997, 2001a,b), and models using contact networks, such as the FMD studies of Ferguson *et al.* (2001a,b). In these models GIS may have a role in providing data to parameterize models and inform the likely distributions of stochastic processes, but would not be used to display model output.

In spatially explicit models, spatial processes are represented by locations in which the coordinates of, for example, farms represent realistic patterns and separations, but they do not necessarily refer to specific locations. The INTERIBR model described by Noordegraaf *et al.* (1998) is an example of this type of model.

Spatially specific models could be considered as a subgroup of spatially explicit models, where the input variables and simulated model output refer to specific geographical locations. Models in this category are more likely to use GIS to display and interrogate the highly detailed model output. Examples include the FMD models of Keeling *et al.* (2001) and Morris *et al.* (2001), the screwworm fly incursion models (Anaman *et al.*, 1994b; Atzeni *et al.*, 1994, 1997) and the parapox model of Rushton *et al.* (2000). These authors used a GIS (GRASS) to provide data input in the form of habitat information (blocks of aggregated pixels) and display model output. The GIS was linked to a population dynamic model via a Unix shell and the population model was coupled with a parapox disease model.

7.4.2 Approaches to modelling spatial processes

Within these different simulation modelling frameworks, there are also different ways of representing spatial processes. These processes may occur within discrete space lattices, continuous space or multipatch landscapes, or be represented by a contact network. Although many of these structures do not involve the use of GIS, they do illustrate the range of approaches and suggest how GIS could be used to greater advantage in the future.

In discrete space models the spatial arrangement of individuals, groups or surfaces may be represented by a two-dimensional regular array of discrete cells or an irregular arrangement of point locations. Models using regular arrays are often referred to as lattice models, grid cell models or cellular automata. Key processes, such as local disease transmission, can be simulated by considering the state of each cell and its neighbouring cells. *Coupled map lattices* (CML) are models in which the behaviour of the system is expressed by a large number of locally coupled equations describing dynamic change in cells occupied by continuous populations. In contrast, when the behaviour is specified by a set of probabilistic rules that determine the transition of cells from one discrete state to another, the models are termed *probabilistic cellular automata* (for a more detailed description see Keeling, 1999a).

Microparasites are defined as parasites with direct reproduction within the host, usually at a high rate, and include most viral, bacterial and protozoal parasites (Anderson and May, 1991). Models for microparasite infections are often based on the family of SEIR (susceptible, exposed, infected and recovered) models and capture local transmission between neighbouring cells. Each cell within the lattice may represent an individual, or group of individuals, in one of the four states (S, E, I or R). The rate at which the individual changes state (e.g. moves from a susceptible to an exposed animal) is determined by rate parameters and the status of surrounding cells.

Because they incorporate local processes, these models are not subject to the constraint of random mixing often assumed in purely temporal models of disease dynamics. They can be extended to model longer-range transmission, and although most models are based on regular arrays of squares, other shapes and contact structures, in particular hexagons, have also been considered. Most of the discrete space microparasite models reported in the literature appear not to have involved the use of a GIS at any stage of the process and the lattice is usually an abstract representation (i.e. a spatially abstract model).

Macroparasites have no direct reproduction within the host and include most helminths and arthropods (Anderson and May, 1991). Examples of discrete space macroparasite models include studies of the dispersal and damage caused by directly pathogenic parasites, such as the myiasis flies, and ectoparasite vectors such as ticks and biting flies. One example of the application of a lattice-based model (CML) was the use of a weighted grid cell approach to describe the likely scenarios following incursion of screwworm flies into Australia and warble flies into the UK. These models rely on GIS to provide summarized input variables and to display model output and are described in detail later in the chapter.

In contrast to the discrete space models, continuous space models treat space, time and populations as continuous entities. They may be referred to as diffusion or dispersion models whereby changes in populations in space and time are represented by systems of partial differential equations. In essence they describe the rate of change of infected individuals in a continuous host 'carpet'. These systems may be explored analytically or through the use of simulation studies, which are frequently deterministic. An attractive feature of this family of models is their mathematical tractability. Although this has resulted in important theoretical results, their relevance and application to ecological and epidemiological problems is limited. The early reaction–diffusion equations are reviewed by Holmes *et al.* (1994) and later developments include the reproduction and dispersal kernel method (Diekmann, 1978; Vandenbosch *et al.*, 1990); for a review of these methods see Mollison and Levin (1995). Continuous space–time models have been used to estimate the speed of epidemic 'wave-fronts' and the proportion of hosts infected in the wake of an epidemic. They have also been used to describe the importance of host density, movement and random 'long-range' events. However, to date there are few examples of continuous space models using GIS at any stage of model development.

Metapopulation and multipatch models represent spatial variation in host density and contact without considering precise geographical locations or distances. Various configurations are used to describe the pattern of connectedness of populations, often in patches connected by dispersal (coupling). Examples of different structures include island, necklace, loop and spider configurations. There are few examples of veterinary diseases and little reference to the use of GIS to inform these models. To date they have been used mainly to describe human epidemiological processes (e.g. Grenfell *et al.*, 1995) and address ecological problems (Keeling, 1999a). As an example, the role of infectious disease in metapopulation extinction has been considered by combining mathematical epidemiological models with metapopulation models (Hess, 1996). These studies, set in the context of wildlife conservation, highlight the importance of disease in determining metapopulation dynamics and demonstrate the varying behaviour of infectious disease in different spatial configurations. A metapopulation modelling framework was also used by Fulford *et al.* (2002) to investigate the dynamics and control of bovine tuberculosis in possums.

Some of the more recent developments in spatial disease modelling include models that capture the essential spatial characteristics of the system, without explicitly modelling space. In their abstract treatment of space they are similar to lattice models, but rather than modelling potentially thousands of 'sites', the dynamics of pairs of individuals (or farms) are captured by a relatively small number of equations (Keeling, 1999a). For example, these may represent the number or proportion of susceptible–susceptible, infected–infected or susceptible–infected pairs. The dynamics of each pair depends upon knowledge of the status of triples, quadruples and other higher-order 'moments'. This could potentially lead to a large number of intractable equations, but in many situations it is feasible to 'close' the system by using an approximation that fixes the highest moment under consideration. For epidemics of medium density, it is considered sufficient to consider the behaviour of singles, pairs and triples in order to represent transmission within the system, but this may be inappropriate for higher local densities (Keeling, 1999a; Kao, 2002). When applied to a fixed network, such models have considerable potential for modelling communicable diseases and have recently been used to represent spatial heterogeneity in animal disease transmission. One of the epidemic models used in the UK FMD outbreak in 2001 represented local transmission by modelling the spread between farms on a local network of interconnected nodes (Ferguson *et al.*, 2001b). This approach is described and compared with other modelling approaches at the end of this chapter.

A greater understanding of the contact structure of populations of animals will help to refine our understanding of the role of local and global transmission in driving the dynamics of infectious disease. Graph theory and social network theory, previously used to model sexually transmitted disease in humans (Gupta *et al.*, 1989; Ghani *et al.*, 1997), have also been applied to animal populations with the aim of developing a truer picture of their contact structure (Webb and Sauter-Louis, 2002). In this study, risk-potential networks were developed describing the potential spread of infection in a population of sheep. Contact at shows, local contact, and a combination of these two, were compared using path-length analysis (an indication of how closely two farms are connected) and an estimate of the number of disconnected graphs (an indication of the likely scale of an epidemic following a random introduction of an infected animal). These methods require a comprehensive understanding of the direct and indirect contacts between farms. Although this information could be stored, interrogated and displayed using a GIS, such a system is not essential for this type of analysis.

7.5 The use of spatial approaches and GIS in understanding microparasite infections in wildlife: rabies and bovine tuberculosis

7.5.1 Discrete and continuous space models for rabies in foxes

Rabies is the most frequently modelled wildlife disease and accounted for 15 of the 35 wildlife disease models discussed by Barlow (1995). The fox rabies models developed by Mollison and Kuulasmaa (1985) were based on a two-dimensional array of square territories which could be in one of four states: unoccupied (*E*) or occupied by an individual which was susceptible (*X*), incubating the disease (*I*) or infectious (*Y*). This is an example of a probabilistic cellular automaton. An epidemic was simulated stochastically from the instantaneous transition rates:

Event	Change	Transition rate
Infection	$XY \rightarrow IY$	$\beta/4$
Becoming infective	$I \rightarrow Y$	σ
Death	$Y \rightarrow E$	α
Recolonization	$EX \rightarrow XX$	$r/4$

where β is the overall rate at which an infectious individual makes contacts (and transmits infection), σ is the rate at which infected individuals become infective and α is the rate at which infective individuals die. It follows that $1/\sigma$ is the average incubation period and $1/\alpha$ is the average time between becoming infective and dying, and both of these event times are exponentially distributed. The recolonization term represents population regrowth, net of natural mortality.

The models were used to determine threshold criteria for disease invasion and persistence and to test whether control strategies could produce fade-out of disease. Importantly, the threshold criteria for these models, determined by the basic reproduction number (R_0, defined as the number of secondary cases arising from a single infected individual in a totally susceptible population) are different from non-spatial deterministic models. Generally, the threshold for invasion is not $R_0 > 1$, but some value greater than 1. The models have also been used to calculate velocities of disease spread, which are dependent on the contact distribution, and the role of new susceptibles and infectivity in maintaining an endemic state. The model of Mollison and Kuulasmaa (1985) also showed for the first time how clusters of infection arose, even in a homogeneous environment, and that they moved in time and space. These 'wandering patches' of infection were also later obtained from the model of Tischendorf *et al.* (1998), and show how rabies can persist in a landscape despite very low rates of overall prevalence. The models of Jeltsch *et al.* (1997) and Tischendorf *et al.* (1998) have shown that the spatial processes of long-range dispersal and short-range intergroup contact are critical for replicating the wave-like pattern of rabies epizootics.

Extensions to the fox rabies lattice model include the following: incorporating group size (Ball, 1985); a variable incubation period, culling and vaccination (Voigt *et al.*, 1985); heterogeneity in the urban fox population (Trewhella and Harris, 1988; Smith and Harris, 1991); and incorporating field-derived contact rate data (White *et al.*, 1995). The models of Smith and Harris and White *et al.* were location-specific; they simulated the spread in four UK cities. A similar approach was adopted in Germany (Thulke *et al.*, 1999, 2000), where the problem of scaling and postvaccination resurgence was addressed. Deal *et al.* (2000) used a GIS to combine parameters relating to fox biology with geographical characteristics of the landscape to create a spatially specific model for fox rabies in Illinois, USA. This study suggested that disease entering the fox population from a pet source would spread from east to west across the state in waves and become endemic within about 15 years. Smith *et al.* (2002) have used a similar approach to investigate spatial variation in rabies transmission rates in relation to human and landscape features in Connecticut, USA.

The behaviour of fox rabies has also been studied using continuous space diffusion models (Murray *et al.*, 1986; Murray and Seward, 1992). The speed of propagation of the rabies epidemic, the periodicity of epidemics and the distance between epidemics were estimated using a system of differential equations incorporating a diffusion coefficient. Furthermore, using a map of estimated fox densities in England and Wales, the model was used to make quantitative predictions of the spread of rabies from an incursion point on the south coast of England (Murray *et al.*, 1986) (Fig. 7.1). The impact of vaccination 'breaks' was explored using this approach and later models incorporated natural immunity (Murray and Seward, 1992).

The European applications of spatial models and GIS to rabies in foxes have been useful in contributing to the understanding of observed patterns of spread of the disease in specific landscapes, and also the importance of the behaviour of the host in driving some of these patterns. In Britain, the absence of rabies means that the predictions of the models cannot be validated. Nevertheless, the spatial realism of the more recent models means that they can be applied rapidly to specific locations, and they have been used as the basis for rabies contingency planning in Britain (Harris *et al.*, 1992).

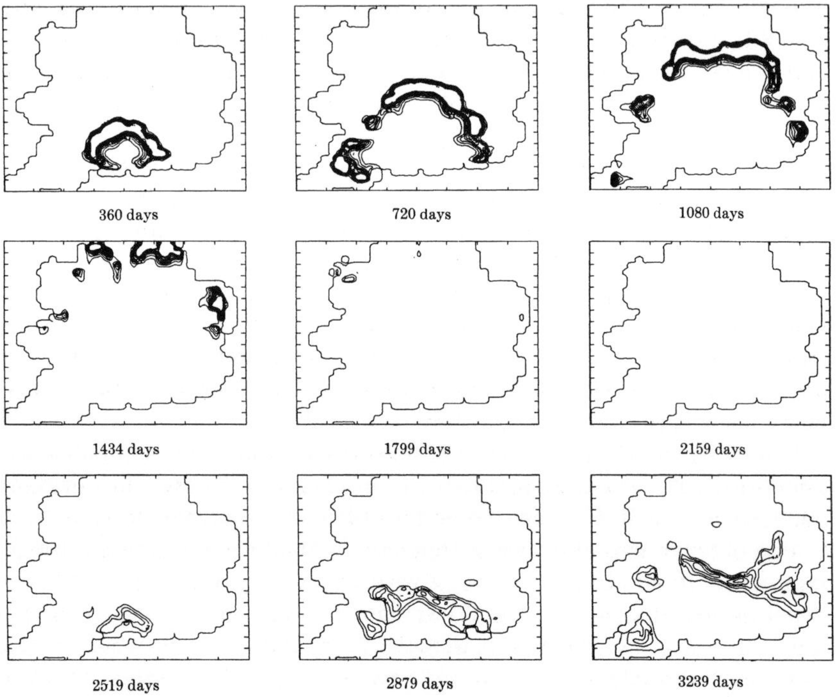

Fig. 7.1. Predicted output of a simulated epidemic front of rabies in foxes as it moves through the southern part of England, following an initial introduction at Southampton (top left). Reproduced with permission from Murray *et al.* (1986), Fig. 12, page 136, with permission of the Royal Society.

7.5.2 Lattice models for bovine tuberculosis in badgers

Bovine tuberculosis (TB) in badgers has been modelled in a variety of ways (Smith, 2001), including discrete space approaches within coupled map lattices (White and Harris, 1995b; Smith *et al.*, 1997). In these models, both inter- and intra-group infection processes are simulated on a regular grid of cells representing territories. The models have been used to assess the impact of control strategies such as culling, vaccination and fertility control (White and Harris, 1995a; White *et al.*, 1997; Smith *et al.*, 2001b).

The original Fortran model of White and Harris (1995b) has since been rewritten in C++ and modified using GIS to a spatially specific form to represent real landscapes (unpublished work, M.T. Bulling, P.C.L. White, L. Garland and S. Harris). This has been done in two ways. First, data from ground surveys have been used within a GIS (ArcInfo) to configure badger and habitat grids representing two 10 × 10 km study areas, one in Gloucestershire and one in Wiltshire, UK. Both study areas were divided into contiguous 500 × 500 m square cells to reflect an average badger territory size at moderate to high densities (Doncaster and Woodroffe, 1993) and to enable a match of the badger and habitat data with the structure of the badger TB model. Badger densities for each cell were then derived from the number of active holes per main sett, after G. Wilson ((1998) Patterns of population change in the Eurasian badger *Meles meles* in Britain 1988–1997. Unpublished PhD thesis, University of Bristol). Secondly, the GIS was used to process Landsat satellite data, which comprise seven bands of reflectance measurements at a spatial resolution of 30 × 30 m. The GIS was trained to recognize the reflectance patterns associated with different habitat types, using a multiple linear regression model. These habitat types were allocated to the 500 × 500 m cells in the model and badger numbers were obtained from badger–habitat relationships derived from the ground survey data.

The new models have shown patterns of space–time clustering of infection that are very similar to those observed in reality. The approach has also demonstrated the importance of heterogeneity in host distribution in determining patterns of space–time clustering of disease. Colour Plate 16 contrasts the pattern of disease clustering arising from a homogeneous host distribution with that from a heterogeneous one, based on one of the study sites. It is clear that the spatially specific heterogeneous distribution results in much greater space–time consistency of patches of infection than the homogeneous model. These models also now incorporate an economic component, which has demonstrated the fundamental importance of spatial patterns of host distribution and disease status in determining the most cost-effective disease control strategy for a specific location (unpublished work, M.T. Bulling, P.C.L. White, L. Garland and S. Harris). The use of GIS in these models to enable them to generate realistic badger population distributions and densities, and hence disease dynamics, in 'real' landscapes makes them potentially a very powerful tool for policy makers in relation to bovine tuberculosis control.

7.6 The use of GIS for providing input and displaying output: myiasis in livestock

Although GIS can be used to provide input variables and to display model output, to date it has rarely been used in veterinary applications to gather and summarize data and seamlessly provide simulations and output for interrogation by the end user. The myiasis examples provided here used a GIS to provide summarized input variables (host density) for a space–time simulation model. In both examples, space was represented by an overlay of interacting grid cells that described fly population growth, dispersal, and the impact of infestation on livestock hosts.

They are essentially large CMLs with edges representing sea-boundaries, and the outputs from these 'whole country' lattice models were displayed using a GIS.

7.6.1 Bioeconomic analysis of a screwworm invasion of Australia

Myiasis is infestation of animals with the maggot larvae of dipteran flies and is a major cause of morbidity and mortality, particularly in ruminants, worldwide. Concern about the invasion of Australia by the screwworm fly, particularly the Old World screwworm *Chrysomya bezziana*, was the stimulus for the development of a space–time simulation model that predicted the likely pattern of fly dispersal and assisted in the formulation of cost-effective control strategies (Mayer *et al.*, 1994). The model considered a number of issues, including the probability of invasion and likely spread of the fly population (following incursion in different places and at different times of the year) and the likely effectiveness of control and eradication strategies. In outline, the model combined data generated from a GIS with a number of Fortran programs that simulated biological and economic aspects of a screwworm invasion. There were three distinct components: population growth, dispersal and economic impact.

The models were populated and parameterized by data from a number of sources, relying heavily on the use of GIS. For example, interpolated long-term monthly climatic averages, adjusted for altitude, were generated using the ESOCLIM package. These were combined with weekly temperature, moisture and growth indices for screwworm flies generated from the CLIMEX package (Sutherst and Maywald, 1985; Mayer *et al.*, 1992, 1994; Sutherst *et al.*, 1989) and vegetation indices generated from NOAA (National Oceanic and Atmospheric Administration, USA) satellite images to drive the whole-population model described below. Other data stored in the GIS included the livestock population (cattle and sheep), the densities of feral and wildlife populations and the estimated wounding rate. The number of fresh, open wounds available for a fly strike was estimated from surveys and knowledge of current management practices, such as surgical husbandry procedures (e.g. mulesing, castration and tail-docking), birth and natural wounding. The GIS package SPANS was used both to store and manipulate input data, such as vegetation and livestock data, and to interpret and interrogate the model output (Butler *et al.*, 1991).

There are a number of approaches to modelling the dynamics of invertebrate populations, ranging from the detailed, mechanistic models (e.g. day-degree and development fraction models) to simple indices of population growth and decline. For screwworm flies, a whole-population model was shown to be a practical and adequate substitute for a detailed cohort life cycle model and was used in all subsequent analyses (Atzeni *et al.*, 1994). The basic model combined information on soil moisture and temperature to produce a weekly growth index. This was simply the product of the soil and temperature indices, each ranging from 0 to 1. Further modifications allowed for local microclimate effects, such as soil moisture around watercourses, by including details derived from vegetation indices. The output was an estimate of the proportionate weekly change in the female population in each grid cell. By using this simple growth index approach, calculated by CLIMEX, computation time was considerably reduced.

Population growth in each grid cell was followed by dispersal – both local natural dispersal of adult flies and long-range outbreaks arising from stock movements. Initially, two approaches to modelling natural fly dispersal were compared: stochastic Monte Carlo simulations and deterministic realizations from an appropriate dispersal probability distribution (Mayer *et al.*, 1993). The two-parameter form of the Cauchy distribution was shown to describe well the patterns of dispersal observed in recapture studies (Mayer and Atzeni, 1993; Mayer *et al.*, 1995) and was used for both the deterministic and stochastic simulations. The deterministic model used a 5 × 5 grid of square cells, each 20 × 20 km. The proportion dispersing into each grid cell was derived by simulating the release of a large number of flies, each with a randomly generated distance (from a Cauchy distribution), and direction (based on a uniform distribution from 0 to 360) from a central cell. The number of flies dispersing into each cell at each time step was calculated from this 5 × 5 matrix of proportions. Further directional movement was provided by weighting the dispersal according to the vegetation index and host density. This also ensured that there was no movement into unfavourable cells, such as desert, lakes and the sea. Although there was some concern about the ability of the deterministic model to predict extreme 'far movers', this was much easier to implement in large-scale simulations.

The information on fly population growth and dispersal was used to calculate the number of infested or 'struck' hosts in each grid cell. The number of fly strikes depended on the number of flies, the rate of ovarian development (related to ambient temperature) and the number of available wounds in the host population. If insufficient wounds were available, this limited the population growth of the fly population, providing a dynamic interaction between the host and fly population. Chemical treatments were also considered by the inclusion of a 'prophylactic protection factor', derived from the rate at which animals would be gathered for treatment, the effectiveness and residual protection afforded by the treatment. Death rates were calculated for each class of livestock under different treatment regimes. The weekly strike rates and mortalities for each class of livestock constituted the input into the economic model, which included losses due to infertility, delayed sales and wool downgrading.

Screwworm outbreaks could be simulated from any port of entry in Australia. Colour Plate 17 shows the estimated dispersal patterns of screwworm flies under a number of different scenarios. The extent and distribution of female screwworm 2 years after incursions on 1 January in Sydney, Cairns, Darwin and Fremantle are shown for an average year (Colour Plate 17a) and a wet year (Colour Plate 17b). The estimated range in an endemic situation (unhindered growth for 10 years) is shown for summer (Colour Plate 17c) and winter (Colour Plate 17d). Although there was limited spread after 2 years around the Sydney and Fremantle invasions compared with the more northerly incursions, the endemic pattern revealed contiguity of spread and a large population north of Sydney in the summer months. The outputs were used to inform detailed economic analyses of the impact of an invasion (Anaman, 1994; Anaman *et al.*, 1994a,b) and the feasibility and cost-effectiveness of eradication through a programme of sterile male release.

7.6.2 Hypodermosis in space and time: the return of warbles to the UK

A similar approach was used to assess the impact of the return of the warble fly to the UK. A weighted grid cell approach, based on dispersal described by the Cauchy distribution, combined with population growth models was used to model the dispersal of gravid flies (French, 1997, 2000). However, there were a number of differences between the two models. First, there were few experimental data on warble fly dispersal distances and therefore a greater reliance on expert opinion. The grid cell sizes were much smaller (1.5 × 1.5 km), to reflect the much shorter estimated median dispersal distances, and the only source of landscape heterogeneity was variability in the host population. Secondly, the more simple population dynamics of warble flies compared with screwworm flies (single host and one generation per year) meant that a density-dependent life cycle model could be used to model population growth. Thirdly, the prevalence of infection and distribution of lesions was estimated using a macroparasite model (Anderson and May, 1991) based on a negative binomial distribution with a variable aggregation parameter (Burillon and Messean, 1982). The economic impact of infestation with warbles largely depends on the extent of hide damage, and this in turn depends on the distribution of warbles among the cattle population. Using these approaches, the distribution of warbles amongst the cattle population could be estimated and used to inform the economic analyses. The underlying cattle population was derived from census data held on a GIS.

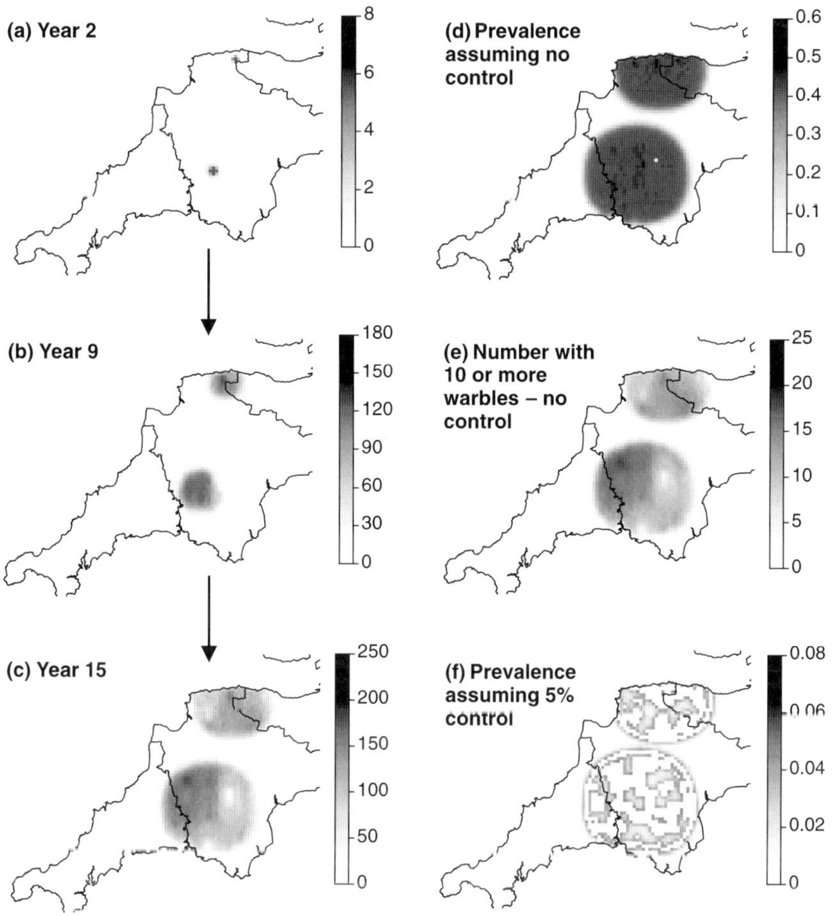

Fig. 7.2. The estimated dispersal of *Hypoderma* spp. following a single incursion and a secondary 'spark' in the south-west of England after (a) 2, (b) 9 and (c) 15 years. The key indicates the number of adult female flies per km^2. The right-hand column shows (d) the estimated prevalence assuming no control, (e) the number of animals with more than 10 warbles after 15 years assuming no control, and (f) the prevalence after 15 years assuming control was implemented if 5% of animals had lesions.

The model generated the number of female flies and cattle lesions ('warble' holes produced by emerging larvae) in each grid cell following incursions into a high-density cattle area (Fig. 7.2). The output was displayed as raster images using macro language files (.iml) in IDRISI. A number of control options were considered, including keeping the existing policy of statutory control, no statutory control assuming no voluntary treatment, no statutory control assuming voluntary treatment, and statutory control with compulsory treatment if the prevalence of infected cattle exceeded 5%.

The myiasis models were developed with the aim of providing decision support to policy makers on the likely impact and control options following the incursion of exotic pests. Their detailed, spatially specific outputs seem readily interpretable by users with a limited understanding of modelling. However, unless they are accompanied by a comprehensive catalogue of assumptions and an understanding of the effects of uncertainty and variability (in both the choice of model and model parameters), they can be highly misleading and give a false impression of the reliability and precision of the model predictions. By their nature, exotic incursion models are difficult to validate; unless a well-monitored invasion has occurred, no data are available for comparison with model output. However, even in the absence of external validation and the presence of uncertainty in model predictions, they give a more informed impression of likely scenarios and indicate areas where data are lacking.

7.7 Modelling the UK FMD epidemic of 2001: contrasting approaches to the same problem

The examples above have highlighted the contributions that spatial approaches and GIS can make to disease models. However, it is frequently difficult to assess the real value of these contributions because different models often have different underlying objectives. They may also be developed at different times and hence have access to differing levels of information for testing and validation. The 2001 FMD epidemic in the UK provided a rare example of a situation in which it was possible to make comparisons between different modelling approaches to the same problem, and therefore to question the usefulness of more complex spatial approaches compared with more simplistic, spatially abstract ones. Spatial simulation models of local transmission were constructed following the 1967/68 UK epidemic (Hugh-Jones, 1976). However, a remarkable feature of the 2001 UK epidemic was the speed with which mathematical models were constructed, parameterized and published, providing information for policy makers in real time as the epidemic was progressing.

7.7.1 A spatially abstract model based on mass action with contact networks

Three months after the onset of the FMD epidemic Ferguson *et al.* (2001a) published a model of the predicted spread of FMD in the UK under different scenarios. The model was deterministic and the output was the scale of the epidemic over time but not the likely spatial pattern. The results were used to inform policy decisions concerning national control measures, in particular the speed and extent of culling and the feasibility of ring vaccination. The model was based on a mathematical mass-action epidemic model, incorporating multiple infectious states, combined with a spatial correlation structure. Initial long-range transmission was modelled using traditional mass action terms, under the assumption of random homogeneous mixing. In contrast, local transmission was captured by a fixed network in which contact and transmission between pairs of farms was represented by a dynamic system of coupled equations. The dynamics of pairs of farms depended upon the status of triples in the network, and the system was closed at the level of triples by an approximation that incorporated a measure of connectedness (the proportion of triples in the network that were triangles) (Keeling, 1999b).

The model was fitted to, and accurately described, data from the early part of the epidemic and provided information about the likely behaviour following a range control strategies. This was achieved with relatively few parameters and a model that was neither location-specific nor linked to a GIS. However, farm locations were used to calculate distance between infectious contacts, effective neighbourhood size and the proportion of long-range contacts, and this information was extracted from GIS-linked databases. Whilst the model predicted the early part of the epidemic well, it was less good at predicting the longer-term temporal pattern, and suggested that the epidemic would be over more quickly than was the case in reality. Because of its spatially abstract nature, the model was not used to predict patterns of disease spread or to identify areas at risk.

7.7.2 A spatially specific approach based on a per-farm hazard model

Eight months into the epidemic, a more detailed analysis of the determinants of the evolution of the epidemic in space and time was conducted using disease, culling and census data (Ferguson *et al.*, 2001a). Risk maps of Great Britain at a 5-km scale were generated from a per-farm hazard model incorporating information on the relative infectiousness of different farm types (based on their type, species mix and size), their susceptibility (incorporating farm type, fragmentation and location of other farms) and time-varying transmission rates.

The model accurately described the temporal pattern of disease at the national scale, including the long tail of cases. It also accurately described the temporal pattern of disease at a local scale for Cumbria and Devon, showing the much higher number of cases in Cumbria. The risk maps indicated the areas most susceptible to the disease, specifically Cumbria, Dumfries and Galloway, the Derbyshire Dales, mid-Wales, South Wales and Devon. However, a map of predicted cases was not produced, and in the event the infection did not significantly affect the Derbyshire Dales, mid-Wales or South Wales. There was also a cluster of infection in south Essex, which the model failed to predict as a high-risk area. The model highlighted the importance of both livestock density and the fragmentation of land parcels on a farm in increasing its susceptibility to FMD and determining the observed spatial patterns. The model was used to examine different control strategies, and demonstrated the importance of rapid culling of both infected and contiguous premises in ensuring the quick and effective control of disease.

7.7.3 A spatially specific, stochastic, individual-based farm model incorporating a transmission kernel

Although the contact network studies that inspired the model of Ferguson *et al.* (2001a) were developed by Keeling (1999b), this author chose an alternative, stochastic approach to modelling the 2001 FMD epidemic (Keeling *et al.*, 2001). Instead of considering a network of farms, the model operated at the individual farm level, and the probability of specific farms becoming infected on a given day was determined by the species composition and associated susceptibility and transmissibility of both the host farm and all infected farms. The likelihood of transmission between farms was determined by their spatial separation and a distance kernel. The kernel was estimated from contract tracing performed during the epidemic and described the relationship between spatial separation and the likelihood of transmission (by any route). The shape of the kernel was assumed to be independent of absolute location and time and isotropic (i.e. it was the same in all directions). Each day the probability of infection was calculated for every farm, and this was used to determine, by Monte Carlo simulation, whether the event happened. The probability that a susceptible farm was infected on any given day was:

$$P_i = 1 - \exp\left[- SN_i \sum_{j \in Infectious(t)} TN_j \, K(d_{ij}) \right]$$

where N_i is the vector of the number of livestock (cattle and sheep) on farm i, S and T are the vectors of susceptibility (representing the risk of catching the disease) and transmissibility (the rate of spreading the disease) for cattle and sheep, and $K(d_{ij})$ is the transmission kernel estimate for the spatial separation d between farms i and j.

The model provided accurate descriptions of the temporal nature of the epidemic, including the long tail of cases, which Keeling *et al.* (2001) believed could only be explored in detail using their individual-based stochastic approach. Colour Plate 18 shows an R_0 map summarizing the estimated number of secondary infections arising from all UK farms. The model was also used to produce a map of predicted cases, and therefore represented an advance on the models of Ferguson *et al.* (2001a,b) in terms of its potential practical application. It accurately predicted the hotspots of infection in Cumbria, Dumfries and Galloway, mid-Wales and Devon and also the small cluster in Essex. As with the model of Ferguson *et al.* (2001a), this model also showed the importance of rapid culls on both infected and contiguous premises. However, because of the more detailed structure, incorporating different species of livestock explicitly, it was also able to demonstrate that intensive culling of both cattle and sheep would have led to more rapid disease control than the more extensive sheep-only culls actually implemented in some regions.

The model showed that ignoring any heterogeneity attributable to the species composition had little effect on the accuracy of temporal predictions but was important for predicting spatial patterns. Only a model that considered both the numbers and variable transmissibility and susceptibility of species on farms captured both the spatial and temporal dynamics of the epidemic.

7.7.4 A spatially specific, stochastic approach based on multiple transmission pathways

Morris *et al.* (2001) populated an existing spatial FMD modelling program, InterSpread (Sanson *et al.*, 1999), with UK geographical and farm livestock data. Unlike the study of Ferguson *et al.* (2001a), but in common with the models of Ferguson *et al.* (2001b) and Keeling *et al.* (2001), the model was location-specific and predicted both the scale and spatial pattern of the epidemic. There was considerable detail in the model and a GIS was an integral part of the system; spatial location of farms (and boundaries) and markets were represented and each was populated with a number of animals of different species. The model used Monte Carlo simulation to track the likely spread from farm to farm. The probability that each infected farm would transmit to any other farm on a given day was determined by a set of single parameter values and samples from probability distributions. Each distribution described the variability in a parameter or process (e.g. the number of days to onset of clinical signs, distance of movements). Four mechanisms of transmission were simulated: local spread to nearby farms via fomites or personnel, spread by the movement of animals to farms or markets, long-distance wind-borne spread, and dairy tanker movements.

Morris *et al.* (2001) did not include a time series plot of disease progression, focusing instead on the spatial aspects of alternative disease control strategies. The model predicted that, even with the least effective control strategy considered, the disease would not have spread throughout the whole of Britain. In common with the predictions of the other models, the model showed that rapid neighbourhood culling was essential for efficient disease control, and that this would effectively contain the infection within the hotspot areas of Cumbria, Dumfries and Galloway, mid-Wales and Devon. However, unlike the model of Keeling *et al.* (2001), this model did not clearly indicate the difference in the level of infection between areas such as Cumbria and Devon. Also in common with the other models, this model showed that the use of vaccination alone would have been much less effective. Moreover, the use of vaccination in addition to culling as part of an integrated strategy caused only a relatively small reduction in the number of cases for a large investment cost.

The detailed description of the 54 parameters contained in the paper of Morris *et al.* (2001) highlights both the complexity of the model and the potential advantages and disadvantages of this approach. Clearly, a large number of interventions could be considered by changing the model parameters, and the sensitivity of the model to changes in each detailed component could be calculated. However, unlike the models of Ferguson and Keeling, it was not clear how the parameter values were estimated or to what extent they had been modified for the UK situation. Furthermore, although many parameters were given probability distributions rather than a single mean value, the choice of distribution, although critical, was not clearly specified.

7.7.5 The contribution of GIS to FMD management via disease modelling

Despite its very considerable assumptions and simplifications of reality, the spatially abstract model of Ferguson *et al.* (2001a) was able to replicate the temporal spread of the UK FMD epidemic of 2001 well, at least in the short term. The predictions regarding the efficacy of different control strategies were also fairly close to those of later, more complex models. If the predictions of simple and more complex models are similar, are increased spatial realism and the use of GIS really necessary for effective modelling for disease control?

The answer to this question depends on the infectivity of the disease agent and the importance of the heterogeneities in the system in affecting transmission. Where infections are spread quickly between hosts, the addition of spatial detail in the modelling structure may make little difference, especially for strategic, broad-scale approaches. However, where infections are spread only slowly and hosts display significant heterogeneity in their distribution or behaviour, the choice of modelling structure and the appropriate representation of spatial processes become much more important. One probable reason for the similarity between the predictions of the simple and more complex models of the FMD epidemic is the high level of infectiousness of the virus. Although heterogeneities did exist in the FMD system, principally regarding farm structure and herd movements, the incorporation by Ferguson *et al.* (2001a) of a simple spatial correlation structure reflecting the contact network of farms was sufficient to compensate for the heterogeneities that were effectively ignored by the model structure. Similarly, Pech and McIlroy (1990) were able to use a basic diffusion to adequately represent the spatial component of a model for the spread of FMD in feral pigs in south-eastern Australia. Nevertheless, the model of Ferguson *et al.* (2001a) did show a higher peak of cases than was predicted by later, more complex models, and also a more rapid fade-out of the disease. The later model of Ferguson *et al.* (2001b) and those of Keeling *et al.* (2001) and Morris *et al.* (2001) were consistent in indicating a lower peak of cases and a longer tail to the outbreak. Indeed, the long tail of infections could only be replicated by including a large amount of detail about spatial structure in the models. The models of Keeling *et al.* (2001) and Morris *et al.* (2001) also highlighted the importance of heterogeneity in determining spatiotemporal patterns of disease spread and control. This is particularly important when making predictions at the fine scale, where FMD models not incorporating heterogeneity in the farm landscape were unable to replicate the observed number and pattern of cases in specific areas (Kao, 2001).

The model of Ferguson *et al.* (2001a) was the one that essentially defined the FMD control strategy, and, because of the nature of the infection, the broad predictions of this model were not greatly different from those of the later, spatially specific models. For these models, there were also clearly trade-offs between complexity and accuracy, and the 'off-the-shelf' model of Morris *et al.* (2001) and that of Ferguson *et al.* (2001b) were less accurate in the details of their predictions than that of Keeling *et al.* (2001). However, all three models were a significant development beyond that of Ferguson *et al.* (2001a), especially in terms of the understanding they contributed to the outbreak and its control. GIS played an essential role in these more complex models, even though it was employed as a tool for handling spatial data rather than as an integral part of the modelling setup.

7.8 Conclusions

Advances in computing hardware and software, coupled with recent developments in epidemic modelling, have placed space–time simulation models at the centre of national disease control policy and decision support. This was particularly evident in the control of the 2001 epidemic of FMD in the UK. GIS has played an important role in providing raw and summarized input data and displaying summarized outputs. However, despite the potential, there are few examples of space–time simulation models that have been seamlessly linked to a GIS. Further developments in GIS technology will aid the process of building dynamic spatial simulation models, particularly detailed location-specific models (e.g. IDRISI32 release 2 contains a cellular automata module). Given the current developments in technology, it is highly likely that we will see examples of fully integrated systems whereby data are gathered in real time, summarized, and used to drive simulations and scenario analysis for decision making.

There are already examples of more integrated systems using both statistical and mathematical models, and the advances in mathematical methods may enable some of the new models to retain a degree of the tractability of deterministic model structures. This development should be welcomed, given the concerns regarding the perceived gap between theory and reality in disease modelling. However, it is important not to lose sight of the practical goals of animal disease modelling, and the complexity of reality needs to be seen as a challenge rather than a problem for modellers if the relevance of models to policy is to be enhanced.

Acknowledgements

The authors wish to thank Dr R. Glanville (Department of Primary Industries, Queensland, Australia) for providing information and outputs from the screwworm fly studies, Dr M. Bulling for providing output from the bovine tuberculosis modelling work, Dr S. Ashworth, G. Gunn and Dr A. Stott (Scottish Agricultural College) and Dr P. Durr (Veterinary Laboratories Agency, UK).

References

Anaman, K.A. (1994) Input–output analysis of the secondary impact of a screwworm fly invasion of Australia on the economy of Queensland. *Preventive Veterinary Medicine* 21, 1–18.

Anaman, K.A., Atzeni, M.G., Mayer, D.G. and Stuart, M.A. (1994a) Benefit–cost analysis of the use of sterile insect technique to eradicate screwworm fly in the event of an invasion of Australia. *Preventive Veterinary Medicine* 20, 79–98.

Anaman, K.A., Atzeni, M.G., Mayer, D.G. and Walthall, J.C. (1994b) Economic-assessment of preparedness strategies to prevent the introduction or the permanent establishment of screwworm fly in Australia. *Preventive Veterinary Medicine* 20, 99–111.

Anderson, R.M. and May, R.M. (1991) *Infectious Diseases of Humans: Dynamics and Control.* Oxford University Press, Oxford, UK.

Anderson, R.M. and Trewhella, W. (1985) Population dynamics of the badger (*Meles meles*) and the epidemiology of bovine tuberculosis (*Mycobacterium bovis*). *Philosophical Transactions of the Royal Society of London, Series B* 310, 327–381.

Anderson, R.M., Jackson, H.C., May, R.M. and Smith, A.M. (1981) Population dynamics of fox rabies in Europe. *Nature* 289, 765–771.

Atzeni, M.G., Mayer, D.G., Spradbery, J.P., Anaman, K.A. and Butler, D.G. (1994) Comparison of the predicted impact of a screwworm fly outbreak in Australia using a growth index model and a life-cycle model. *Medical and Veterinary Entomology* 8, 281–291.

Atzeni, M.G., Mayer, D.G. and Stuart, M.A. (1997) Evaluating the risk of the establishment of screwworm fly in Australia. *Australian Veterinary Journal* 75, 743–745.

Ball, F.G. (1985) Spatial models for the spread and control of rabies incorporating group size. In: Bacon, P.J. (ed.) *Population Dynamics of Rabies in Widllife.* Academic Press, London, pp. 197–222.

Barlow, N.D. (1991a) Control of endemic bovine TB in New Zealand possum populations: results from a simple model. *Journal of Applied Ecology* 28, 794–809.

Barlow, N.D. (1991b) A spatially aggregated disease/host model for bovine Tb in New Zealand possum populations. *Journal of Applied Ecology* 28, 777–793.

Barlow, N.D. (1995) Critical evaluation of wildlife disease models. In: Grenfell, B.T. and Dobson, A.P. (eds) *Ecology of Infectious Diseases in Natural Populations.* Cambridge University Press, Cambridge, UK, pp. 230–259.

Barlow, N.D. (1996) The ecology of wildlife disease control – simple models revisited. *Journal of Applied Ecology* 33, 303–314.

Burillon, G. and Messean, A. (1984) Comparison of two methods of estimation of the warble fly infestation rate. In: Boulard, C. and Thornberry, H. (eds) *A Symposium in the EC Programme of Coordination of Research on Animal Pathology, Brussels, 16–17 September 1982.* A.A. Balkema, Rotterdam, pp. 131–140.

Butler, D.G., Atzeni, M.G. and Mayer, D.G. (1991) GIS as a data manager for national epidemiological models. In: *Proceedings of the 9th Biennial Conference on Modelling and Simulation, Greenmount Resort Hotel, Gold Coast, Qld, December, 1991*, pp. 410–415.

Deal, B., Farello, C., Lancaster, M., Kompare, T. and Hannon, B. (2000) A dynamic model of the spatial spread of an infectious disease: the case of fox rabies in Illinois. *Environmental Modeling and Assessment* 5, 47–62.

Diekmann, O. (1978) Thresholds and travelling waves for the geographical spread of infection. *Journal of Mathematical Biology* 6, 109–130.

Doncaster, C.P. and Woodroffe, R. (1993) Den site can determine shape and size of badger territories: implications for group living. *Oikos* 66, 88–93.

Ferguson, N.M., Donnelly, C.A. and Anderson, R.M. (2001a) The foot-and-mouth epidemic in Great Britain: pattern of spread and impact of interventions. *Science* 292, 1155–1160.

Ferguson, N.M., Donnelly, C.A. and Anderson, R.M. (2001b) Transmission intensity and impact of control policies on the foot and mouth epidemic in Great Britain. *Nature* 413, 542–548.

French, N.P. (1997) A model of warble fly infestation (hypodermosis) in space and time. In: *Proceedings of the VIII International Symposium on Veterinary Epidemiology and Economics, Paris, 8–11 July, 1997*, pp. 13.16.1–13.16.3.

French, N.P. (2000) Models of mange and myaisis: the use of mathematical and computer simulation studies to understand the ecology and epidemiology of ectoparasites of veterinary importance. In: Good, M., Hall, M., Losson, B., O'Brien, D., Pithan, K. and Sol, J. (eds) *COST Action 833. European Cooperation on Scientific and Technical Research 'Mange and Myiasis in Livestock'*, pp. 32–48.

Fulford, G.R., Roberts, M.G. and Heesterbeek, J.A.P. (2002) The metapopulation dynamics of an infectious disease: tuberculosis in possums. *Theoretical Population Biology* 61, 15–29.

Ghani, A.C., Swinton, J. and Garnett, G.P. (1997) The role of sexual partnership networks in the epidemiology of gonorrhea. *Sexually Transmitted Diseases* 24, 45–56.

Grenfell, B.T., Bolker, B.M. and Kleczkowski, A. (1995) Seasonality and extinction in chaotic metapopulations. *Proceedings of the Royal Society of London, Series B* 259, 97–103.

Gupta, S., Anderson, R.M. and May, R.M. (1989) Networks of sexual contacts – implications for the pattern of spread of HIV. *AIDS* 3, 807–817.

Harris, S., Cheeseman, C., Smith, G. and Trewhalla, W. (1992) Rabies contingency planning in Britain. In: O'Brien, P. and Berry, G. (eds) *Wildlife Rabies Contingency Planning in Australia: National Wildlife Rabies Workshop, 12–16 March 1990*. Australian Government Publishing Service, Canberra, pp. 63–67.

Hess, G. (1996) Disease in metapopulation models: implications for conservation. *Ecology* 77, 1617–1632.

Holmes, E.E., Lewis, M.A., Banks, J.E. and Veit, R.R. (1994) Partial differential equations in ecology: spatial interactions and population dynamics. *Ecology* 75, 17–29.

Hugh-Jones, M.E. (1976) A simulation spatial model of the spread of foot-and-mouth disease through the primary movement of milk. *Journal of Hygiene, Cambridge* 77, 141–153.

Jeltsch, F., Muller, M., Grimm, V., Wissel, C. and Brandt, R. (1997) Pattern formation triggered by rare events: lessons from the spread of rabies. *Proceedings of the Royal Society of London, Series B* 264, 495–503.

Kao, R. (2001) Landscape fragmentation and foot and mouth transmission. *Veterinary Record* 148, 746–747.

Kao, R. (2002) The role of mathematical modelling in the control of the 2001 FMD epidemic in the UK. *Trends in Microbiology* 10, 279–286.

Keeling, M.J. (1999a) Spatial models of interacting populations. In: McGlade, J. (ed.) *Adanced Ecological Theory: Principles and Applications*. Blackwell Science, Oxford, UK, pp. 64–99.

Keeling, M.J. (1999b) The effects of local spatial structure on epidemiological invasions. *Proceedings of the Royal Society of London, Series B* 266, 859–867.

Keeling, M.J., Woolhouse, M.E.J., Shaw, D.J., Matthews, L., Chase-Topping, M., Haydon, D.T., Cornell, S.J., Kappey, J., Wilesmith, J. and Grenfell, B.T. (2001)

Dynamics of the 2001 UK foot and mouth epidemic: stochastic dispersal in heterogeneous landscape. *Science* 294, 813–817.
May, R.M. (1974) *Stability and Complexity in Model Ecosystems.* Princeton University Press, Princeton, New Jersey.
Mayer, D.G. and Atzeni, M.G. (1993) Estimation of dispersal distances for *Cochiomyia hominivorax* (Diptera: Calliphoridae). *Environmental Entomology* 22, 368–374.
Mayer, D.G., Atzeni, M.G. and Butler, D.G. (1992) Adaptation of CLIMEX for spatial screwworm fly population dynamics. *Mathematics and Computers in Simulation* 33, 439–444.
Mayer, D.G., Atzeni, M.G. and Butler, D.G. (1993) Spatial dispersal of exotic pests – the importance of extreme values. *Agricultural Systems* 43, 133–144.
Mayer, D.G., Atzeni, M.G., Butler, D.G., Anaman, K.A., Glanville, R.J., Stuart, M.A., Walthall, J.C. and Douglas, I.C. (1994) Biological simulation of a screwworm fly invasion of Australia. Project Report Series Q094005. Department of Primary Industries, Brisbane.
Mayer, D.G., Atzeni, M.G., Swain, A.J. and Stuart, M.A. (1995) Models for the spatial dispersal of insect pests. *Environmetrics* 6, 497–503.
Mollison, D. and Kuulasmaa, K. (1985) Spatial epidemic models: theory and simulations. In: Bacon, P.J. (ed.) *Population Dynamics of Rabies in Wildlife.* Academic Press, London, pp. 291–309.
Mollison, D. and Levin, S.A. (1995) Spatial dynamics of parasitism. In: Grenfell, B.T. and Dobson, A.P. (eds) *Ecology of Infectious Diseases in Natural Populations.* Cambridge University Press, Cambridge, UK, pp. 384–398.
Morris, R.S., Wilesmith, J.W., Stern, M.W., Sanson, R.L. and Stevenson, M.A. (2001) Predictive spatial modelling of alternative control strategies for the foot-and-mouth disease epidemic in Great Britain, 2001. *Veterinary Record* 149, 137–144.
Murray, J.D. and Seward, W.L. (1992) On the spatial spread of rabies among foxes with immunity. *Journal of Theoretical Biology* 156, 327–348.
Murray, J.D., Stanley, E.A. and Brown, D.L. (1986) On the spatial spread of rabies among foxes. *Proceedings of the Royal Society of London, Series B* 229, 111–150.
Noordegraaf, A.V., Buijtels, J.A.A.M., Dijkhuizen, A.A., Franken, P., Stegeman, J.A. and Verhoeff, J. (1998) An epidemiological and economic simulation model to evaluate the spread and control of infectious bovine rhinotracheitis in the Netherlands. *Preventive Veterinary Medicine* 36, 219–238.
Pech, R.P. and McIlroy, J.C. (1990) A model of the velocity of advance of foot and mouth disease in feral pigs. *Journal of Applied Ecology* 27, 635–650.
Pfeiffer, D.U. and Hugh-Jones, M. (2002) Geographical information systems as a tool in epidemiological assessment and wildlife disease management. *Revue Scientifique et Technique Office International des Epizooties* 21, 91–102.
Rushton, S.P., Lurz, P.W.W., Gurnell, J. and Fuller, R. (2000) Modelling the spatial dynamics of parapoxvirus disease in red and grey squirrels: a possible cause of the decline in the red squirrel in the UK? *Journal of Applied Ecology* 37, 997–1012.
Sanson, R.L., Morris, R.S. and Stern, M.W. (1999) EpiMAN-FMD: a decision support system for managing epidemics of vesicular disease. *Revue Scientifique et Technique Office International des Epizooties* 18, 593–605.
Smith, D., Lucey, B., Waller, L., Childs, J. and Real, L. (2002) Predicting the spatial

dynamics of rabies epidemics on heterogenous landscapes. *Proceedings of the National Academy of Sciences USA* 99, 3668–3672.

Smith, G.C. (2001) Models of *Mycobacterium bovis* in wildlife and cattle. *Tuberculosis* 81, 51–64.

Smith, G.C. and Harris, S. (1991) Rabies in urban foxes (*Vulpes vulpes*) in Britain: the use of a spatial stochastic simulation model to examine the pattern of spread and evaluate the efficacy of different control regimes. *Philosophical Transactions of the Royal Society of London, Series B* 334, 459–479.

Smith, G.C., Cheeseman, C.L. and Clifton-Hadley, R.S. (1997) Modelling the control of bovine tuberculosis in badgers in England: culling and the release of lactating females. *Journal of Applied Ecology* 34, 1375–1386.

Smith, G.C., Cheeseman, C.L., Clifton Hadley, R.S. and Wilkinson, D. (2001a) A model of bovine tuberculosis in the badger *Meles meles*: an evaluation of control strategies. *Journal of Applied Ecology* 38, 509–519.

Smith, G.C., Cheeseman, C.L., Wilkinson, D. and Clifton Hadley, R.S. (2001b) A model of bovine tuberculosis in the badger *Meles meles*: the inclusion of cattle and the use of a live test. *Journal of Applied Ecology* 38, 520–535.

Sutherst, R.W. and Maywald, G.F. (1985) A computerised system for matching climates to ecology. *Agriculture, Ecosystems & Environment* 13, 281–299.

Sutherst, R.W., Spradberry, J.P. and Maywald, G.F. (1989) The potential geographical distribution of the Old World screw-worm fly, *Chrysomya bezziana*. *Medical and Veterinary Entomology* 3, 273–280.

Thulke, H.H., Grimm, V., Muller, M.S., Staubach, C., Tischendorf, L., Wissel, C. and Jeltsch, F. (1999) From pattern to practice: a scaling-down strategy for spatially explicit modelling illustrated by the spread and control of rabies. *Ecological Modelling* 117, 179–202.

Thulke, H.H., Tischendorf, L., Staubach, C., Selhorst, T., Jeltsch, F., Muller, T., Schluter, H. and Wissel, C. (2000) The spatio-temporal dynamics of a post-vaccination resurgence of rabies in foxes and emergency vaccination planning. *Preventive Veterinary Medicine* 47, 1–21.

Tischendorf, L., Thulke, H.-H., Staubach, C., Muller, M.S., Jeltsch, F., Goretzski, J., Selhorst, T., Muller, T., Schuter, H. and Wissel, C. (1998) Chance and risk of controlling rabies in large-scale and long-term immunized fox populations. *Proceedings of the Royal Society of London, Series B* 265, 839–846.

Tompkins, D. and Wilson, K. (1998) Wildlife disease ecology: from theory to policy. *Trends in Ecology and Evolution* 13, 476–478.

Trewhella, W.J. and Harris, S. (1988) A simulation model of the pattern of dispersal in urban fox (*Vulpes vulpes*) populations and its application for rabies control. *Journal of Applied Ecology* 25, 435–450.

Vandenbosch, F., Metz, J.A.J. and Diekmann, O. (1990) The velocity of spatial population expansion. *Journal of Mathematical Biology* 28, 529–565.

Voigt, D.R., Tinline, R.R. and Broekhoven, L.H. (1985) A spatial simulation model for rabies control. In: Bacon, P.J. (ed.) *Population Dynamics of Rabies in Wildlife*. Academic Press, London, pp. 311–349.

Webb, C.R. and Sauter-Louis, C. (2002) Investigations into the contact structure of the British sheep population. In: Menzies, F.D. and Reid, S.W.J. (eds) *Proceedings of the Society for Veterinary Epidemiology and Preventive Medicine, University of Cambridge, 3–5 April, 2002*, pp. 10–20.

White, P.C.L. and Harris, S. (1995a) Bovine tuberculosis in badger (*Meles meles*) populations in southwest England: the use of a spatial stochastic simulation model to understand the dynamics of the disease. *Philosophical Transactions of the Royal Society of London, Series B* 349, 391–413.

White, P.C.L. and Harris, S. (1995b) Bovine tuberculosis in badger (*Meles meles*) populations in southwest England: an assessment of past, present and possible future control strategies using simulation modelling. *Philosophical Transactions of the Royal Society of London, Series B* 349, 415–432.

White, P.C.L., Harris, S. and Smith, G.C. (1995) Fox contact behaviour and rabies spread: a model for the estimation of contact probabilities between urban foxes at different population densities and its implications for rabies control in Britain. *Journal of Applied Ecology* 32, 693–706.

White, P.C.L., Lewis, A.J.G. and Harris, S. (1997) Fertility control as a means of controlling bovine tuberculosis in badger (*Meles meles*) populations in south-west England: predictions from a spatial stochastic simulation model. *Proceedings of the Royal Society of London, Series B* 264, 1737–1747.

8 The Use of GIS in Companion Animal Epidemiology

Dominic Mellor, Giles Innocent and Stuart Reid

8.1 Introduction

Companion animal species – principally horses, dogs and cats, but including small caged pets and exotic species – present unique challenges in the application of epidemiological methods in general and in GIS in particular. In contrast to production animal species, companion animals interact far more intimately, and over a longer time span, with a larger proportion of the human population. Many companion animal species share the same environment as their owners and their social dynamics may be much the same. There is significant potential for zoonotic disease as well as the opportunity to study companion animals as sentinels of human exposures, and/or models of human illness, with the benefits of usually much shorter disease generation times. In addition, there is also the potential for companion animal species to harbour and transmit diseases of importance to production animal species.

A search of the scientific literature published over the last quarter of the 20th century identifies very few studies using GIS in the study of companion animals. O'Brien *et al.* (1999) reported using GIS to investigate the spatial and temporal distribution of canine cancers in Michigan, USA, and Mellor *et al.* (1999, 2001) used GIS in demographic and epidemiological studies of the equine population of northern Britain. Gregory *et al.* (2004) used GIS to study associations between pet ownership and socioeconomic variables. Other studies have recorded demographic and other details of companion animal populations without making use of GIS (Nassar *et al.*, 1984; Thrusfield, 1989; Nassar and Mosier, 1991; Wright and Cation, 1996; Kaneene *et al.*, 1997; Centers for Epidemiology and Animal Health, USDA:APHIS:VS, 1998) and there have been studies that have explored spatial structure in companion animal populations in relation to disease prevalence without using GIS (Fromont *et al.*, 1996; Paré *et al.*, 1996; Barwick *et al.*, 1998). The nature and structure of companion animal populations as well as the role of these animals in society may in part explain the limited use of GIS.

In studies involving production animal species, the focus is naturally on relatively large groups of animals managed in a relatively small area and, for most epidemiological purposes, the point location of the premises where animals are kept is usually a suitable reference point for all the animals on the premises. Movements of these animals, except relatively rare movements to and from market, tend to be over very short distances. The focus of spatial epidemiological studies in these species is largely on the spread and control of economically important infectious diseases. In contrast, companion animals tend to be kept in smaller groups, with a spatial distribution that more closely follows that of the human population; they frequently move considerable distances away from, and back to, the premises where they are kept. In addition, and importantly from the point of view of studies involving potential zoonoses, the extent and nature of human contact with these animals can be highly variable, and an animal's owner is not always the person who has the greatest contact with it (Poresky and Daniels, 1998). Therefore, in studies on companion animal species, there can be more emphasis on non-infectious diseases and on human demographic and socioeconomic factors that may affect disease prevalence.

Throughout the 20th century, dogs and cats, and more recently other species, became increasingly important pet companions for humans (Council for Science and Society, 1988). Pet ownership for the majority of people appears to involve integrating the animal into daily life, and household pets are frequently perceived almost as family members. In the majority of developed countries, it is estimated that roughly half of all households now own companion animals (Beck and Meyers, 1996). Growing scientific evidence supports the view that companion animal ownership and attachment can improve the physical and emotional well-being of children, adults, the elderly, the socially isolated and those with disabilities (Council for Science and Society, 1988; Beck and Meyers, 1996). Studies of the influence of socioeconomic environment on the likelihood of pet ownership have produced conflicting results. Some researchers have found higher household income to be positively associated with pet ownership (Franti and Kraus, 1974; Troutman, 1988; Teclaw *et al.*, 1992; Wise and Yang, 1992), whereas others have failed to identify income or social class as an important variable (Robertson *et al.*, 1990; Leslie *et al.*, 1994). However, there is some evidence that social class and income level alone are not the only indicators of social disadvantage (Carstairs and Morris, 1991). Consequently, efforts have been made to focus on the multifactorial nature of social disadvantage and social exclusion from society. Deprivation, defined as observable and demonstrable social disadvantage relative to an accepted standard, encompasses various conditions, independent of income, experienced by people who are materially poor. By combining a range of variables from human census returns, a single deprivation score can be calculated for geographical areas as summary output, with a distribution of scores from affluent to deprived (Gibb *et al.*, 1998).

At the fundamental level, there is a considerable need for detailed information on the size, nature and distribution of companion animal populations. In most instances, because these animals are typically not encompassed within agricultural censuses, even the most basic population data for the species of interest do not exist. Furthermore, in most parts of the world, registration of companion animals is not required, data on disease occurrence are not available and there is no surveillance for any other than notifiable diseases.

Perhaps one of the most potentially useful and interesting applications of GIS in companion animal studies is in comparing spatial patterns of disease among different populations. Pet dogs in particular are likely to follow their owners closely and to be subjected to many of the same environmental exposures. In diseases of unknown epidemiology and aetiology, but which are biologically similar between the species, study of the spatial distribution of disease may suggest environmental exposures worthy of further investigation. Furthermore, comparison of the distributions of the disease in companion animals and humans, focusing on areas where these are the same and where they are divergent, may further elucidate important aspects of disease epidemiology and suggest new hypotheses to be investigated.

8.2 Principles

A consideration of how individual companion animals view space and how companion animal populations are structured in space is of great importance. These features vary considerably both between and within companion animal species. Caged pets and birds and exotic pets tend to be kept at the same premises as their owner, tend not to travel with their owners on a regular basis, and rarely have direct contact with animals outside the household. Cats are also likely to be kept in the same household in which their owner resides. Many cats are kept in 'closed' households or flats and never venture outside or have contact with animals outside the household, whilst others have free access to the local neighbourhood through cat-flaps; still others may live almost permanently outdoors in a semi-feral existence. Dogs also tend to be kept at the same premises as their owners, but are more likely to travel from the premises for exercise, may accompany owners to their place of work and on vacation and are generally most likely to share their owners' spatial and environmental experiences. These features may make dogs the most suitable sentinel species for human diseases (Castañera *et al.*, 1998).

In all these species, the location of the owner's residence is likely to be the best single geographical reference point for the animals in question. However, in horses the situation is different. Studies in the UK have shown that approximately 30% of horses are kept at premises away from their owner's place of residence and that approximately 45% of horses are kept on premises shared with horses belonging to other people. Individual horses were reported to travel from the premises where they were kept, mix with other horses at a show or event, and return a median of 12 (range 0–150) times per year (Mellor *et al.*, 2001). Competing horses may travel regularly overseas, and breeding animals may spend prolonged periods of time at stud far from their normal place of residence. Undoubtedly the situation will vary from region to region and country to country, but it serves to demonstrate both the dynamic nature of the equine population and the variation within it. In all epidemiological studies of companion animal populations, as with human populations, it is important to bear in mind that the place at which an animal is kept may be some distance from the place at which it encountered a particular exposure of interest.

Whilst the exploration of spatial relationships is often highly desirable in companion animal epidemiological studies, the application of GIS needs careful consideration. Without accurate data on the size, nature and distribution of companion animal populations it is difficult to make inferences from spatial studies conducted on a sample of animals. Without accurate data on animal territory (e.g. cats) or movement details (e.g. horses) it is difficult to test hypotheses relating to the spatial nature of exposure to risk factors or disease spread. It is therefore usually necessary to collect population data prospectively, and a study may still be limited because of the difficulties of identifying a suitable sampling frame and a lack of knowledge of the underlying population at risk. Veterinary clinic records and pet insurance company databases may be seen as useful sources of data, but data protection legislation and commercial sensitivity often limit their availability. These sources of data have been shown to have good agreement in terms of demographic variables (Egenvall *et al.*, 1998), but the reliability of spatial data has not been evaluated.

Geocoding, the process of locating animals in space for use in a GIS, is of prime concern. This can be done using grid references from maps or by recording locations where animals are kept using GPS (global positioning system) devices. However, more frequently, for large data sets companion animal locations are derived from the owner's address, postcode or zip code by converting this into coordinates that can be recognized by the GIS. For example, in the UK the postcode system divides the country into a number of large 'areas' (e.g. CA, G, LE and so on, usually relating to the nearest postal town), which are subdivided into 'districts' (e.g. G61, G62 and so on), which are further subdivided into 'sectors' (e.g. G61 1, G61 2 and so on); these are finally subdivided into 'units' (e.g. G61 1NY, G61 1QH and so on). Each postcode unit equates to approximately 15 households in the UK, although this figure varies between urban and rural areas. Thus, where full postcode information is available, the coordinates of that postcode unit's centroid can be retrieved as an indicator of an animal's location. There are some problems with using postcode data for geocoding. First, the size of postcode unit areas varies, the centroid of the area will not be the precise point at which an animal is kept, and the amount of error varies between locations. However, this is usually sufficiently accurate for most spatial epidemiological purposes. In addition, postcodes change over time as houses are built or demolished and new areas are developed. This can cause serious problems, particularly when data have been collated over a long period of time: some postcodes may no longer exist, and it can be very difficult to locate these points in a GIS. Clearly, with all species, but especially with horses, it is essential that the postcode recorded is that corresponding to the animal's place of residence.

The availability of digitized boundary data against which to map companion animal data may also prove problematic. Administrative boundary data are readily and freely available to researchers in many parts of the world, and there are often large data sets of potentially useful attributes relating to these areas, particularly in relation to the human population (see Chapter 11). However, from the point of view of the species and disease under study, such a basis for areal division is entirely arbitrary and likely to be meaningless. Nevertheless, some of these difficulties may be overcome by merging numbers of smaller areas to form more meaningful larger areas on the basis of some natural boundary, such as a river or some other property of interest. Further problems may arise when a study needs to explore relationships between data sets recorded at different spatial scales (for example, horse populations by parish and human populations by postcode district), although techniques exist to deal with this. Similarly, the use of data sets collected at different times may pose problems because the size and name of areal units may change over time (Openshaw, 1984). More amenable bases for areal division, such as land use, may be less freely available, and may lack some of the desired attribute data.

The areal scale at which analyses are undertaken also necessitates careful consideration of the system under investigation, and ideally a number of spatial scales should be explored. Smaller areas are more likely to be homogeneous in terms of the distribution of attributes within them. Larger-scale areal aggregation increases the probability that the exposure of an individual associated with that area occurred within the area of interest. Inevitably, the objective must be to conduct the most biologically plausible analyses with the best data available. In all cases, the conceptual and measurement problems arising here have much in common with studies of other animal populations.

8.3 Practice

Here, we consider two examples of the use of GIS in companion animal study. First, we explore the potential application of geodemographics in order to help us understand the social geography of such animals. Next, we consider the use of GIS in exploring the incidence of cancer among such animals.

8.3.1 Using GIS to define populations at risk: companion animal demographics

Demographic data constitute the most crucial baseline reference information for any population and are essential for interpretation of data derived from studies based on samples or subgroups of the population. When considering diseases, especially infectious diseases, among specific groups of animals of the same or other species, knowledge of the size and proximity of reservoir populations is essential for assessments of disease transmission and persistence (Mellor *et al.*, 1999). Furthermore, where companion animal species are concerned, an unfortunate consequence of the increase in pet ownership throughout the 20th century has been a rise in the number of abandoned, unwanted companion animals (Arkow, 1991). Thus, interest in companion animal populations arises from their relationship with humans, their relationship with production animal species and also from the need for pet population regulation and control (Heussner *et al.*, 1978). Concern over the welfare of abandoned animals and awareness of potential pet-associated problems, such as dog bites, zoonoses, pollution and other animal-related nuisances, have increased this need (Anvik *et al.*, 1974; Carding, 1975; Franti *et al.*, 1980; Nassar *et al.*, 1984; Leslie *et al.*, 1994). Many healthy but unwanted dogs and cats inundate animal welfare centres each year and euthanasia of these animals occurs frequently (Posage *et al.*, 1998). In the past, overbreeding was considered to be the major cause of surplus pets and neutering programmes were considered the best means to manage the problem (Alexander and Shane, 1994; Patronek and Glickman, 1994; Digiacomo *et al.*, 1998; Posage *et al.*, 1998). However, recent studies have shown that the majority of animals destroyed are juvenile and adult animals that were intentionally acquired as pets

(Patronek and Glickman, 1994; Digiacomo *et al.*, 1998; Posage *et al.*, 1998). Factors such as employment, age of household head, educational level, household income, family size, number and age of children, type of home, home ownership status and community setting have all been reported to affect the likelihood of pet ownership (Franti and Kraus, 1974; Wise and Kushman, 1984; Troutman, 1988; Teclaw *et al.*, 1992; Wise and Yang, 1992; Leslie *et al.*, 1994).

Demographic data are rarely available for companion animal populations and are notoriously costly and difficult to collect (O'Brien *et al.*, 1999). As part of a major study in northern Britain designed to determine the relative prevalence and importance of diseases affecting the equine population of this region, demographic data, including geographical distribution, were derived from questionnaire surveys of veterinary practitioners and horse owners. Initially, a census of all first-opinion veterinary practices providing care for horses was undertaken to obtain a crude estimate of population size and geographical distribution. Locations of veterinary practices were geocoded from postcodes and mapped using GIS, and this was used to direct sampling stratified by location to ensure geographically representative data for more detailed studies. Point locations for premises where horses were kept were also geocoded from postcode data collected in subsequent surveys of horse owners registered with the sample veterinary practices. A GIS was used to produce a map of the distribution of veterinary practices and premises where horses were kept against a background of administrative boundaries (regions in Scotland, counties in northern England). Choropleth maps of equine population density were created by extrapolating from the sample total to an estimated population total for each region using standard sampling theory (Levy and Lemeshow, 1991). It was possible not only to demonstrate that the equine population of this part of Britain was more than three times larger than official figures suggested (derived from DEFRA (formerly MAFF) and Scottish Office agricultural census data) but also, by using GIS, to define the regional level geographical distribution of the population (Fig. 8.1) (Mellor *et al.*, 1999). Whilst this map is clearly a very crude representation of the true distribution of the equine population, it represents the first step in a demographic study and was used to guide more detailed studies.

In subsequent studies, GIS was used to explore some of the effects of human population density on equine management practices. Using both digitized boundary data and human population attribute data from the 1991 Population Census, and overlaying on this the point locations of a representative sample of premises where horses were kept, the influence of human population density on equine management was investigated. Given the number and geographical distribution of horse owners in the study, census districts were chosen as a medium-resolution level

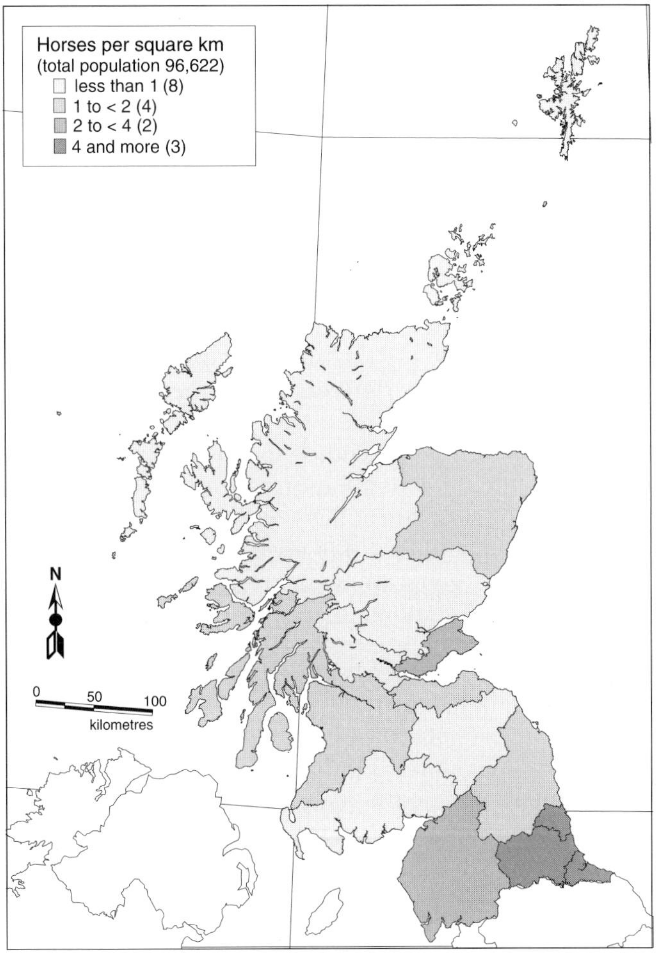

Fig. 8.1. The distribution and density of the estimated equine population of Scotland and northern England derived from a spatially representative stratified random sample of veterinary practices and horse owners. The numbers in parentheses in the figure legend refer to the numbers of administrative regions in the different classes.

for aggregating human population data, and gave a median of three premises where horses were kept per census district (range 0–25). Census district digital boundary and population attribute data were mapped using the GIS, and this was used to calculate the population density in each census district (Fig. 8.2). In the absence of universally accepted standard cut-off points for data aggregation at this resolution, a cut-off point of a population density of 200 persons per square kilometre was chosen to give roughly equal numbers of census districts

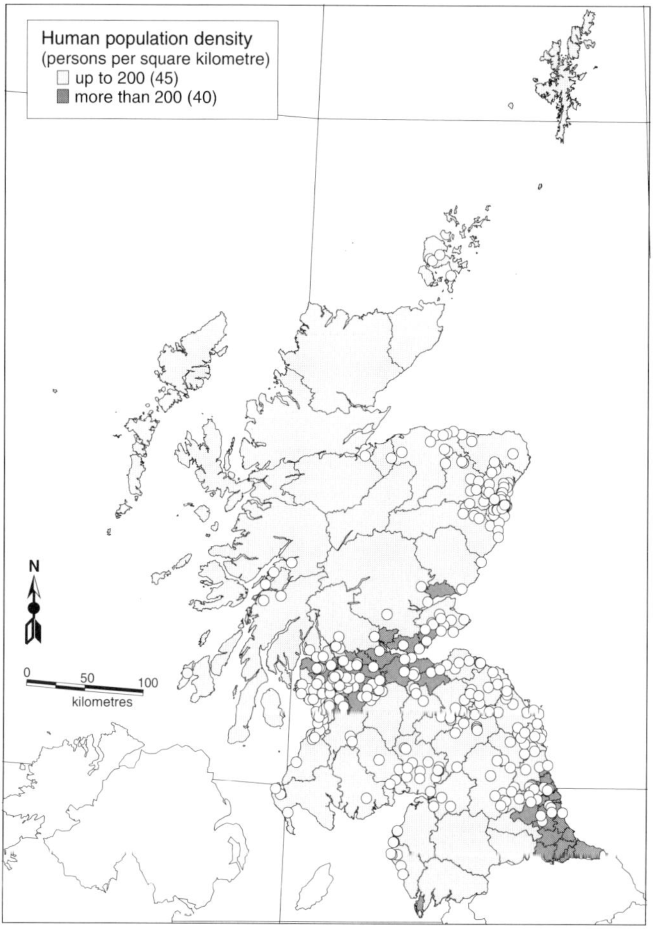

Fig. 8.2. The location of sampled premises (open circles) where horses were kept against a background of more and less densely populated census districts in northern Britain. The numbers in parentheses in the figure legend refer to the numbers of administrative regions in the different classes. This work is based on data provided with the support of the ESRC and JISC and uses boundary material that is copyright of the Crown and the Post Office. Source: The 1991 Census, Crown Copyright. ESRC purchase.

above and below this figure. Point locations, derived from postcodes, of all the sample of premises where horses were kept were overlaid on the choropleth background (Fig. 8.2). The GIS was then used to query the database of horse premises on the basis of whether they were located in more densely populated census districts (more than 200 persons per square kilometre) or less densely populated census districts (up to 200 persons per square kilometre) for the purposes of further analysis.

These studies revealed that horses kept in more densely populated areas were significantly more likely to be kept on shared premises away from the owner's residence and spend less time outside grazing and consequently more time housed (Mellor *et al.*, 2001). Thus, the hypothesis that horses kept in areas of more dense human population may be at greater risk from diseases or problems associated with housing, such as respiratory disease and stable vices, could be proposed, and such information would be of great relevance to horse owners, the veterinary profession and equine insurance companies. This type of approach has many potential applications and could be used to characterize the demographics of the client bases of different veterinary clinics, which may become interesting variables in comparisons of animal disease profiles between them. The use of GIS gives such investigations the potential to consider and identify risk factors for disease that have not been considered previously.

Gregory *et al.* (2004) used a GIS to investigate the association of pet ownership with population density and deprivation in a random telephone survey of 1727 households in the Strathclyde region, UK. Population census data and digitized boundary data were selected at the postcode sector level. This scale of areal aggregation was chosen as a compromise between homogeneity of the areal units in terms of the variables of interest (population density and deprivation) and there being a reasonable number of pet-owning households in each areal unit (median 4, range 0–17). Figure 8.3 shows the spatial distribution of pet ownership (point locations of households which did and did not own a pet) in relation to postcode sector deprivation (deprivation is a composite score derived from a number of human census variables both related and unrelated to income and social class). The association between pet ownership and area deprivation was assessed using the Pearson χ^2 test for independence, which showed a significantly higher proportion of pet owners residing in areas of minimum deprivation score and of lower population density compared with non-pet owners. When analysed at the level of pet species, this relationship held true for dog owners, but for cat owners there was no effect of population density. Owners of pets other than dogs and cats were considered together, and these were more likely to reside in areas of lower population density, but there was no effect of deprivation score. However, these results must be interpreted with care, given the likelihood of heterogeneity within the areas considered and the potential for misclassification at the boundary between two areas with different values for deprivation or population density. Nevertheless, this type of approach offers the opportunity to investigate numerous important determinants of pet ownership and the human–animal bond.

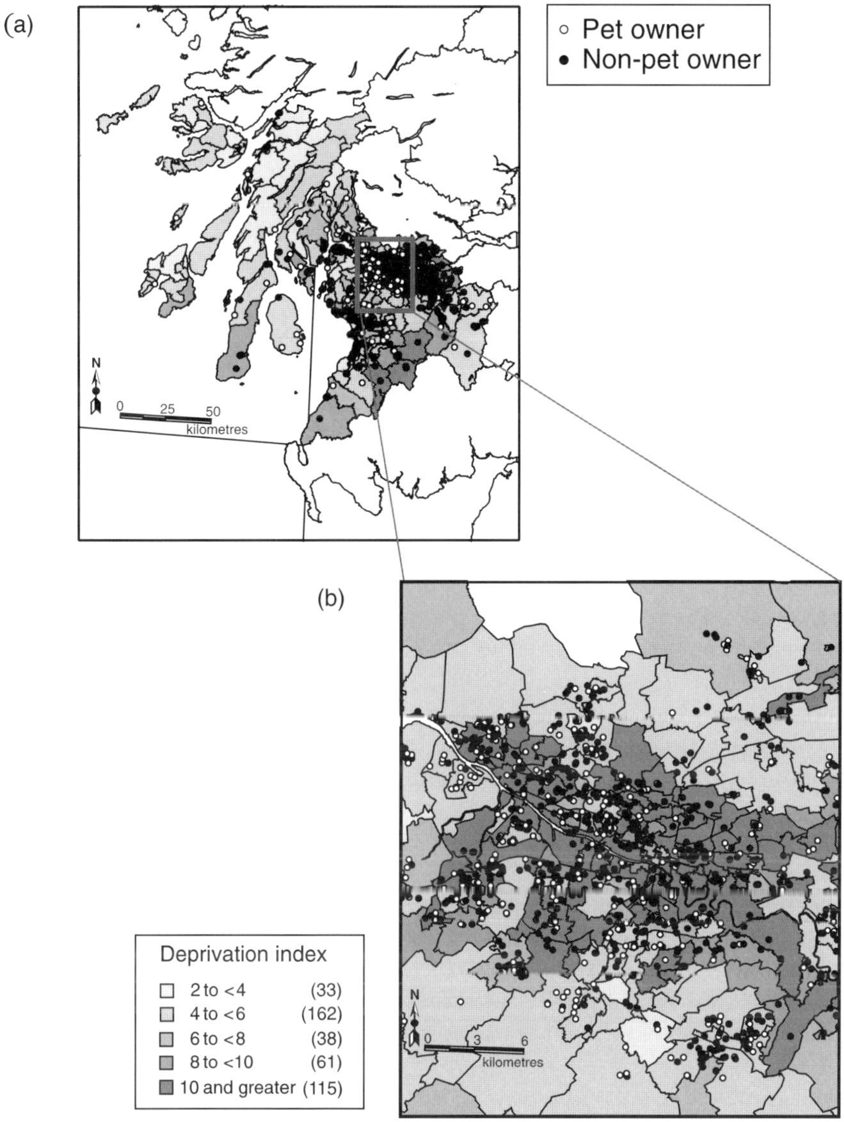

Fig. 8.3. (a) The spatial distribution of sampled households in which a pet or pets of any kind were and were not owned, in relation to postcode sector deprivation in the Strathclyde region of Scotland. (b) Enlargement showing part of the city of Glasgow in more detail. This work is based on data provided with the support of the ESRC and JISC and uses boundary material that is copyright of the Crown and the Post Office. Source: The 1991 Census, Crown Copyright. ESRC purchase.

8.3.2 Using GIS in cancer epidemiology: companion animals as sentinels

The concept of using sentinels for human disease risks is by no means new, and may date back to before the practice of using canaries in mines to detect the presence of dangerous gases. The study of companion animal populations as sentinels of human diseases is not confined to cancer studies; indeed, there is a considerable body of literature on dogs as sentinels for human Lyme borreliosis (Lindenmayer *et al.*, 1991; Olson *et al.*, 2000; Goossens *et al.*, 2001; Guerra *et al.*, 2001). However, it is in cancer studies that most work has been done and most use of GIS has been made. Animal cancer registries have been in existence since the 1960s and, although there are relatively few examples, many of which ran for only a few years, they generated a huge amount of useful data on (mainly) canine and feline neoplasia diagnosed in various university veterinary hospitals. In terms of analytical approaches to these data, attention has focused on various cancers that have similar biological features in dogs and humans (Glickman, 1993; Knapp and Waters, 1997; O'Brien *et al.*, 1999). O'Brien *et al.* (1999) used a GIS to geocode and display point patterns of the residence of dog owners. Locations of owners presenting dogs diagnosed with cancers to a referral clinic in Michigan were derived from street addresses recorded in patient files at the clinic using a combination of proprietary US mailing address software and a GIS. The authors used *K* function analysis within the GIS (Diggle, 2003; see Chapter 5 in the present book) to identify significant spatial clustering of lymphosarcoma, mammary adenocarcinoma, melanoma and spindle cell sarcoma in specific locations. Despite the fact that interpretation of these findings was limited by a lack of knowledge of the distribution of the population at risk, such apparent clustering could not have been detected without the use of GIS and spatial analytical techniques, and would clearly be worthy of further investigation.

Richards *et al.* (2000) reported epidemiological investigations of canine cancer by studying biopsy submissions to veterinary histopathological services from veterinary practices. Attempts to define the spatial distribution of canine neoplasia and subsequently to compare patterns to biologically similar human cancers were hampered by the fact that the only geographical reference available for each biopsy was the veterinary practice from which it was submitted (again, geocoded from the postcode of the veterinary practice using proprietary mailing address software and GIS). Thus, cluster analysis methods, based on individual case location and directed at identifying hotspots of canine cancer, were difficult to apply because the data are already artificially clustered at the level of the veterinary practice. Not surprisingly, using practice location as a surrogate for case location resulted in veterinary practices that submitted large numbers of biopsies being identified as clusters. However, data from the equine demographic study (see Section 8.3.1) have shown that horse owners reside a median of 9 miles (semi-interquartile range 4.25 miles) from the veterinary practice centre that provides care for their animals. Thus, it is reasonable to assume that dog (and cat) owners will be at least as close as, if not nearer than, this. Hence, studies on these practice data may well provide crude indicators of areas at greater (and lesser) cancer risk, and these areas are worthy of greater study. Using GIS to identify clusters of veterinary practices submitting higher (and lower) than expected numbers of neoplastic biopsies may be a suitable compromise (Fig. 8.4), but such findings need very careful interpretation because of the variable factors that influence biopsy submission within and between veterinary practices. In addition, cases associated with a particular veterinary practice may be closer to another practice because factors other than geographical proximity may influence an animal owner's choice of practice. However, there can be no doubt that the application of GIS and spatial analytical techniques to these data offers a much more rigorous and potentially informative approach than would otherwise be the case.

8.4 Conclusions

The small number and relatively crude nature of the studies referred to in this chapter are testament to the embryonic status of companion animal epidemiological studies employing GIS and spatial statistical analysis. Undoubtedly, GIS has a great deal to offer to epidemiological studies involving companion animals, particularly in highlighting interesting relationships worthy of more detailed investigation. However, a historic lack of interest in companion animal epidemiology and a lack of resources for studies in these species have limited the development of this field. As a result, specific analytical techniques have not been developed for spatial analysis of data derived from such studies. Fortunately, there are well-developed techniques in human spatial epidemiology, many of which can readily be applied to companion animal data and which comprise the majority of the analytical approaches taken. Given the dynamic nature of dog populations in particular, area-based analytical approaches may often be more appropriate than the analysis of point patterns of the raw data. Careful consideration, on a case-by-case basis, of the scale and basis for areal division is needed before applying the standard analytical techniques described for this type of data (Bailey and Gatrell, 1995).

It is to be hoped that heightened epidemiological interest in companion animal species, both in their own right and in their interaction with humans, will see an increase in resources dedicated to studies in these species. In the first instance there is a need to establish the basic

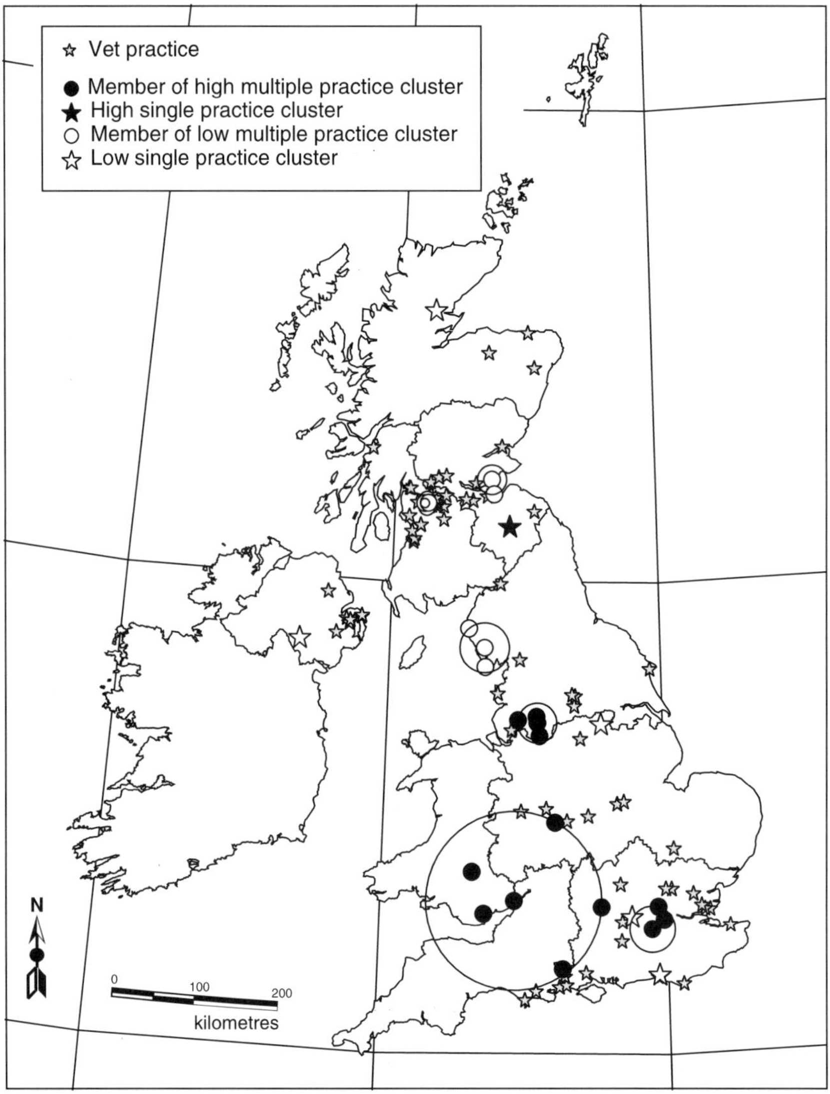

Fig. 8.4. Membership and locations of significant clusters of participating veterinary practices in the UK submitting high and low proportions of neoplastic biopsies from dogs to diagnostic laboratories. Circles show the extent of the clusters. Cluster analysis conducted using SaTScan (NCI, USA).

demographic parameters of these populations. It is important that subsequent studies are designed with the explicit intent of exploring the spatial nature of companion animal disease and interaction with humans to ensure that suitable data are collected, with particular awareness of the limitations of the data.

Rapid developments in information and communications technology mean that powerful and sophisticated analytical techniques are widely available to a well-connected community of scientists and interested parties. Communications provide an essential and previously limiting infrastructure to facilitate the collection of large volumes of information on companion animals. Information technology provides the power to manage and appropriately analyse the data in a timely fashion to produce meaningful results with the potential to effect change for the better. Thus, the study of companion animals is empowered in a way never possible before and in which the exploration of spatial relationships both within and among populations is and will be compelling and informative.

Acknowledgements

Dominic Mellor and Giles Innocent are funded by the Wellcome Trust. The authors would like to thank Professor George Gettinby (Department of Statistics and Modelling Science, University of Strathclyde), Professor Max Murray, Fiona Gregory and Heather Richards (Department of Veterinary Clinical Studies, University of Glasgow) for their contributions, assistance and advice.

References

Alexander, S.A. and Shane, S.M. (1994) Characteristics of animals adopted from an animal control centre whose owners complied with a spaying/neutering program. *Journal of the American Veterinary Medical Association* 205, 472–476.

Anvik, J.O., Hague, A.E. and Rahaman, A. (1974) A method of estimating urban dog populations and its application to the assessment of canine faecal pollution and endoparasitism in Saskatchewan. *Canadian Veterinary Journal* 15, 219–223.

Arkow, P. (1991) Animal control laws and enforcement. *Journal of the American Veterinary Medical Association* 198, 1164–1172.

Bailey, T.C. and Gatrell, A.C. (1995) *Interactive Spatial Data Analysis*. Longman, Harlow, UK.

Barwick, R.S., Mohammed, H.O., McDonough, P.L. and White, M.E. (1998) Epidemiologic features of equine *Leptospira interrogans* of human significance. *Preventive Veterinary Medicine* 36, 153–165.

Beck, A.M. and Meyers, N.M. (1996) Health enhancement and companion animal ownership. *Annual Review of Public Health* 17, 247–257.

Carding, A.H. (1975) The growth of pet populations in Western Europe and the implications for dog control in Great Britain. In: Anderson, R.S. (ed.) *Pet Animals and Society: A BSAVA Symposium*. Baillière Tindall, London.

Carstairs, V. and Morris, R. (1991) *Deprivation and Health in Scotland*. Aberdeen University Press, Aberdeen, UK.

Castañera, M.B., Lauricella, M.A., Chuit, R. and Gürtler, R.E. (1998) Evaluation of dogs as sentinels of the transmission of *Trypanosoma cruzi* in a rural area of north-western Argentina. *Annals of Tropical Medicine and Parasitology* 92, 671–683.

Centers for Epidemiology and Animal Health, USDA:APHIS:VS (1998) *National Animal Health Monitoring System Equine '98 Report.* Fort Collins, Colorado, USA. http://www.aphis.usda.gov/vs/ceah/cahm

Council for Science and Society (1988) Companion animals in society: report of a working party of the Council for Science and Society. Oxford University Press, Oxford, UK.

Diggle, P.J. (2003) *Statistical Analysis of Spatial Point Patterns*, 2nd edn. Edward Arnold, London.

Digiacomo, N., Arluke, A. and Patronek, G. (1998) Surrendering pets to shelters: the relinquisher's prospective. *Anthrozoös* 11, 41–51.

Egenvall, A., Bonnett, B.N., Olson, P. and Hedhammar, A. (1998) Validation of computerized Swedish dog and cat insurance data against veterinary practice records. *Preventive Veterinary Medicine* 36, 51–65.

Franti, C.E. and Kraus, J.F. (1974) Aspects of pet ownership in Yolo county, California. *Journal of the American Veterinary Medical Association* 164, 166–171.

Franti, C.E., Kraus, J.F., Borhani, N.O., Johnson, S.L. and Tucker, S.D. (1980) Pet ownership in rural northern California (El Dorado county). *Journal of the American Veterinary Medical Association* 176, 143–149.

Fromont, E., Artois, M. and Pontier, D. (1996) Cat population structure and circulation of feline viruses. *Acta Œcologica* 17, 609–620.

Gibb, K., Kearns, A., Keoghan, M., Mackay, D. and Turok, I. (1998) Revising the Scottish Area Deprivation Index. Central Research Unit, The Scottish Office, Edinburgh.

Glickman, L.T. (1993) Natural exposure studies in pet animals: sentinels for environmental carcinogens. *Veterinary Cancer Society Newsletter* 17, 5–7.

Goossens, H.A.T., van den Bogaard, A.E. and Nohlmans, K.E. (2001) Dogs as sentinels for human Lyme borreliosis in The Netherlands. *Journal of Clinical Microbiology* 39, 844–848.

Gregory, F., Mellor, D.J. and Reid, S.W.J. (2004) The demographics of pet ownership. Part II: Area based socio-economic analysis of pet ownership. *Veterinary Record* (in press).

Guerra, M.A., Walker, E.D. and Kitron, U. (2001) Canine surveillance system for Lyme borreliosis in Wisconsin and northern Illinois: geographic distribution and risk factor analysis. *American Journal of Tropical Medicine and Hygiene* 65, 546–552.

Heussner, J.C., Flowers, A.I., Williams, J.D. and Silvy, N.J. (1978) Estimating dog and cat populations in an urban area. *Animal Regulation Studies* 1, 203–212.

Kaneene, J.B., Saffell, M., Fedewa, D.J., Gallagher, K. and Chaddock, H.M. (1997) The Michigan equine monitoring system. I. Design, implementation and population estimates. *Preventive Veterinary Medicine* 29, 263–275.

Knapp, D.W. and Waters, D.J. (1997) Naturally occurring cancer in pet dogs: important models for developing improved cancer therapy for humans. *Molecular Medicine Today* 3, 8–11.

Leslie, B.E., Meek, A.H., Kawash, G.F. and McKeown, D.B. (1994) An epidemiological investigation of pet ownership in Ontario. *Canadian Veterinary Journal* 35, 218–222.

Levy, P.S. and Lemeshow, S. (1999) *Sampling of Populations: Methods and Applications*, 3rd edn. John Wiley & Sons, New York, pp. 121–189.

Lindemayer, J.M., Marshall, D. and Onderdonk, A.B. (1991) Dogs as sentinels for Lyme disease in Massachusetts. *American Journal of Public Health* 81, 1448–1455.

Mellor, D.J., Love, S., Gettinby, G. and Reid, S.W.J. (1999) Demographic characteristics of the equine population of northern Britain. *Veterinary Record* 145, 299–304.

Mellor, D.J., Love, S., Walker, R.P., Gettinby, G. and Reid, S.W.J. (2001) Sentinel practice-based survey of the management and health of horses in northern Britain. *Veterinary Record* 149, 417–423.

Nassar, R. and Mosier, J. (1991) Projections of pet populations from census demographic data. *Journal of the American Veterinary Medical Association* 198, 1157–1159.

Nassar, R., Mosier, J.E. and Williams, L.W. (1984) Study of the feline and canine populations in the Greater Las Vegas area. *American Journal of Veterinary Research* 45, 282–287.

O'Brien, D.J., Kaneene, J.B., Getis, A., Lloyd, J.W., Rip, M.R. and Leader, R.W. (1999) Spatial and temporal distribution of selected canine cancers in Michigan, USA, 1964–1994. *Preventive Veterinary Medicine* 42, 1–15.

Olson, P.E., Kallen, A.J., Bjorneby, J.M. and Creek, J.G. (2000) Canines as sentinels for Lyme disease in San Diego County, California. *Journal of Veterinary Diagnostic Investigation* 12, 126–129.

Openshaw, S. (1984) *The Modifiable Areal Unit Problem*. Geo Books, Norwich, UK.

Paré, J., Carpenter, T.E. and Thurmond, M.C. (1996) Analysis of spatial and temporal clustering of horses with *Salmonella krefeld* in an intensive care unit of a veterinary hospital. *Journal of the American Veterinary Medical Association* 209, 626–628.

Patronek, G.J. and Glickman, L.T. (1994) Development of a model for estimating the size and dynamics of the pet dog population. *Anthrozoös* 7, 25–42.

Poresky, R.H. and Daniels, A.M. (1998) Demographics of pet presence and attachment. *Anthrozoös* 11, 236–241.

Posage, J.M., Bartlett, P.C. and Thomas, D.K. (1998) Determining factors for successful adoption of dogs from an animal shelter. *Journal of the American Veterinary Medical Association* 213, 478–482.

Richards, H.G., McNeil, P.E., Thompson, H. and Reid, S.W.J. (2000) An epidemiological analysis of a canine biopsies database compiled by a diagnostic histopathology service. In: Thrusfield, M.V. and Goodall, E.A. (eds) *Proceedings of the Society for Veterinary Epidemiology and Preventive Medicine, University of Edinburgh, 29th–31st March, 2000*, pp. 204–212.

Robertson, I.D., Edwards, J.R., Shaw, S.E. and Clark, W.T. (1990) A survey of pet ownership in Perth. *Australian Veterinary Practitioner* 20, 210–214.

Teclaw, R.F., Mendlein, J.M., Garbe, P.L. and Mariolis, P. (1992) Characteristics of pet populations and households in the Purdue Comparative Oncology Program catchment area 1988. *Journal of the American Veterinary Medical Association* 201, 1725–1729.

Thrusfield, M.V. (1989) Demographic characteristics of the canine and feline populations in the UK in 1986. *Journal of Small Animal Practice* 30, 76–80.

Troutman, C.M. (1988) Veterinary services market for companion animals. *Journal of the American Veterinary Medical Association* 193, 920–922, 1056–1058, 1217–1219, 1362–1363, 1490–1491.

Wise, J.K. and Kushman, J.E. (1984) Pet ownership by life group. *Journal of the American Veterinary Medical Association* 185, 687–690.

Wise, J.K. and Yang, J.-J. (1992) Veterinary service market for companion animals. *Journal of the American Veterinary Medical Association* 201, 990–992, 1174–1176.

Wright, R.G. and Cation, J. (1996) *Ontario Horse Industry Report.* Ontario Ministry of Agriculture and Food, Guelph, Ontario, Canada, pp. 1–36.

The Use of GIS in Epidemic Disease Response

9

Robert L. Sanson

9.1 Introduction

The magnitude of the potential economic impact of epidemic animal disease events has been highlighted in recent years through outbreaks such as the foot-and-mouth disease (FMD) epidemics in Taiwan in 1997 and the UK during 2001, and the classical swine fever epidemic in The Netherlands in 1997. For instance, the direct losses due to the Dutch classical swine fever outbreak were estimated at US$2.3 billion (Horst *et al.*, 1999). The use of any tool that can aid the decision makers and potentially reduce the size of the epidemic by providing better understanding of the epidemiology of the disease, assist with the implementation of disease control measures, facilitate the rapid identification of new 'hotspots' and help communicate the 'war effort' to major stakeholders and trading partners must be considered for adoption. Geographical information systems (GIS) are one such technology that can contribute in multiple ways.

Maps have always played a huge role in the management of disease emergencies. Historically, different-coloured pins stuck into large-scale paper maps allowed strategists to track a given epidemic and debate the various control options. The advent of GIS has led to far more sophisticated uses of spatial data, including the prediction of the airborne spread of FMD, web-based reporting, spatial analysis (during and after the event), better deployment of human resources and the optimization of control methods through simulation modelling.

This chapter will outline different ways in which GIS can be incorporated in the epidemic disease response effort, from simple mapping of cases through to complex spatial analyses; it will then discuss the use of GIS during two recent epidemics, and will finally attempt to present the essential components of a state-of-the-art, integrated and fully featured emergency disease response GIS.

9.2 Use of GIS during epidemics

Perhaps the simplest use of GIS is in the production of point maps of cases. Sergeant *et al.* (1997) described a low-cost solution for mapping disease outbreaks in Laos using a combination of EpiInfo and EpiMap, public domain software programs that can run on IBM-compatible microcomputers. This system relies on the recording of the geographical coordinates of villages, so that village-based data can be visualized together with the outlines of regions, districts or provinces.

More sophisticated uses of GIS involve the production of maps that show derived measures based on a combination of multiple layers of data. Figure 9.1 illustrates an application developed on behalf of the Department of Livestock Development, Thailand, to monitor and predict FMD outbreaks at various administrative scales.

9.2.1 Operational uses

There are many operational activities during an emergency response that can benefit from a GIS. These include the following:

- Controlled area delineation and reporting.
- Semi-automated digitization of surveillance zones.
- Production of routine summary maps for controllers, government ministers and the media.
- Searching for likely sources of infection for new infected premises (IPs).
- Identifying immediate neighbours and farms within a given distance of IPs.
- Estimating resources required for farm visits.
- Allocating at-risk farms to patrol veterinarians, including route optimization.
- Monitoring the visiting of at-risk farms.

Fig. 9.1. (Opposite.) (a) ArcView application used by the Department of Livestock Development, Thailand, to monitor foot-and-mouth disease outbreaks at various administrative scales. (b) Cumulative incidence of foot-and-mouth disease in selected provinces in Thailand. (c) Probability of a foot-and-mouth disease outbreak in a selected area of Thailand based on a number of risk factors.

(a)

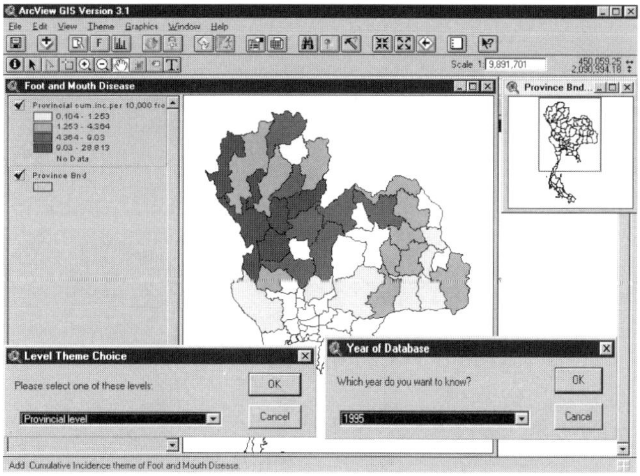

ArcView GIS Version 3.1
Foot and Mouth Disease
Provincial cum.inc.per 10,000 fro
0.104 - 1.253
1.253 - 4.364
4.364 - 9.03
9.03 - 28.813
No Data
Province Bnd
Level Theme Choice
Please select one of these levels:
Provincial level
OK
Cancel
Year of Database
Which year do you want to know?
1995
OK
Cancel
Add Cumulative Incidence theme of Foot and Mouth Disease

(b)

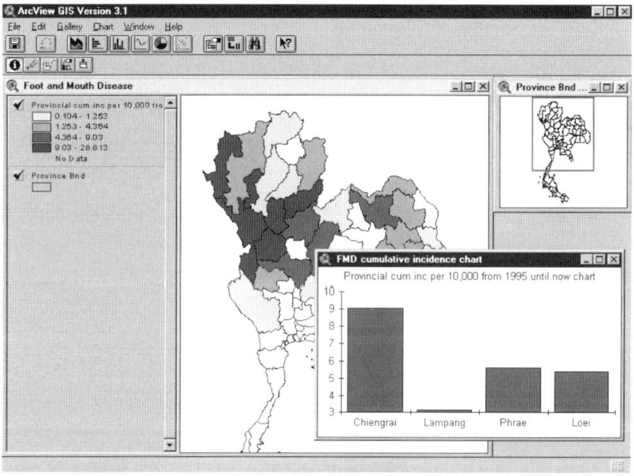

ArcView GIS Version 3.1
Foot and Mouth Disease
Provincial cum.inc.per 10,000 fro
0.104 - 1.253
1.253 - 4.364
4.364 - 9.03
9.03 - 28.813
No Data
Province Bnd
FMD cumulative incidence chart
Provincial cum.inc.per 10,000 from 1995 until now chart
Chiengrai
Lampang
Phrae
Loei

(c)

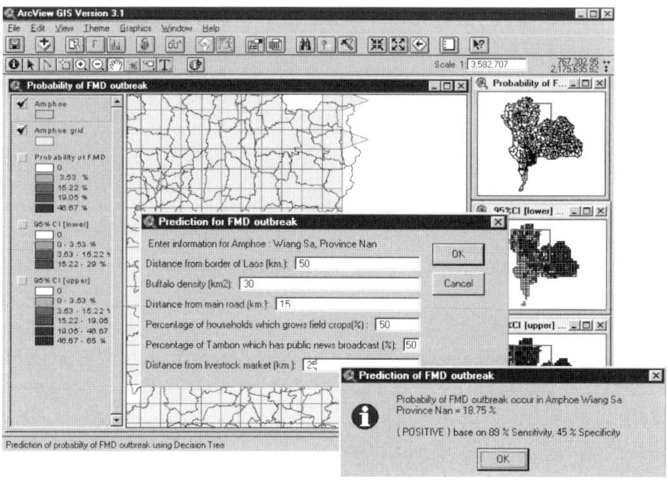

ArcView GIS Version 3.1
Probability of FMD outbreak
Amphoe
Amphoe grid
Probability of FMD
95% CI [lower]
95% CI [upper]
Prediction for FMD outbreak
Enter information for Amphoe : Wiang Sa, Province Nan
Distance from border of Laos (km.): 50
Buffalo density (km2): 30
Distance from main road (km.): 15
Percentage of households which grows field crops(%): 50
Percentage of Tambon which has public news broadcast (%): 50
Distance from livestock market (km.):
OK
Cancel
Prediction of FMD outbreak
Probabilty of FMD outbreak occur in Amphoe Wiang Sa Province Nan = 18.75 %
(POSITIVE) base on 89 % Sensitivity, 45 % Specificity
OK
Prediction of probability of FMD outbreak using Decision Tree

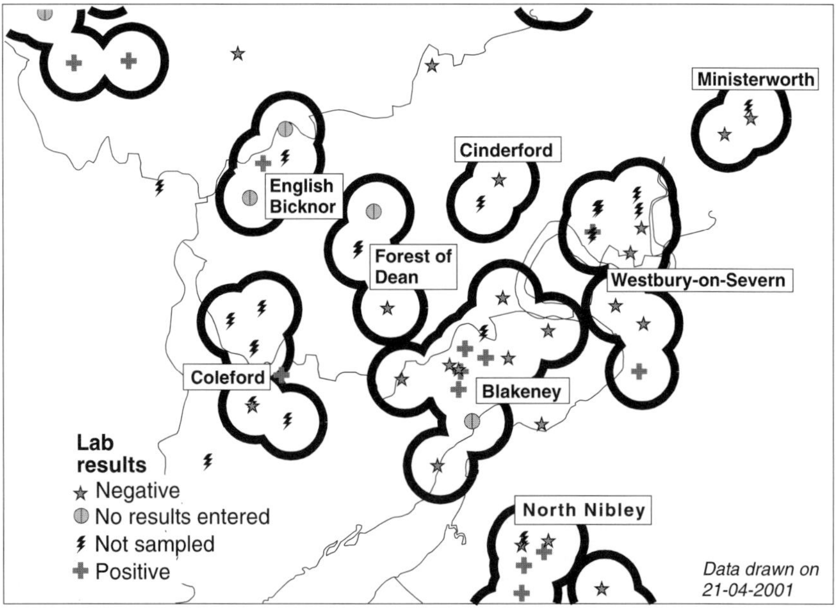

Fig. 9.2. Map showing serological sampling results for infected premises in the 2001 foot-and-mouth disease epidemic in the UK, centred upon the Forest of Dean in Gloucestershire. Data are from DEFRA.

- Surveillance planning, including random selection of farms.
- Monitoring of sero-surveillance results (Fig. 9.2).
- Vaccination programme planning.
- Feral or wild animal control planning.
- Pre-emptive slaughter planning.
- Checking locations of farms requesting movement permits.

For any protracted epidemic with large numbers of IPs, automating as many of these functions as possible via the use of scripting (available in most commercial desktop GIS packages) can lead to substantial efficiency gains. Staff with little or no GIS-specific training can then be used for much of this routine work, freeing up the available GIS professionals to concentrate on more complex mapping and analysis tasks.

9.2.2 Prediction of airborne spread

The massive epidemic of FMD in the UK in 1967/68 revealed the significance of airborne spread of the virus in a way not previously appreciated (Henderson, 1969; Smith and Hugh-Jones, 1969; Hugh-Jones and Wright, 1970; Tinline, 1970; R. Tinline (1972) A simulation study of the 1967–68 foot-and-mouth epizootic in Great Britain. Unpublished PhD thesis, University of Bristol). Simultaneous research into virus excretion by infected livestock (Sellers and Parker, 1969; Donaldson *et al.*, 1970), minimum infective doses and virus survival (Donaldson, 1972; Donaldson and Ferris, 1975) led to the development of computerized techniques for predicting airborne spread using estimates of FMD virus production and dispersion modelling based on weather data recorded during the outbreak (Gloster *et al.*, 1981, 1982). The outputs of this modelling, in terms of plume maps, are of particular value in the prompt identification of exposed premises. Colour Plate 19 illustrates a plume map generated during the UK 2001 FMD epidemic to investigate spread off the presumed index case.

9.2.3 Spatial analysis

Spatial analysis can provide insights into the epidemiology of the disease, assist the identification of regionally important risk factors, quantify costs and benefits in economic analyses, and permit the effectiveness of the control activities to be monitored closely throughout the infected area(s).

Figure 9.3 illustrates the use of survival analysis to investigate the probability of farms avoiding infection, given the distance from IPs. A subset of all farms within 3 km of any IP was first created using a spatial query. The GIS was then used to calculate the distance from each farm to the earliest IP within 3 km, as a method of classifying farms into distance bands. Finally, the data relating to infection status and date of infection were submitted to the survival routines. Information from this type of analysis can be used to determine optimal patrol zone size.

It is beyond the scope of this chapter to provide an exhaustive list of spatial analysis techniques, other than to reinforce the power of GIS in helping various facets of an epidemic disease response. Such methods are considered and illustrated in other chapters in this book.

9.2.4 Spatial simulation modelling

Modelling is a powerful tool for conducting 'what-if?' scenarios prior to implementation of alternative control or eradication strategies. Realistic spatial models were pioneered by researchers such as Saarenmaa and his co-workers (Saarenmaa *et al.*, 1988), using artificial intelligence techniques. INTERSPREAD (Sanson *et al.*, 1994) is an example of a fully spatial inter-farm spread model. It was used extensively during the UK 2001 FMD epidemic (Morris *et al.*, 2001). Figure 9.4 illustrates one of the types of maps produced. Although designed originally to model FMD, it is

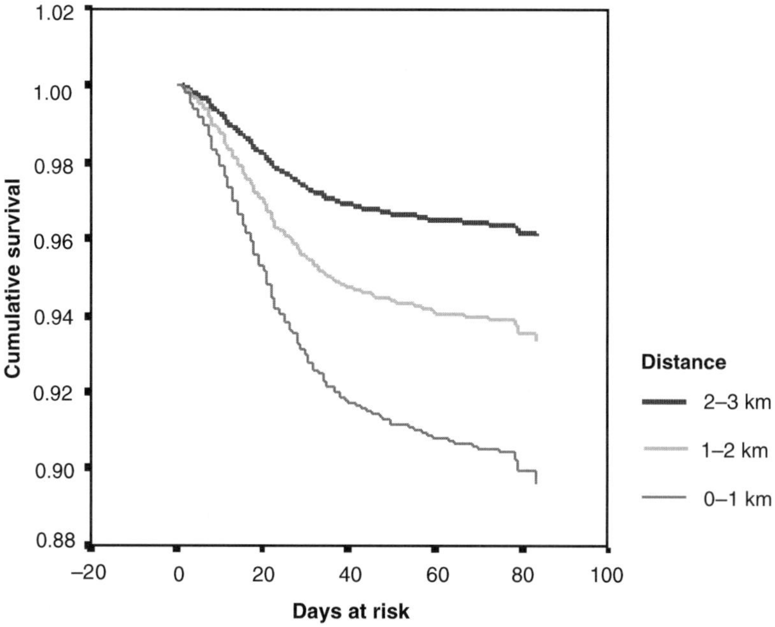

Fig. 9.3. Kaplan–Meier survival curves showing the cumulative probability of at-risk farms avoiding infection during the UK foot-and-mouth disease epidemic in 2001 by distance from the first infected premises within 3 km. Figure used with permission of the Epidemiology Unit, DEFRA, London.

relatively generic in the sense that the model represents the underlying livestock population and the mechanisms of spread that are common to many infectious diseases. By modifying the disease-specific parameters, the model can be used to provide decision support for other epidemic diseases, as was the case during the Dutch 1997 classical swine fever epidemic (Jalvingh *et al.*, 1999; Nielen *et al.*, 1999).

9.3 Availability of geographical data

In order to conduct the types of analyses and the mapping tasks outlined above, a range of different map layers (at various scales) will be required. The time needed to digitize the required spatial layers or the cost of purchasing geographical data in digital form used to be a limiting factor in the implementation of many GIS. Fortunately, in recent years there has been an explosion in the amount of digital spatial data that has been captured and amassed globally. For the purpose of epidemic disease mapping, we need to consider both the unit of interest (typically farms or villages) and ancillary or contextual data.

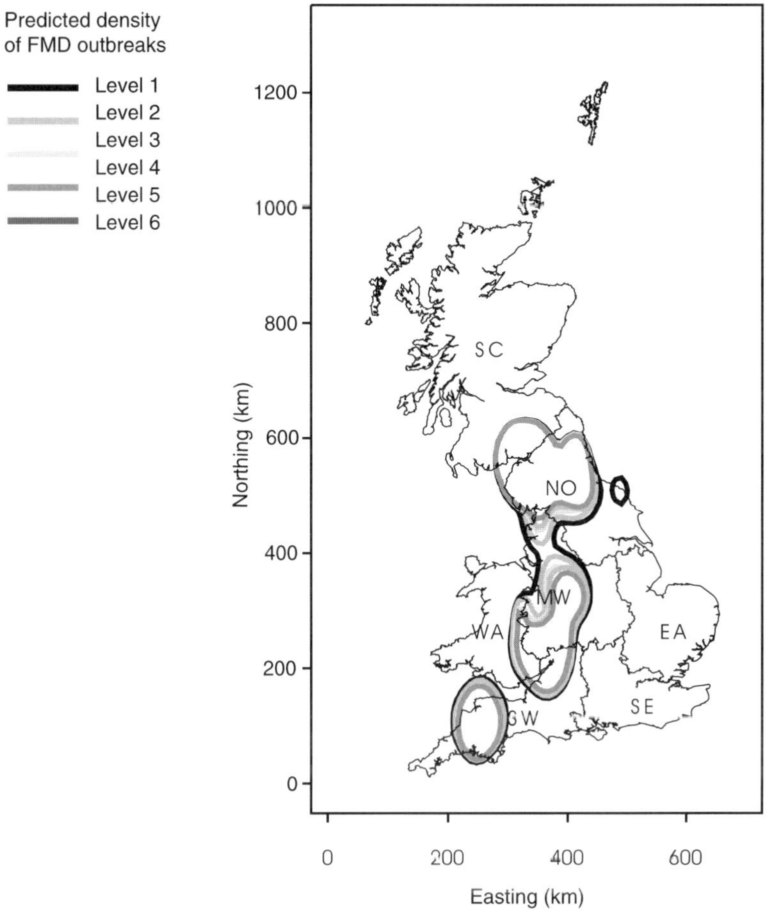

Fig. 9.4. Predicted density of outbreaks of foot-and-mouth disease using different sizes of contiguous cull zones around infected premises, simulated with the InterSpread model during the UK 2001 epidemic. Isolines indicate areas within which the density of simulated infected premises exceeds 50 per 100 km^2 for each of the different culling strategies. The two-letter abbreviations represent the five DEFRA regions of England, plus Scotland and Wales.

9.3.1 Spatially referenced farm databases

The availability of a national spatial farm or village database is vital. However, in order to be useful during an emergency, such a database needs to be extensively validated through regular operational use in 'peacetime'. The units of interest for disease control purposes must be represented in the database (i.e. herds, flocks, etc.), in addition to the contact details of key personnel associated with the enterprises.

The New Zealand AgriBase system (Sanson and Pearson, 1997), despite having a national biosecurity focus, is largely funded by the private sector to support a wide range of programmes, including rescue helicopter missions, environmental studies, network route optimization and precision farming. Because of the regular use of AgriBase and the particular methods used to geocode farms, farms will never fall 'out to sea'. Linking farm records directly to land parcels in the national cadastral database creates farm boundaries. Farm centroids are computed algorithmically. Specific point features (e.g. gate locations) are captured through Web-mapping technology, where users click on a point on a map of the farm on screen. These techniques ensure the locational accuracy of the data.

Computer printouts of the grid references of all case farms in the UK 1967/68 FMD epidemic were fortuitously preserved by Dr Martin Hugh-Jones, then at the Central Veterinary Laboratory, Weybridge. This data set has been used by a number of researchers to look at various aspects of that epidemic (Hugh-Jones and Wright, 1970; Sanson and Morris, 1994; R. Tinline (1972) A simulation study of the 1967–68 foot-and-mouth epizootic in Great Britain. Unpublished PhD thesis, University of Bristol). However, the lack of a control data set (non-infected farms in the outbreak areas) has proved a major challenge in the calculation of true rates and probabilities. Sanson *et al.* (2000) had to simulate a control data set in their re-analysis of the start of the FMD epidemic near Oswestry in order to estimate the probability of infection due to airborne spread, based on distance and direction from the source farm (Colour Plate 20). A complete spatial farm database, available from the outset and linked to the operational activities, will ensure that these types of analyses can be readily conducted throughout the epidemic.

It is not necessary to have a 100% complete and up-to-date farm database at all times. Spatial accuracy is important, however. Mackereth (1998) investigated the level of completeness required to support a range of spatial analysis techniques. His findings indicated that spatial completeness of 80% or greater would support the majority of uses of the data, provided spatial location and farm type were correctly recorded. Experience from simulation exercises using the EpiMAN decision-support system for FMD has shown that considerable time savings can be made for tasks such as using the GIS to identify and print visit forms for at-risk farms within a 3 km radius of IPs, once spatial completeness exceeds 70%.

Farm locations can be stored as point locations (latitude and longitude, or easting and northing coordinate pairs) or as bounding polygons. The former are much simpler to store in a standard database. Common desktop GIS packages can read these points straight from the database and convert them to a 'live' point theme. Bounding polygons are technically more difficult to store and use, although considerable developmental effort has been and is being undertaken to develop methods for achieving this (see discussion below).

Table 9.1. Relative merits of point versus polygon representation of farms.

Issue	Farms as points	Farms as bounding polygons
Data capture	Easy	Requires cadastral database
Missing data	Difficult to identify	Relatively obvious
Database storage	*x*, *y* fields	More complicated
Database access by common desktop GIS	Easy – using ODBC connection	Need either programming or more advanced system (e.g. ArcSDE)
Appropriate map scales	National (small scale)	Much more informative at large scale
Simulation modelling	Fast, but can under-estimate epidemic size	Slow
Spatial analysis	Neighbourhood techniques – estimates only	True contiguity matrices

There is some debate as to whether farms should be represented as points or as area features. Table 9.1 lists some of the advantages and disadvantages of the two formats.

Clearly, points are simple abstractions of the actual areas occupied by farms. Accurate identification of neighbours is one of the most important deficiencies of point locations, particularly if farms comprise several non-contiguous blocks of land. Where the farm area is known, Mackereth (personal communication, G.F. Mackereth) has suggested a locally adaptive radius adjustment around points to identify neighbours, using the recorded area of each farm, plus the mean area of all farms in the locality to compute an appropriate search radius around each farm. In effect, farms are converted from simple points to variable-sized circles. This may yield a more accurate contiguity matrix than Thiessen polygon techniques, which fail to account for non-agricultural land.

9.3.2 Ancillary geographical data

In terms of supporting or contextual data sets, there are three types of spatial data. *Vector data* include point, line or polygon representations of geographical features such as coastlines, roads (at various scales), cities and places, administrative boundaries (e.g. counties and parishes), lakes and other topographical features. Generally, this type of data is easy to acquire. A number of the GIS software companies include substantial world-wide data sets when their software is purchased. There are also a number of public-domain or low-cost data sets available on the Internet, such as the Digital Chart of the World (DCW). For further details about this and other online resources, see Chapter 11, this volume.

Raster (cell-based) data can be sourced either from scans of existing paper maps at various scales (e.g. Ordnance Survey topographical maps) or from pixel-based images from satellite or airborne sensors. Scanned paper maps are generally used as visual backdrops to other map data, whereas remotely sensed images can be processed in various ways to extract useful information, such as differing ground cover or disease in crops. With increasing world-wide interest in remote sensing to monitor the state of the environment, satellites carrying digital sensors have proliferated. The following site, maintained by the United Nations Environment Programme (UNEP) is a rich source of data: http://www-cger.nies.go.jp/grid-e/griddl-e.html. Some of the new satellites can provide very high-resolution images suitable for the 'heads-up' digitizing of farms or village locations. For instance, the Quickbird satellite can produce images with a pixel resolution of 0.7 m on the ground (see http://www.digitalglobe.com).

Spatially continuous data (such as terrain or rainfall) are typically stored in one of three ways: (i) as vector contours (isolines) with an attached *z* value; (ii) a regular array of heights known as a digital elevation model (DEM); or (iii) a triangulated irregular network (TIN) that uses triangular facets to represent the surface. Real elevation data can be further processed to derive variables such as slope and aspect, for instance south-facing versus north-facing slopes. Sanson *et al.* (2000) analysed the terrain in the vicinity of the index farm of the UK 1967/68 FMD outbreak to see whether farms located on slopes facing the index farm were any more likely to be infected by airborne spread than farms on the lee side (Fig. 9.5).

Many countries, such as New Zealand and the USA, provide national or localized data sets without cost. In other countries, the cost of digital data can still be quite high. Nevertheless, data availability is much better than even a decade ago, so that implementing a GIS today is not in general hindered by lack of suitable data.

9.4 Use of GIS during two recent epidemics

9.4.1 The 2000 New Zealand response to *Varroa destructor*

The presence of *Varroa destructor* (Asian honey bee mite) was discovered in the upper North Island of New Zealand in April 2000. The New

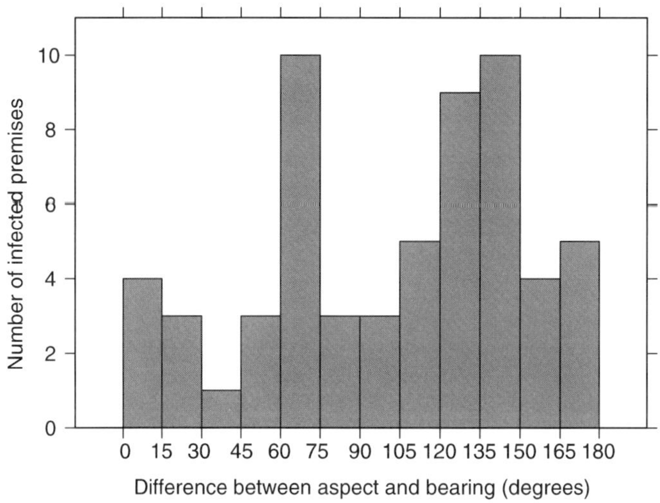

Fig. 9.5. Histogram of the difference (in degrees) between aspect of the land at the location of farms infected downwind and the bearing from each infected farm back to the source farm. If there was a relationship, one would expect the histogram to show a clustering close to zero degrees. From Sanson *et al.* (2000) with permission from the Ordnance Survey. Crown Copyright (NC/00/724).

Zealand Ministry of Agriculture and Forestry (MAF) launched an immediate response. The headquarters were established close to the initial finding in South Auckland. The primary focus of activity was to delimit the extent of the infestation, using Apistan miticidal strips and sticky base boards to diagnose infected hives.

A GIS team was established to aid in mapping the extent of infection. The MapInfo and ArcView software packages were both used. In New Zealand, an apiary register is maintained by AgriQuality Limited on behalf of MAF. Map sheet references of registered apiaries are stored in the database. These were converted to full NZ map grid coordinates using conversion scripts written at the time. A substantial number of grid references were found to be incorrect. Some of the errors were due to inadvertent transposition of the easting and northing values and were relatively easy to fix. Other errors were rectified manually using topographical maps at 1:50,000 scale.

As the investigation proceeded, a number of epidemiological questions were addressed using spatial analysis techniques (Mackereth and King, 2000), including kernel estimation (Fig. 9.6). Of particular interest was the feasibility of eradication. A stochastic spatial simulation model, Varroa_sim (Sanson and King, 2000), was programmed in ArcView using the Avenue programming language. This model used the 9229 registered apiaries in the North Island with valid map grid coordinates (as at May

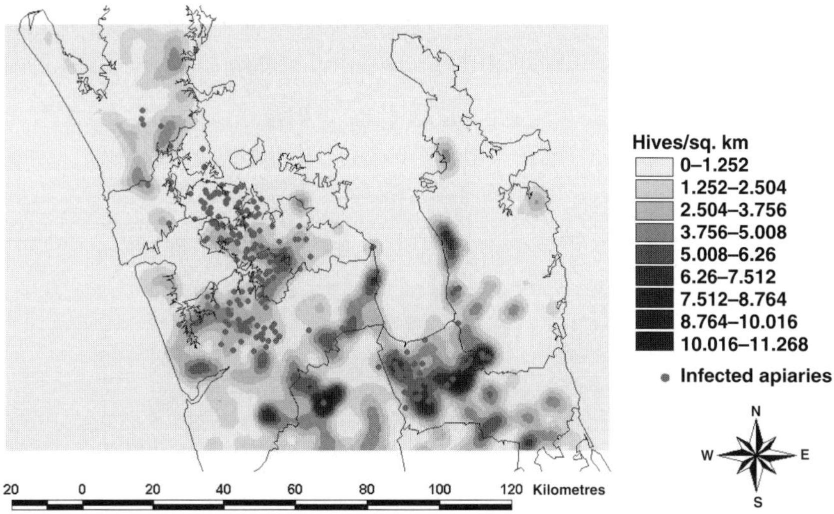

Fig. 9.6. Locations of infected apiaries overlaid on an interpolated surface map of hive densities in part of the North Island, New Zealand, as determined during the *Varroa destructor* delimiting survey during 2000.

2000) as the population at risk. Model runs were initialized with two infected hives in South Auckland and allowed to run for a number of years. Three spread mechanisms were represented: (i) local spread (approximately 5 km per year); (ii) beekeeper spread (spread within a particular beekeeper's operations); and (iii) pollination events (inter-hive spread, which may occur when large numbers of hives are brought into kiwi fruit orchards for pollination during the spring in the major horticultural areas). Transmission rates were derived from the epidemiological analyses. All spread mechanisms and eradication options were presented as menu options within the map-viewing interface. This allowed individual scenarios to be simulated interactively, and results following each time-step were immediately visible. The model showed that eradication was technically feasible. The ultimate decision by MAF not to proceed with an eradication attempt was made on the basis of various other considerations. Following the delimiting survey of the North Island, a number of programming changes were made to the Apiary database, to automatically convert map sheet references to full NZ map grid and to ensure that only valid locations are inserted.

GIS was also used in the planning of a South Island *Varroa* survey, the first round of which failed to detect any infection (as at January 2002) (Sanson, 2002). A mapping website was established to aid in the selection of apiaries for investigation (Fig. 9.7).

This was the first major disease or pest response in New Zealand to

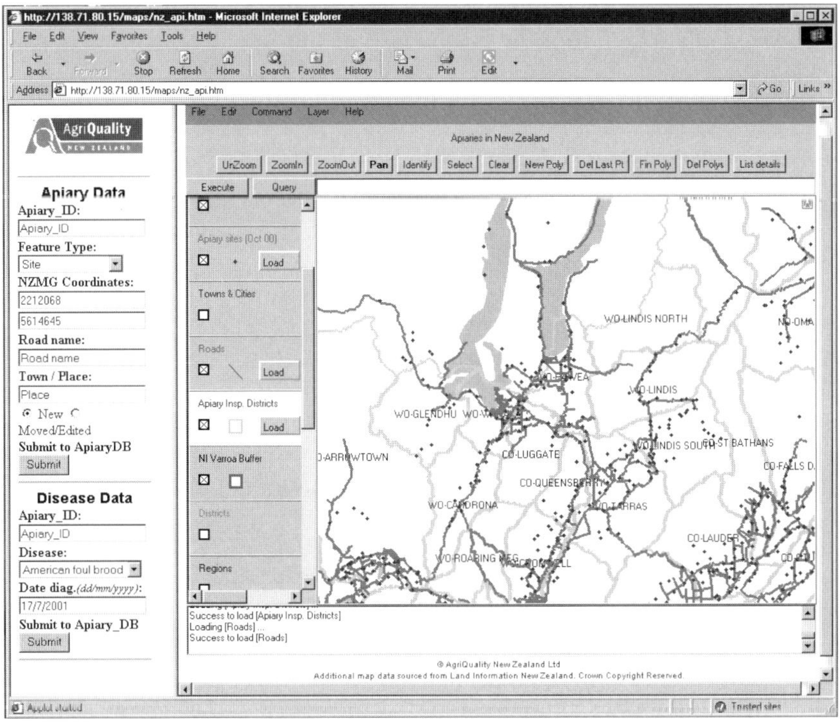

Fig. 9.7. Screen shot from the map-based Internet site established to aid surveillance activities for *Varroa destructor* in New Zealand.

use GIS as a key operational and planning tool, and any doubts concerning the usefulness of GIS in such roles were dispelled. However, it did reinforce the importance of a spatially accurate 'population of interest' database.

9.4.2 The 2001 UK foot-and-mouth disease epidemic

When FMD was confirmed in the UK on 20 February 2001 (Scudamore, 2001), the British Ministry of Agriculture, Fisheries and Food (MAFF, subsequently renamed the Department of Environment, Food and Rural Affairs, or DEFRA) quickly assembled in London a mapping team comprising 13 GIS professionals to assist with the eradication effort. Most regional Disease Control Centres also had GIS teams. In addition, various GIS consultants were employed from time to time to develop specific applications to facilitate some of the mapping tasks. In all, between 70 and 80 GIS staff were employed full-time for much of the epidemic (personal communication, L. Smith).

Farm data were based on a compilation of the Agricultural Census,

VetNet and the Scottish Executive Rural Affairs Department (SERAD) databases. The locations of holdings had historically been stored as Ordnance Survey grid references. These had to be converted to the full British map grid before they could be used within a GIS. Early versions of the combined data set contained many spatial errors and omissions. Given that the main farm identifier was the county/parish/holding number, it was possible to check whether each pair of farm coordinates fell within the correct county and parish boundary. This allowed erroneous data to be identified, and either eliminated or rectified.

To aid field staff in locating farms, a large number of global positioning system (GPS) receivers were purchased by MAFF. Ordnance Survey grid references of farms were recorded from these units on to paper-based forms, which were then entered into the disease control system (DCS), a web-based recording system. Unfortunately, the use of this technology was not able to prevent at least some transcription errors entering the system, which meant that maps drawn at headquarters level sometimes showed the incorrect location of infected premises. GPS units were also used to identify at-risk farms destined for pre-emptive slaughter at the height of the epidemic. The importance of accurate recording was certainly highlighted by the media when mistakes were made!

The main desktop GIS package used for map production was ArcView 3.2. Throughout the epidemic, a huge range of maps was produced for the Minister, the Chief Veterinary Officer and his decision makers, the field teams, the media and the public. Every IP and every controlled area was mapped. Much of the effort was spent in digitizing the controlled areas, which tended to change frequently as the epidemic evolved. Contract programmers were employed to write Avenue extensions to simplify many of the repetitive tasks. An Arc IMS web-mapping system was implemented to provide access to the locations of IPs and spatial extents of controlled areas.

The public were also given access to a range of maps on the MAFF website (http://www.defra.gov.uk/footandmouth). These included regularly updated static summary maps, an interactive map that permitted spatial searching, and ArcView shape files of infected areas that could be downloaded.

Spatial modelling of the epidemic using InterSpread (Morris *et al.*, 2001) played an important role in investigating the relative merits of the various control options. One of the findings was that introducing ring or protective band vaccination programmes would offer little improvement over the basic stamping-out strategy.

Given the quantity of data captured, much of which was georeferenced to farm locations, a number of spatial analyses were conducted. King (personal communication, C.B. King) conducted survival analysis on the breakdown rate of farms within various distance bands around

IPs (Fig. 9.3). Survival analysis has two major strengths: it copes with censored data, and shows how the probability of a given event occurring (or not occurring) varies over time. Used in a spatial context, it can provide powerful insights into the patterns of infection (Sanson and Morris, 1994). Mackereth (personal communication, G.F. Mackereth) quantified the risk of infection with FMD with respect to distance from IPs. The risk was found to diminish with increasing distance from IPs and during the course of the epidemic. Regional differences in the dynamics of the epidemic were explored. He also demonstrated how GIS could be used to monitor various aspects of the operational activities, such as patrol visits of at-risk farms and sero-surveillance (Fig. 9.2).

Wind-borne spread was modelled using a number of different models at various scales. Meso-scale modelling was used to assess the probability of viral spread from the UK to the European continent (Sorenson *et al.*, 2000). Farm-scale modelling was conducted both retrospectively – in the case of the presumed index case to investigate possible explanations for spread to neighbouring sheep farms (Colour Plate 19) – and in a predictive sense, as a means of prioritizing patrol veterinarian visits to exposed farms (Sanson *et al.*, 1999). Although it is possible that some airborne spread of the virus did occur, expert opinion was that this mechanism of transmission did not play a significant role in the overall epidemiology of the outbreak (Gibbens *et al.*, 2001). The possibility of spread from funeral pyres was also considered (Gloster *et al.*, 2001).

Spatial analyses using data originating from the epidemic will no doubt continue to be reported in the future, as DEFRA and the British government debate appropriate measures to reduce the risk of future epidemics and plan eradication and/or control strategies.

9.5 Towards a spatial decision-support system

The simplest use of GIS during an emergency entails point mapping of disease outbreak locations. To achieve this, the minimum requirements are a data set of point coordinates of the outbreak locations (obtained using GPS or from a map) plus some software for displaying the data. The software can be free (such as EpiMap, available from the World Health Organization or the Centers for Disease Control) or low-cost (e.g. Manifold, http://www.manifold.net).

However, to derive the maximum benefit from GIS technology a more integrated approach is required. There are various levels of integration and completeness of functionality that can be achieved, and these will be described below. However, the core components of a mapping solution are a database to record key events relating to the outbreak itself, a spatial data set representing the epidemiological units of interest, some mapping software that can link to the database, and obviously staff who know how to process the data. If each of the epidemiological units has a unique identifier and the identifier is used as a primary key in the database, it is relatively straightforward to produce current maps as the outbreak evolves.

9.5.1 EpiMAN

The EpiMAN-FMD project (Sanson *et al.*, 1991, 1999), which began in late 1988, set out to create a full-function spatial emergency response system. It developed a number of spatial capabilities, including:

- Printing up-to-the-minute overview maps of IPs and at-risk properties.
- Plotting large-scale maps of individual at-risk properties so that patrol veterinarians would know how to get there, and so that they could mark the locations of infected groups of animals if disease was discovered.
- Modelling and mapping airborne plumes of FMD virus, to enable the identification of at-risk farms (WindSpread model).
- Automatic identification of farms within a user-defined radius of IPs plus printing of visit forms.
- Checking the location of farms from which movement permits have been requested to see if the properties are inside or outside the controlled area.
- The building of a fully spatial model of FMD that would permit the testing of 'what-if?' scenarios (InterSpread model).
- Facilities for conducting spatial analyses of the outbreak.

The original design used a single licence of ArcInfo (ESRI) running on a Sun workstation, linked to a second Sun workstation running the oracle database management system (DBMS). Spatial processes, such as producing maps of outbreak sites and plotting airborne FMD virus plumes, were queued as batch processes. However, this structure was not amenable to rapid implementation in other countries due to the specific hardware and software licensing costs, and the proprietary nature of the spatial data sets required. The system would also not scale well without incurring large costs.

Subsequently, research effort was undertaken to embed spatial data directly into the database server. A spatial search and mapping engine was programmed as a dynamic link library that could be linked within the client software (Microsoft access). This design automated many of the spatial processes, such that they were largely invisible to the operator and required very little user training. It was amenable to scaling up – additional PCs could readily be added to the network in the emergency headquarters (HQ) – and required no expensive third-party licensing fees. Import routines were written to allow geographical data to be imported into the database server from a range of GIS software packages. This design effectively removed the requirement for a commercial GIS within the HQ.

Spatial data in EpiMAN are stored in standard database tables. Farm locations can be represented as point features (centroids of farms) or as polygons (one or more rings defining the outlines of farm boundaries). Points are simply stored in two fields in a table as an *x,y* coordinate pair. Coordinates have to be in a Cartesian (projected) coordinate system, such as the New Zealand Map Grid or British National Grid.

Polygons are a little more complicated, but are stored in a table with the following data items:

- Unique farm identifier.
- Centroid *x*.
- Centroid *y*.
- Lower left *x* coordinate of the feature minimum bounding rectangle (MBR).
- Lower left *y* coordinate of the MBR.
- Upper right *x* coordinate of the MBR.
- Upper right *y* coordinate of the MBR.
- Actual polygon coordinates (text field) with *x,y* coordinate pairs within a ring delimited by commas, and multiple rings delimited by semicolons, with the last ring terminated by two semicolons. The last coordinate pair within a ring is a repeat of the first coordinate pair.

This format is very similar to that specified by the Open GIS (OGIS) Consortium with their Well Known Text (WKT) format, and this means that any OGIS-compliant software can read and write data stored in this manner. The inter-farm simulation model (InterSpread) uses data in either point or polygon format to represent the spatial location of farms and saleyards.

This design has meant that automatic or semi-automatic spatial routines have performed very well. At the same time, desktop GIS, such as ArcView 3.x (ESRI) and recent MapInfo versions that support ODBC, can link directly to the database tables in the server, and map at least the point locations of IPs and at-risk farms. In ArcView, this requires creating an 'Event Theme', while MapInfo requires a MAPINFO_MAPCATALOG table that contains projection information for the relevant tables. This means that these 'bolt-on' desktop GIS can be used to supplement the spatial functionality of EpiMAN, in particular the *ad hoc* production of cartographic maps and spatiotemporal analyses. Further developments are seeking to exploit remote-access technology (citrix) to provide wider access to the centralized data, including remote insert and update capabilities.

Various parts of EpiMAN were used during the UK 2001 FMD epidemic: InterSpread for predictive modelling; WindSpread for investigating possible airborne spread, particularly in the early stages of the response; and EpiMAN's facilities for manipulation of data relating to IPs to produce a range of useful reports, such as epidemiological timelines and networks of spread. The lack of prior implementation and non-familiarity by operational personnel throughout the realm meant that the full suite of facilities was not exploited. This highlights the requirement for prior planning and training in use of systems like EpiMAN if disease control personnel are going to make optimal use of these advanced tools.

A number of countries have committed to the development of systems based on EpiMAN. For example, Stärk *et al.* (1998) reported on a version of EpiMAN to manage swine fever epidemics.

9.5.2 Key components of a response GIS

On the basis of EpiMAN experience, it is proposed that a modern, comprehensive, fully integrated GIS-based emergency response system should combine the components depicted in Fig. 9.8.

A large epidemic can generate a huge volume of data. Central to the whole system is therefore a multi-user DBMS that includes a complete subsystem for storing the locations of farms (or villages) as well as key contact details and livestock denominator data. Not only is the farm database required to support the operational activities in the field, but it is also of immense importance in permitting robust statistical analyses during and after the epidemic. There should be a clear set of procedures for maintaining the farm data throughout the epidemic. These should be able to operate independently of the epidemic-specific tools so that, if necessary, separate staff can be dedicated to the different tasks.

Substantial effort has been made to find ways to store spatial data in back-end mainstream DBMS, in an open and accessible manner. The benefits of doing this are seen to be several:

- Spatial data are stored with the rest of an agency's data, resulting in rationalization of database hardware, software and back-up systems.
- There is one current copy of the data with agency-wide access.
- Different client systems may be able to access the data simultaneously.
- It permits mixed spatial and non-spatial queries.

There are three main approaches to storing spatial data in database servers. The Environmental Systems Research Institutes's Spatial Database Engine (SDE) offers a layered approach. The spatial coordinates are stored in the underlying database (in a manner supported by the partic-

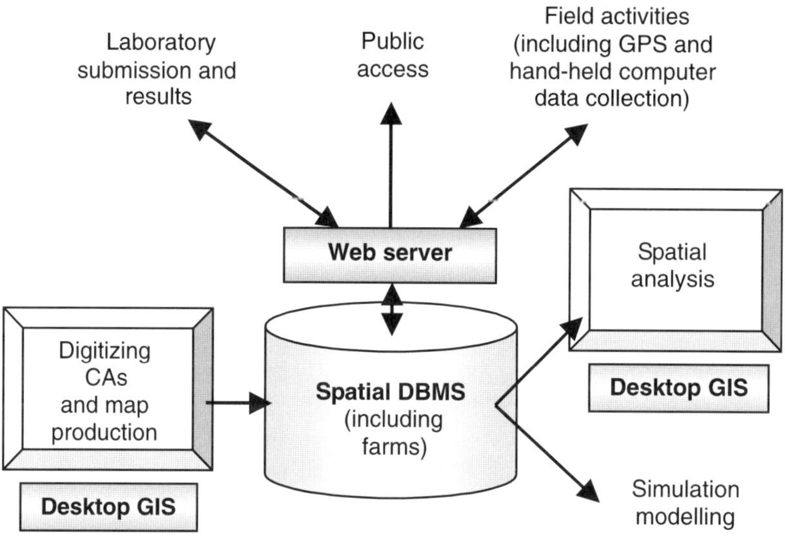

Fig. 9.8. Suggested structure of a state-of-the-art, comprehensive and fully integrated spatial epidemic response system. CA, controlled area.

ular database system) and SDE provides the spatial query functionality and presents the data to the client application (be it ArcView, ArcExplorer or a web server such as ArcIMS). The second method, adopted by object-oriented or object-extended relational DBMS such as PostgreSQL and ORACLE 8*i*, is the creation of specific spatial data types. Access to the data is by way of a spatially extended structured query language (SQL), or via an application programming interface (API). The third approach is arguably the most open, and is based on storing the spatial data in standard relational databases, in conformity with a set of specifications proposed by the OGIS consortium (http://opengis.org/). This system is not reliant on any proprietary software.

The response database should record all activities, including information on properties that are exposed but do not succumb. This will permit true rates and proportions to be elucidated. There should only be one live version of the data, which should be accessible to everyone involved in the control effort. Where possible, data should be entered close to source, to minimize delays in data entry and to allow local resolution of any discrepancies.

In order to facilitate live access to the database, both for data entry and reporting purposes, a web server is now regarded as essential. The web server should have live access to the central epidemic database and should include a mapping engine. The web server needs to support several different user interfaces, some of which will be accessible to the public, whilst others will require password access. These include:

- Providing forms-based access to the central database server for field staff, to support remote data entry.
- Providing up-to-the-minute epidemic status information for decision makers.
- Providing summary information for the media, the public and trading partners.
- The laboratory submission and reporting system should be completely web-based, so that multiple laboratories can handle the testing and results can be made accessible immediately tests are completed.

The Web can be considered as basically a very wide area network (VWAN). Its technologies have been optimized for linking diverse computers and the efficient transmission of information between remote users. Disease response systems can exploit these attributes.

Browser-based mapping is the ultimate in thin-client GIS. In some ways, it is a return to the old days of dumb terminals linked to mainframe computers. The modern equivalent, however, is far more interactive, and the ubiquitous nature of the Web means that the client browser can be anywhere in the world with an Internet connection and can run on any type of computer with any operating system. The quality of maps that can be printed from the browser is still somewhat inferior to that achieved with a desktop GIS package, as the image is usually rendered only at screen resolution.

Most web-mapping systems are based around the provision of visual access to existing data, and hence tend to support view-only applications. There is still much development to be realized and limited ability to edit or create new spatial data. The AGRIBASE programme (Sanson and Pearson, 1997) has recently developed a Java class extension to the JSHAPE applet (JSHAPE software) that permits on-screen digitizing of point, line and simple polygon features. Live database access can be incorporated using server side extension software, such as Allaire's COLD FUSION.

Even with a web-mapping interface, it is still likely that desktop GIS will be required: for digitizing controlled areas, *ad hoc* cartographic map production, and spatial analyses of the outbreak. Mapping systems should be able to plot the current state of the epidemic straight out of the database using a live database connection.

9.6 Further technological considerations

9.6.1 Global positioning systems

In a disease response context, GPS primarily have a role in recording the location of infected premises (IPs) and at-risk farms where no national farm database exists, or else in checking locations where errors are known to be present. GPS rely on a hand-held receiver decoding time-stamp signals from a constellation of 24 orbiting satellites, launched and maintained by the US Defence Force. Provided signals can be received from at least three satellites via direct line of sight, triangulation techniques are used to calculate the location of the receiver anywhere on the earth in two-dimensional space. Four satellites are required to calculate an altitude – specifically, height above the spheroid. The spheroid is the particular model of the shape of the earth and, in the case of GPS, is based on the GRS80 spheroid, and the datum (which 'ties' the surface of the earth to the spheroid) is known as 'WGS84'. Coordinates are reported in latitude and longitude, although some hand-held GPS can convert these coordinates into various national grid formats.

The accuracy achievable from consumer-quality hand-held receivers is theoretically in the order of 2–5 m. However, in practice the horizontal accuracy is often in the 10–15 m range, with vertical error typically twice that of horizontal error. Inaccuracies are caused by atmospheric interference, multipath signals (where the receivers pick up direct and bounced signals from the same satellites), lack of line-of-sight access to satellites, satellites low on the horizon, or insufficient satellites in the field of view. Differential systems that use a second GPS unit at a known surveyed location can be used to remedy some of the above issues.

9.6.2 Hand-held computers

Relatively powerful hand-held computers (such as the Compaq iPAQ) can now be linked to a GPS receiver plus appropriate mapping software to provide a complete map-based field recording system. For example, ESRI have released ArcPad software that allows data collection forms to be designed. Suitable background maps can be downloaded from a desktop computer to the unit. When the GPS is activated, the maps constantly re-centre, so that the user can always see where he or she is. When a GPS location is captured or a spot on the displayed map is tapped, the geographical feature is stored and the data collection form opens. In this way, data can be stored digitally, to be downloaded to a central database when the user returns to the office. This system ensures that data are captured at source and removes the likelihood of recording errors, subject to the accuracy of the GPS unit as discussed above.

In the future, wireless communications from the field to the central database server will become the norm. Already, there are Wap-enabled cellular phones that are capable of displaying simple maps, which can direct the user to the nearest restaurant, for example. These developments will aid real-time data capture and transmission, which could be of critical value in managing fast-spreading diseases such as FMD.

9.7 Conclusions

The evolution of GIS and computer technology in general is now at a stage when building the type of integrated GIS-based response system proposed (Fig. 9.8) is quite feasible. Web technology means that remote staff and headquarters-based decision makers alike can access critical data stored in a central repository. The ease of linking computer components means that much can be achieved even in the face of an epidemic, as was demonstrated during the UK 2001 FMD epidemic. However, the lack of a single, centralized database meant that much effort was wasted on re-entering data into multiple systems, files had to be transferred between databases, and it was likely that many 'islands' of data were formed, which will limit or hinder the ability to conduct a full range of epidemiological analyses.

The UK response also showed how expensive (particularly in personnel terms) an inefficient GIS design could be as a result of the lack of integration. Assembling the spatial data layers, dealing with errors in the farm database, the constant transfer of files between systems and sites and the lack of automation contributed to the inefficiencies. In other words, modern GIS capabilities were not fully exploited.

Clearly, creating a complete and spatially accurate farm database is difficult in the face of an outbreak. Developing a system that can meet a range of 'peacetime' objectives is worthwhile. The experience in New Zealand with AgriBase has shown that paying users are the best critics of the quality of data in a database. Having a real-world data model, which innately knows where things are and permits the behaviours of various objects in the system to be modelled realistically, is fundamental to an intelligent decision-support system. For instance, highly structured industries like the poultry industry often have networks of routine movements, such as the delivery of feed trucks on certain days and the pick-up and distribution of eggs through well-defined nodes. It should be possible to document many of these during 'peacetime' so that, in the event of an emergency, much of the knowledge required to make early decisions in terms of controlled area delineation or who to inform should be available to the decision-makers. The database should therefore permit the storage of all types of entities that need to be investigated or controlled in a response – locations such as saleyards, abattoirs and dairy factories – as well as more abstract entities, such as well-defined routes.

The EpiMAN system, which was designed in the early 1990s, was ahead of its time. It demonstrated most of the aspects of the system proposed. What was considered a technical challenge then has now become much more routine as GIS, computer hardware, programming environments and the Web have evolved. Nevertheless, assembling such a system in the midst of a large epidemic is inadvisable. There should be a proper data store available from the outset, kept constantly up to date, from which all personnel can access the required information. Furthermore, operators need training so that all users are thoroughly familiar with the available tools, and consistency of data input can be assured throughout a protracted campaign. Although new operators can be recruited during the epidemic, having a core of trained staff who can be mobilized from the outset should be part of contingency planning. Any system developed should be highly scaleable, so that epidemics that involve large regions can still be managed.

It behoves State veterinary services in countries where disease control and eradication is important to harness the power of GIS technology to aid their programmes. Computers promised us a better world, but, as always, it is what we do with the opportunities presented to us that makes the real difference.

Acknowledgements

The author would like to thank the Epidemiology Team at DEFRA headquarters, London, the EpiCentre, Massey University, and the National Centre for Disease Investigation, New Zealand for providing a number of the example maps.

References

Donaldson, A.I. (1972) The influence of relative humidity on the aerosol stability of different strains of foot-and-mouth disease virus suspended in saliva. *Journal of General Virology* 15, 25–33.

Donaldson, A.I. and Ferris, N.P. (1975) The survival of foot-and-mouth disease virus in open air conditions. *Journal of Hygiene, Cambridge* 74, 409–416.

Donaldson, A.I., Herniman, K.A.J., Parker, J. and Sellers, R.F. (1970) Further investigations on the airborne excretion of foot-and-mouth disease virus. *Journal of Hygiene, Cambridge* 69, 557–564.

Gibbens, J.C., Sharpe, C.E., Wilesmith, J.W., Mansley, L.M., Michalopoulou, E., Ryan, J.B.M. and Hudson, M. (2001) Descriptive epidemiology of the 2001 foot-and-mouth disease epidemic in Great Britain: the first five months. *Veterinary Record* 149, 729–743.

Gloster, J., Blackall, R.M., Sellers, R.F. and Donaldson, A.I. (1981) Forecasting the airborne spread of foot-and-mouth disease. *Veterinary Record* 108, 370–374.

Gloster, J., Sellers, R.F. and Donaldson, A.I. (1982) Long distance spread of foot-and-mouth disease virus over the sea. *Veterinary Record* 110, 47–52.

Gloster, J., Hewson, H., Mackay, D., Garland, T., Donaldson, A., Mason, I. and Brown, R. (2001) Spread of foot-and-mouth disease from the burning of animal carcases on open pyres. *Veterinary Record* 148, 585–586.

Henderson, R.J. (1969) The outbreak of foot-and-mouth disease in Worcestershire. An epidemiological study: with special reference to spread of the disease by wind-carriage of the virus. *Journal of Hygiene, Cambridge* 67, 21–33.

Horst, H.S., Meuwissen, M.P.M., Smak, J.A. and Van der Meijs, C.C.J.M. (1999) The involvement of the agriculture industry and government in animal disease emergencies and the funding of compensation in Western Europe. *Revue Scientifique et Technique Office International des Epizooties* 19, 30–37.

Hugh-Jones, M.E. and Wright, P.B. (1970) Studies on the 1967–8 foot-and-mouth disease epidemic: the relation of weather to the spread of disease. *Journal of Hygiene, Cambridge* 68, 253–271.

Jalvingh, A.W., Nielen, M., Maurice, H., Stegeman, A.J., Elbers, A.R.W. and Dijkhuizen, A.A. (1999) Spatial and stochastic simulation to evaluate the impact of events and control measures on the 1997–1998 classical swine fever epidemic in The Netherlands. I. Description of simulation model. *Preventive Veterinary Medicine* 42, 271–295.

Mackereth, G.F. (1998) Spatial data requirements for animal disease management in New Zealand. Unpublished MSc thesis, Massey University, Palmerston North, New Zealand.

Mackereth, G.F. and King, C.B. (2000) Delimiting the geographical extent and associated spread mechanisms of apiaries infected with Varroa jacobsoni in the North Island of New Zealand as at June 2000. National Centre for Disease Investigation, Ministry of Agriculture and Forestry, Upper Hutt, New Zealand. http://www.gisvet.org

Morris, R.S., Wilesmith, J.W., Stern, M.W., Sanson, R.L. and Stevenson, M.A. (2001) Predictive spatial modelling of alternative control strategies for the foot-and-mouth disease epidemic in Great Britain, 2001. *Veterinary Record* 149, 137–144.

Nielen, M., Jalvingh, A.W., Meuwissen, M.P.M., Horst, S.H. and Dijkhuizen, A.A. (1999) Spatial and stochastic simulation to evaluate the impact of events and control measures on the 1997–1998 classical swine fever epidemic in The Netherlands. II. Comparison of control strategies. *Preventive Veterinary Medicine* 42, 297–317.

Saarenmaa, H., Stone, N.D., Folse, L.J., Packard, J.M., Grant, W.E., Makela, M.E. and Coulson, R.N. (1988) An artificial intelligence modelling approach to simulating animal/habitat interactions. *Ecological Modelling* 44, 125–141.

Sanson, R.L. (2002) Detection surveys where disease is clustered: varroa mites as an example. In: Perry, G. and Boland, P. (eds) *Proceedings of the Epidemiology Chapter Programme of the Australian College of Veterinary Scientists Science Week, Gold Coast , 4–6 July 2002* (CD-ROM).

Sanson, R.L. and King, C.B. (2000) VARROA_SIM: a spatial simulation model of *Varroa jacobsoni*. In: *Proceedings of the New Zealand Veterinary Association Epidemiology and Animal Health Management Branch Seminar, Wallaceville, Upper Hutt, New Zealand, 23–24 November 2000*. Foundation for Continuing Education of the NZVA, pp. 71–74.

Sanson, R.L. and Morris, R.S. (1994) The use of survival analysis to investigate the probability of local spread of foot-and-mouth disease: an example study on the United Kingdom epidemic of 1967–1968. In: Rowlands, G.J., Kyule, M.N. and Perry, B.D. (eds) *Proceedings of the 7th International Symposium on Veterinary Epidemiology and Economics, Nairobi, 15–19 August 1994*, pp. 186–188.

Sanson, R. and Pearson, A. (1997) Agribase – a national spatial farm database. In: *Proceedings of the VIII International Symposium on Veterinary Epidemiology and Economics, Paris, 8–11 July, 1997*, pp. 12.16.1–12.16.3.

Sanson, R.L., Liberona, H. and Morris, R.S. (1991) The use of a geographical information system in the management of a foot-and-mouth disease epidemic. *Preventive Veterinary Medicine* 11, 309–313.

Sanson, R.L., Stern, M.W. and Morris, R.S. (1994) INTERSPREAD: A spatial stochastic simulation model of epidemic foot-and-mouth disease. In: Rowlands, G.J., Kyule, M.N. and Perry, B.D. (eds) *Proceedings of the 7th International Symposium on Veterinary Epidemiology and Economics, Nairobi, 15–19 August 1994*, pp. 493–495.

Sanson, R.L., Morris, R.S. and Stern, M.W. (1999) EpiMAN-FMD: a decision support system for managing epidemics of vesicular disease. *Revue Scientifique et Technique Office International des Epizooties* 18, 593–605.

Sanson, R.L., Morris, R.S., Wilesmith, J.W. and Mackay, D.K.J. (2000) A re-analysis of the start of the United Kingdom 1967–8 foot-and-mouth disease epidemic to calculate transmission probabilities. In: Salmon, M.D., Morley, P.S. and Ruch-Gallie, R. (eds) *Proceedings of the 9th Symposium of the International Society for Veterinary Epidemiology and Economics, Breckenridge, Colorado, August 6–11, 2000.* http://www.gisvet.org

Scudamore, J.M. (2001) Foot-and-mouth disease outbreak (letter). *Veterinary Record* 148, 250.

Sellers, R.F. and Parker, J. (1969) Airborne excretion of foot-and-mouth disease virus. *Journal of Hygiene, Cambridge* 67, 671–677.

Sergeant, E.S.G., Cameron, A.R., Baldock, F.C. and Vongthilath, S. (1997) An animal health information system for Laos. In: More, S. (ed.) *Proceedings of the Epidemiology Programme of the 10th Federation of Asian Veterinary Associations Congress, Cairns, Australia, 25–28 August 1997*, pp. 157–160.

Smith, L.P. and Hugh-Jones, M.E. (1969) The weather factor in foot and mouth disease epidemics. *Nature* 223, 712–715.

Sorenson, J.H., Mackay, D.K.J., Jensen, C.O. and Donaldson, A.I. (2000) An integrated model to predict atmospheric spread of foot and mouth disease virus. *Epidemiology and Infection* 124, 577–590.

Stärk, K.D.C., Morris, R.S., Benard, H.J. and Stern, M.W. (1998) EpiMAN-SF: a decision support system for managing swine fever epidemics. *Revue Scientifique et Technique Office International des Epizooties* 17, 682–690.

Tinline, R.R. (1970) Lee wave hypothesis for the initial pattern of spread during the 1967–8 foot and mouth epizootic. *Nature* 227, 860–862.

The Use of GIS in the Management of Wildlife Diseases

10

Joanna S. McKenzie

10.1 Introduction

There is growing awareness amongst the veterinary profession of the importance of diseases in wildlife populations (Bengis, 2002). Interest has predominantly focused on diseases of wildlife that are transmitted to humans, domestic animals and livestock populations. The most notable of these is rabies, but the list also includes Lyme disease, classical swine fever, echinococcosis, hantavirus and, most recently, West Nile virus (Roehrig *et al.*, 2002) and viral infections in bats such as Lyssa, Nipah, Hendra and Menangle viruses (Halpin *et al.*, 1999). A number of sylvatic foci of diseases have emerged in recent decades and have threatened to undermine national control programmes in livestock, including bovine tuberculosis (TB) in New Zealand, the UK and Ireland, bovine brucellosis in North America and possibly rinderpest (Bengis *et al.*, 2002). More recently there has been an increased awareness of the need for surveillance activities to include wildlife species, to support country or regional claims of freedom (Bengis *et al.*, 2002). There has also been increased interest in the potential involvement of wildlife species in outbreaks of highly contagious diseases of livestock, such as foot-and-mouth disease, giving rise to the need to better understand the distribution of these species and the areas of contact between livestock and wildlife populations. At the same time, there is increasing awareness of the cultural and conservation value of wildlife species and the potential impact of disease on these populations (Mbassa *et al.*, 2000; Deem *et al.*, 2001).

Veterinary epidemiologists face special challenges in detecting and managing diseases in wildlife species. The artificial management boundaries that define the distribution of livestock species are not present for wildlife, making it difficult to define the location and number of animals in populations of interest. An even greater challenge is the detection of infected wild animals, due to the logistics of capturing and testing animals and the lack of validation of many tests in wildlife species. Geographical information systems (GIS) provide a range of tools that can assist the research and management of disease in wildlife. The increasing availability of digital data sets of environmental factors, particularly via satellite imagery, and the more accessible and accurate technology for recording the locations of animals in the wild using global positioning systems (GPS) and satellite tracking technology (see Chapter 11) mean that epidemiologists are able to make more extensive use of this technology. Spatial database management systems available within GIS are important for managing location data of wild animals that are observed or captured, plus attribute data for each location. Mapping the data provides a strong visual means of conveying information on the distribution of known disease cases and the population at risk. GIS can be used to manipulate the data into a format suitable for spatial analyses and to display the results of the analyses, enabling patterns of disease to be explored and hypotheses to be developed about routes of transmission and risk factors. A major strength of GIS is the ability to overlay multiple layers of environmental data in conjunction with geographical data, such as animal locations and disease cases, facilitating the development of hypotheses about environmental risk factors and the development of habitat models associated with the disease and/or the population of interest. GIS are used to build spatial simulation models of disease in wildlife which are likely to reflect more accurately the spatial heterogeneity of populations and disease. GIS are also beginning to be incorporated into information systems and decision-support systems with simple user interfaces which enable them to be used by decision makers who are not familiar with GIS technology, taking this technology to a wider group. The aim of this chapter is to review the way in which GIS have been applied to research and management of diseases in wildlife populations.

10.2 Spatial distribution of wildlife disease

To represent the spatial distribution of disease in wildlife species, case and population data must be georeferenced, either to a single point location (a set of *x,y* coordinates) or to a geographical area which is defined by a digital boundary map, the latter being the only option when point coordinates are not available for data but the area from which it originated is known. A major challenge in spatially representing measures of disease, such as prevalence and incidence, in wildlife populations is obtaining an underlying distribution of the population at risk. Such population data are most commonly recorded by the government departments responsible for managing a country's natural resources, using government administrative boundaries such as regions, districts and census areas. However, these may not have any relationship to disease or environmental issues, and in the case of wildlife populations boundaries of national parks or river catchments may be more useful if digital boundary data and population data are available for such areas. For example, ecological zones were used by Barling *et al.* (2000) as the area unit in a study to identify the relationship between the prevalence of *Neospora caninum* in cattle in Texas and the density of wild canids.

The scale of interest will influence the precision of the spatial data, i.e. how accurately the recorded spatial data represent the location of the object of interest in the field. This in turn will influence how the data are georeferenced and the way in which they are displayed within a GIS. Representing disease over large geographical areas usually entails enlargement of the spatial grain, i.e. enlarging the spatial unit of interest, which is associated with less spatial precision and loss of fine-scale detail. Where fine-scale detail is required, i.e. the spatial grain is small, the geographical area that is covered is usually small in order to accommodate the logistical challenges of obtaining such detailed spatial information. Because the ways in which the spatial data can be used vary with the spatial quality of the data, the discussion on the application of GIS to represent the spatial distribution of disease in wildlife is divided into the two areas of broad-scale and fine-scale patterns.

10.3 Georeferenced data sources to represent broad-scale disease patterns

The challenging logistics and expense of capturing wild animals and testing them for disease make it difficult to apply direct capture methods over large geographical areas. As a result, studies to estimate broad-scale disease patterns in wildlife often use: (i) animals that are captured by hunters; (ii) measurements of disease in in-contact predator/scavenger species that are susceptible to the disease of interest; or (iii) measurement of disease in in-contact domestic animal/human populations, which are more accessible for testing.

Hunters provide a convenient source of samples for assessing wildlife disease distribution for species that are hunted on a commercial or recreational basis, by means of either field collection points or game packing houses, where wildlife carcases are processed for human consumption (Lugton *et al.*, 1998; Tackmann *et al.*, 1998; Bengston and Rogers, 2000; Kaneene *et al.*, 2000; Kramer *et al.*, 2000). The spatial data are as accurate as the precision with which hunters can recall the location at which they shot or captured the animal(s) and the precision with which this can be located on a digital map. As a result of these challenges, capture locations are often generalized to a county or region, or to a particular forest or wildlife park area.

In some cases, direct capture of wild animals is used, for example as a part of the North Australian Quarantine System. There are large areas of the north of Australia where no livestock are farmed and the wildlife population is monitored to identify any incursion of exotic disease along the northern coast. Because vastly extensive areas are involved, helicopters and fixed-wing planes are used to locate and capture animals for testing and GPS are used to record the geographical location of each animal sampled. This enables maps showing the location of tested animals to be drawn and to be combined with other geographical data, which may help stratify surveillance activities on the basis of the most likely location of populations of interest. In the large forest areas of New Zealand, where wild animals do not have direct contact with farmed animals, surveys for TB in feral deer (*Cervus elaphus*) and pigs (*Sus scrofa*) are conducted using direct capture methods. Helicopters are used to capture animals for testing and GPS units are used to record the capture locations. This enables accurate recording of the location of animals, which can then be mapped over aerial photographs or topographic maps of the forests to visualize the spatial distribution of samples. Having adequate spatial distribution of samples throughout the forest areas is extremely important in these surveys, as they are being used to determine the distribution of infected populations as a means of targeting disease control measures.

Creative use has been made of other sources of wild animal samples, such as animals killed by vehicles on roads, where the data are georeferenced using road maps or GPS. Data on road fatalities of badgers (*Meles meles*) collected by the Ministry of Agriculture, Fisheries and Food (MAFF; now DEFRA) during the mid-1980s has been used to supplement other sources of badger TB data to indicate broad disease patterns in the UK (personal communication, P. Durr).

Species that are higher in the food chain than the wildlife species of interest, such as predator or scavenger species, can often be useful indicators of the presence of disease in certain wildlife populations, particularly if the disease is transmitted by ingestion of infected material and the survival of the predator/scavenger animals is not affected by the disease. In this case the predator species are being used to sample the population of interest, with the advantage that the prevalence of disease is higher as one moves up the food chain. In addition to indicating the presence/absence of disease, data from these sources can indicate the relative abundance of disease in the species of interest. The brushtail possum (*Trichosurus vulpecula*) is the major wildlife reservoir of *Mycobacterium bovis* in New Zealand, but it is difficult to detect the disease in brushtail possums in the wild due to the highly clustered temporal and spatial pattern of the disease. Surveys of species that scavenge on dead brushtail possum carcasses, such as feral pigs and ferrets (*Mustela putorius furo*), have been more effective in identifying the presence or absence of disease in brushtail possums than in surveying possums themselves. Furthermore, the prevalence of disease in ferrets has been shown to reflect the abundance of disease in in-contact brushtail possum populations (Caley *et al.*, 2001).

Data from surveys of predator/scavenger species are georeferenced by: (i) assigning the data to a geographical area for which digital boundary data are available; (ii) using a GPS to record trap or capture locations; or (iii) manually digitizing locations using georeferenced topographic maps or aerial photographs as locational guides. Buffering the capture locations with areas that reflect the home range of the tested species may represent the geographical distribution of disease in the underlying species of interest. The precision with which these species identify the area in which infected animals exist in the underlying population depends on the size of their home range.

In areas where there is contact between the diseased wildlife population of interest and susceptible human or farmed animal populations, evidence of spread of infection to these populations is a useful indirect indication of the location of infected wildlife populations. Logistically, testing these populations is considerably easier than testing wildlife populations and as a result may provide more accurate information on the distribution of the disease in the wildlife population. Although mapping Lyme disease risk in Maryland on the basis of prevalence of infection in ticks was believed to be the most accurate method, tick data are often unavailable, out of date, costly and difficult to collect (Frank *et al.*, 2002). As an alternative, zip-code level data on the incidence of Lyme disease in humans was believed to be the most useful indicator of the risk of Lyme disease in this area. In New Zealand, the patterns of TB in farmed cattle indicate both the presence and the abundance of infection in in-contact brushtail possum populations. Cattle are tested for TB on a regular basis as a part of the TB control programme and these data provide a strong indication of the distribution of tuberculous brushtail possum populations, given that cattle-to-cattle spread of infection is minimal because of the regular testing programme. Cattle TB incidence can be mapped at the farm level using a digital map of farm boundaries (Sanson and Pearson, 1997). Analysis of spatial patterns in the incidence of cattle TB has been used to indicate spatial patterns of TB in possums in New Zealand (J.S. McKenzie (1999) The use of habitat analysis in the control of wildlife tuberculosis in New Zealand. Unpublished PhD thesis, Massey University, Palmerston North, New Zealand, http://epicentre.massey.ac.nz/Information_Theses.htm).

Disease patterns in domestic animal populations may also provide information on possible risks of infection for in-contact wildlife populations. A study of the spatial and temporal patterns of canine distemper virus infections in domestic dogs on the perimeter of Serengeti National Park provided an indication of a possible source of infection for a distemper outbreak in wildlife in the national park (Cleaveland *et al.*, 2000).

10.4 Mapping broad-scale disease data

10.4.1 Point data

At the simplest level, spatial disease data may be presented as points representing diseased cases only, with no information on the population at risk. While such data have limitations, maps of the distribution of cases of disease in wildlife can provide a broad picture of relative abundance of disease in different areas, with little or no consideration of the size of the population at risk. Such a map could be used to indicate broad geographical areas where there is a higher risk of wildlife disease being transmitted to human or farmed animal populations, which in turn could be used to set policy on the surveillance or movement of livestock in such areas. A map of the distribution of classical swine fever in wild pigs in Germany was obtained by serologically testing pigs shot by hunters (Kramer *et al.*, 2000). Tested pigs were georeferenced by allocating them to the municipality in which they had been shot. The data were mapped by representing each case as a point location randomly located within a municipality, indicating the areas of the country where more intensive surveillance for classical swine fever in domestic pigs needs to be conducted because of the risk of transmission from wild pigs (Fig. 10.1).

A sequence of maps showing the point locations of case data during successive time periods may also be used to represent the spatio-temporal changes of a disease. Animating such a temporal sequence of maps by generating TIFF images and displaying them as a movie using media player tools can highlight changes more acutely than viewing static maps (Kramer *et al.*, 2000).

Supplementing maps of point locations of case data with point locations of negative animals indicates the number and distribution of animals tested, providing a graphical representation of the raw data as shown in the map of foxes tested for *Trichinella spiralis* in Brandenburg, Germany (Fig. 10.2) (Wacker *et al.*, 1999).

Mapping the point locations of wild animals that have been tested as a part of a wildlife surveillance programme can support claims of disease freedom by providing a visual representation of the spatial distribution and intensity of testing. Information that indicates the number of animals tested within each location can also be presented using symbols scaled to the number of animals tested. This is illustrated in Fig.

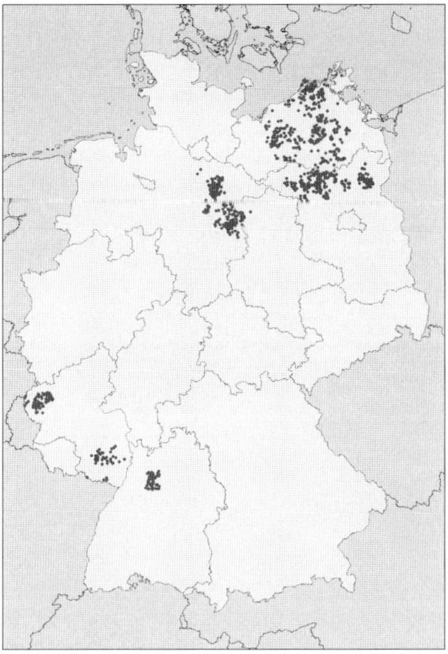

Fig. 10.1. Spatial distribution of classical swine fever (CSF) cases in wild boars in Germany between 1997 and 1999. One dot is equivalent to one CSF case. Reproduced with permission from Kramer *et al.* (2000).

10.3, which shows the spatial distribution of the number of possums captured in a TB survey in an area of New Zealand.

10.4.2 Area data

Mapping of disease measures such as prevalence or incidence requires aggregation of case data and population at-risk data within geographical areas for which digital boundaries exist. The disease measure is used as an attribute of each area, and is mapped as choropleth maps, defined as maps in which areas of equal value are separated from areas of different value by boundaries. Figure 10.2b shows a choropleth map of the prevalence of *T. spiralis* in foxes in Brandenburg, Germany. An important issue associated with analysis of area data is described as the modifiable areal unit problem, which refers to the fact that the map pattern can vary dramatically if the size and shape of the areal units forming the study region are altered. Quite different analytical results can be obtained by changing the configuration of the areal units (Bailey and Gatrell, 1995). Overlaying data from different sources can also be a challenge when the data have been aggregated into different areal units. For example, wildlife disease

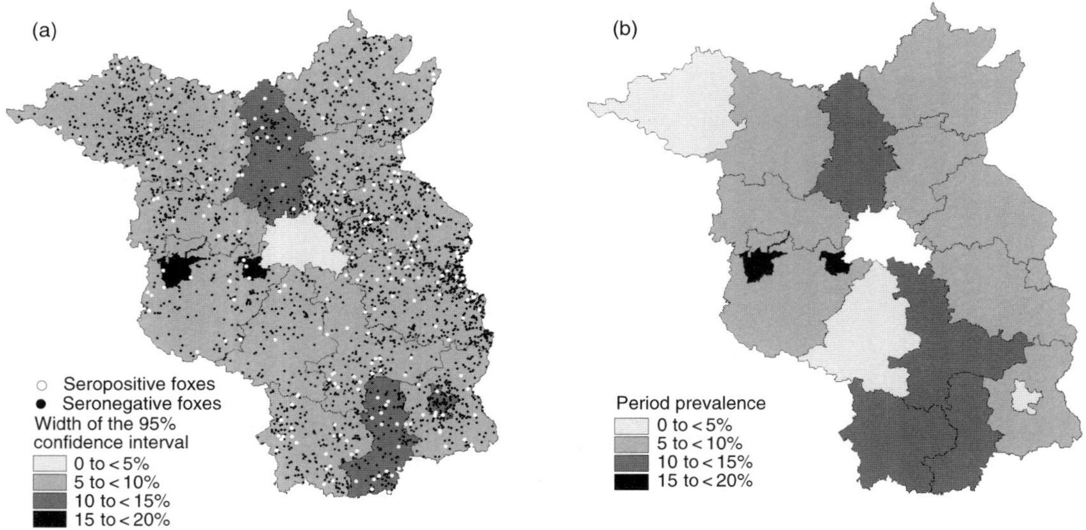

Fig. 10.2. Maps of the seroprevalence of *Trichinella spiralis* in hunter-gathered foxes in municipalities of Brandenburg, Germany. (a) Distribution of foxes serologically tested for *T. spiralis* overlaid on a choropleth map showing the 95% confidence interval for the prevalence estimate at the county level. (b) Seroprevalence of *T. spiralis* by county. Map (a) reproduced with permission from Wacker *et al*. (1999); Map (b) provided by Dr K. Wacker, Federal Research Centre for Virus Diseases of Animals, Institute for Epidemiological Diagnostics, Wusterhausen, Germany.

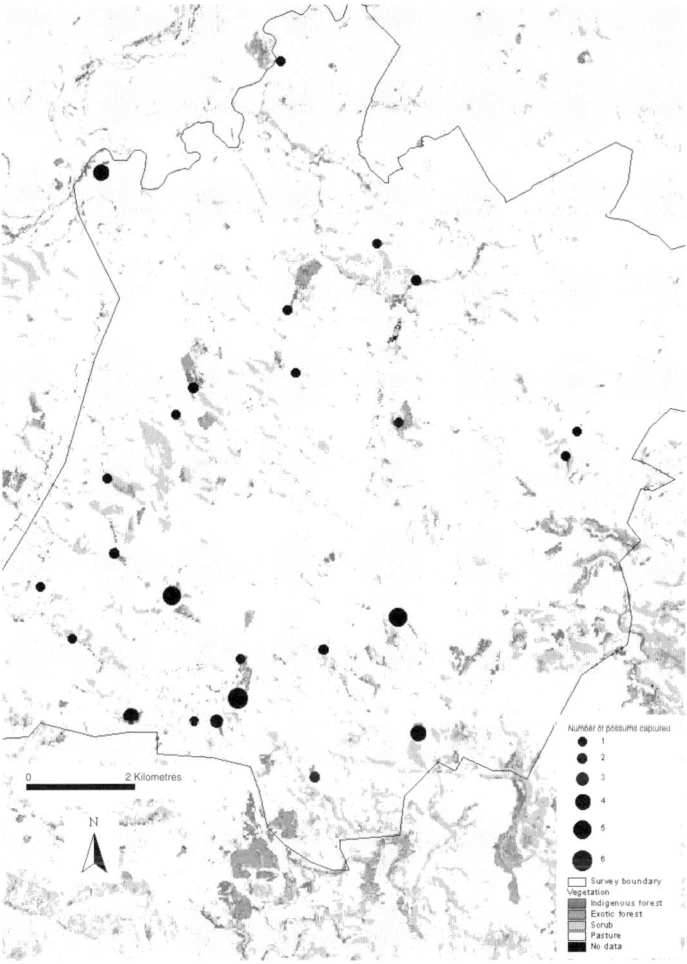

Fig. 10.3. Map of the spatial distribution of possums captured in a tuberculosis survey in the south-eastern North Island, New Zealand.

and population data may be based on government administrative areas, whereas some environmental data may be based on ecological zones. Combining data from different areal units can be challenging and methods to achieve this have been described (Bailey and Gatrell, 1995).

10.5 Data quality issues

Maps can be powerful visual tools but, like any representation of data, the quality of the information that they present is dependent on the quality of the data from which the maps are generated. One of the biggest challenges in obtaining measures of disease in wildlife populations is obtaining information on the size and distribution of the population at risk. The number of animals captured/killed and examined in wildlife surveys is commonly used as a best estimate of the population. However, this is frequently a biased sample, the bias varying with the method of animal collection. In hunter-based surveys, sampling intensity varies across the landscape as hunter effort tends to be focused where there is the best chance of obtaining animals, leading to spatial variation in the accuracy of disease measures. To help readers interpret maps of disease measures it is important to supplement these with maps of the quality of the data. Wacker *et al.* (1999) presented maps of the distribution of *T. spiralis* infection in hunter-gathered foxes in Brandenburg, Germany, together with a map of the width of the confidence interval surrounding prevalence estimates as an explicit indication of the quality of the data (Fig. 10.2a and b).

Hunters may also favour areas with more accessible habitat, resulting in over-representation of samples from certain habitat types and under-representation from others. Staubach *et al.* (2001) tested if the land cover characteristics of locations at which hunters caught foxes were statistically different from those in the study area by comparing the proportions of the different habitat types at a large number of randomly generated locations within 2.5 km buffers surrounding each capture location with proportions of the habitat types in the study area as a whole.

The age structure of hunter-gathered samples varies depending on the time of year, particularly if the hunting season is restricted to certain times of the year. Hunter-gathered samples also frequently under-represent older animals in the population (Pfeiffer and Hugh-Jones, 2002). This can result in a misleading picture of disease prevalence if there is variation in the prevalence within different age groups. For example, the prevalence of *Echinococcus multilocularis* is lower in fox cubs that have not been weaned than in adult foxes; thus, samples collected prior to May could underestimate the prevalence of infection compared with samples taken at other times of the year (Tackmann *et al.*, 1998). Because of the potential confounding effect of different age structures, the authors recommend that prevalence estimation may only be valid in age-stratified random samples, particularly if the age structure of the hunter-gathered sample varies between regions.

Cross-sectional surveys are a common method employed to gather disease information in wildlife. Individual cross-sectional studies have the major disadvantage that they do not account for temporal patterns of the population or of the disease, and reflect the disease situation at only one point in time. This may produce misleading results where there is temporal variation in disease prevalence; this may occur through variation in transmission rates as a result of behavioural aspects of the population, such as mating, juvenile dispersion, population migration and food sources. To obtain a more accurate picture, it is important to conduct repeated cross-sectional surveys or to conduct longitudinal studies where it is possible to identify individual animals and to recapture the animals and monitor their disease status. Where disease is not distributed randomly, it is important that the spatial scale of sampling matches the likely scale of clusters. Tackmann *et al.* (1998) suggest that surveys to estimate the prevalence of *Echinococcus multilocularis* in foxes in areas of low and moderate endemicity in Germany should be conducted using geographical units with a maximum area of 500 km^2, this being the area in which one can expect a homogeneous distribution of infection in foxes.

It may be useful to conduct studies at two levels: a very localized scale and a broader scale. There may be a trade-off between spatial coverage and temporal coverage if limited resources are available, and the aim of the study should be considered seriously so that the results are not compromised on both counts. For example, in a study of Sin Nombre virus (SNV) in deermice (*Peromyscus maniculatus*), Boone *et al.* (2000) opted for an emphasis on spatial coverage with less frequent temporal coverage. The advantage of this wider spatial approach was to capture ecological diversity and provide statistical replicates of sites with similar characteristics. The disadvantage was that there was less certainty in the infection status of each site. The authors note that 'When generalization of results is an important goal, a large replicated data set that has a modest degree of measurement error is statistically preferable to a smaller, more precisely measured but poorly replicated data set'.

10.6 Detailed disease patterns at smaller geographical scales

Exploratory spatial analysis techniques can be used to identify disease and population patterns which help develop hypotheses regarding the epidemiology of the disease (see Chapter 5). These techniques require data with comprehensive spatial coverage at a spatial scale that is fine enough to enable detection of disease clustering if it is present. Patchy data lead to less reliable results. Data sets of suitable quality for space and space–time analysis involve intensive animal capture–mark–recapture techniques and disease testing at time intervals that will capture short-term temporal fluctuation in disease, and should be conducted for a sufficiently long period to capture longer-term temporal patterns. There are very few examples of the application of such exploratory spatial analysis techniques to wildlife disease data, probably as a result of the challenging logistics of conducting such studies in wild animals.

There have been two major longitudinal studies of TB in wildlife populations that have incorporated GIS and spatial analytical techniques: an 11-year study of TB in brushtail possums in New Zealand (B.M. Paterson (1993) Behavioural patterns of possum and cattle which may facilitate the transmission of tuberculosis. MSc thesis, Massey University, Palmerston North, New Zealand, http://epicentre.massey.ac.nz/Information_Theses.htm; D.U. Pfeiffer (1994) The role of a wildlife reservoir in the epidemiology of bovine tuberculosis. Unpublished PhD thesis, Massey University, Palmerston North, New Zealand; R. Jackson (1995) Transmission of tuberculosis (*Mycobacterium bovis*) by possums. Unpublished PhD thesis, Massey University, Palmerston North, New Zealand, http://epicentre.massey.ac.nz/Information_Theses.htm; I.W. Lugton (1997) The contribution of wild animals to the epidemiology of tuberculosis in New Zealand. Unpublished PhD thesis, Massey University, Palmerston North, New Zealand, http://epicentre.massey.ac.nz/Information_Theses.htm; L.A. Corner (2001) Bovine tuberculosis in brushtail possums (*Trichosurus vulpecula*): studies on vaccination, experimental infection and disease transmission. Unpublished PhD thesis, Massey University, Palmerston North, New Zealand, http://epicentre.massey.ac.nz/Information_Theses.htm; S. Norton (2001) Bovine tuberculosis in the brushtail possum (*Trichosurus vulpecula*). Behaviour and the development of an aerosol vaccinator. Unpublished MSc thesis, Massey University, Palmerston North, New Zealand, http://epicentre.massey.ac.nz/Information_Theses.htm) and a 15-year study of TB in badgers (*Meles meles*) in the UK (Cheeseman *et al.*, 1981, 1988; Delahay *et al.*, 2000). Other longitudinal studies have analysed temporal disease patterns but not fine-scale spatial disease patterns (Boone *et al.*, 2000; Hazel *et al.*, 2000; Parmenter *et al.*, 2000).

Animal location data in these studies are principally georeferenced using GPS to record the coordinates of trap locations and other locations that have been identified through radio-tracking, such as den sites. Other options are manually digitizing the locations from georeferenced land cover maps, such as satellite images, aerial photographs and topographic maps, which provide spatial orientation, and reading *x,y* coordinates off topographic maps and manually entering these into a database which can be imported into a GIS. Attribute data representing the identification of the captured animal, disease status, sex, age, reproductive status, etc. are assigned to these locations and are used to map disease and population data. GIS are used to display descriptive spatial data, such as maps of capture locations of diseased and non-diseased animals. Prevalence and incidence measures of disease may be incorporated into maps in a number of ways: using symbols such as pie charts to indicate the magnitude of disease; using colour gradients to reflect different levels of disease; and three-dimensional mapping with the disease measure as the third dimension. Examples of the various ways of mapping data on TB infection in brushtail possums are shown in Pfeiffer and Hugh-Jones (2002). Spatial and temporal patterns of disease incidence may also be represented by incorporating charts of incidence during multiple time periods into a map, such as the map of the spatio-temporal distribution of *M. bovis* infection in badgers at Woodchester Park, Gloucestershire, UK (Delahay *et al.*, 2000) shown in Fig. 10.4. The spatial unit of interest in this study was not the individual animal location but the territory of a badger social group. The distribution of plastic pellets at latrines and field records of boundary runs were used to digitize social group territories on a 1:10,000 raster image of the study area using a GIS.

Maps of capture locations and disease data can be overlaid on various backdrop data, such as satellite images, aerial photographs, contour maps or a three-dimensional representation of the area, to view the data within the context of the environment in which they are located, as shown by Pfeiffer and Hugh-Jones (2002), or they may be schematically drawn to scale with no backdrop data, as shown in Fig. 10.4.

Mapping genetic subtypes of disease agents provides greater insight into patterns of transmission than mapping cases of disease. Michel and Maré (2000) investigated genetic subtypes to gain an insight into the pattern of spread of *M. bovis* through different wildlife species in the Kruger National Park. The authors found a direct correlation between geographical distance from the purported origin of infection and genetic distance, represented by the similarity index of different strains of the organism. They also found that only one genotype was found in the greater kudu, suggesting that a separate infection cycle was maintained within this species, whereas multiple genotypes were found in other animal species.

In the longitudinal study of TB in brushtail possums described above, spatial and space–time analyses of the different subtypes of *M. bovis* showed more tightly clustered temporal and spatial patterns of the spread of TB between brushtail possums, compared with analyses of all *M. bovis* infections (D.U. Pfeiffer (1994) The role of a wildlife reservoir in the epidemiology of bovine tuberculosis. Unpublished PhD thesis, Massey University, Palmerston North, New Zealand; R. Jackson (1995) Transmission of tuberculosis (*Mycobacterium bovis*) by possums. Unpublished PhD thesis, Massey University, Palmerston North, New Zealand, http://epicentre.massey.ac.nz/Information_Theses.htm; I.W. Lugton (1997) The contribution of wild animals to the epidemiology of tuberculosis in New Zealand. Unpublished PhD thesis, Massey University, Palmerston North, New Zealand, http://epicentre.massey.ac.nz/Information_Theses.htm; L.A. Corner (2001) Bovine tuberculosis in brushtail possums (*Trichosurus vulpecula*): studies on vaccination, experimental infection and disease transmission. Unpublished PhD thesis, Massey University, Palmerston North, New Zealand, http://

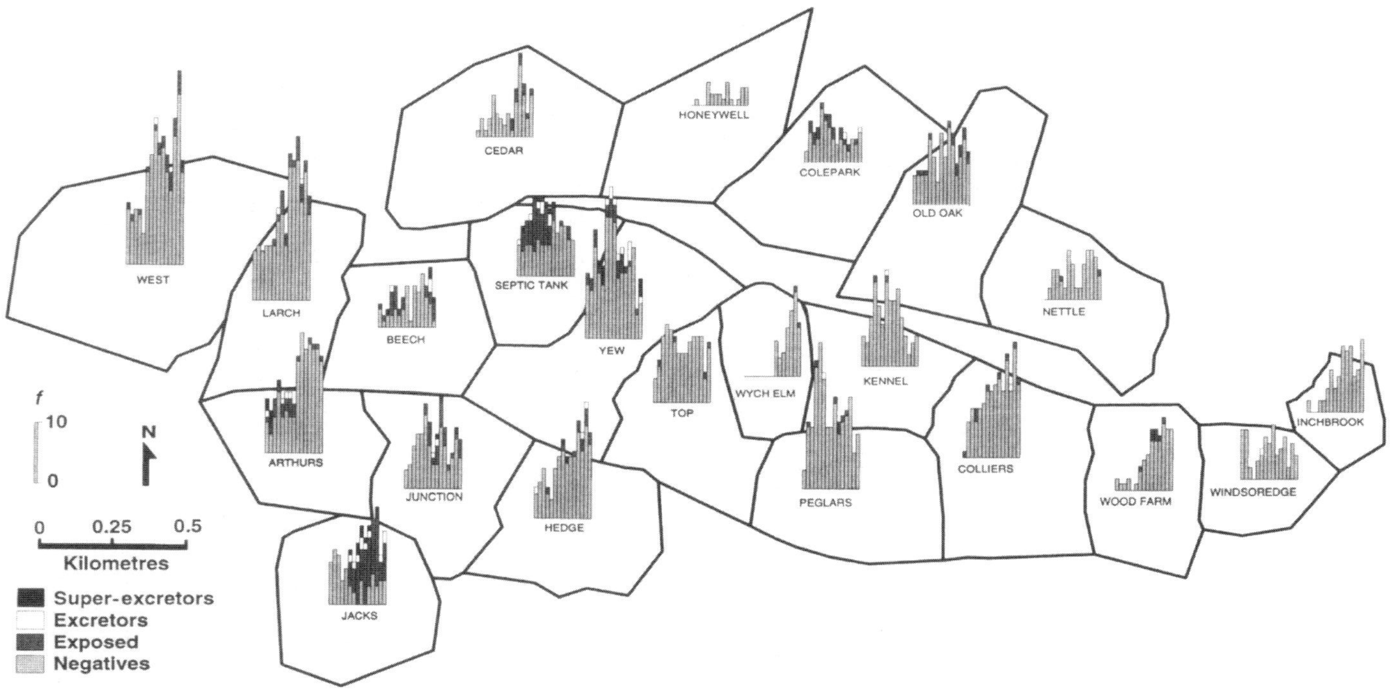

Fig. 10.4. Thematic map showing the spatiotemporal distribution of *Mycobacterium bovis*-infected badgers at Woodchester Park, UK. Graphs show the annual frequencies of badgers (1982–1996) that were negative, exposed to *M. bovis*, *M. bovis* excretors, and super-excretors. The map shows a schematic representation of the boundaries of badger social groups, but accurately reflects the relative positions of groups and distances between groups that persisted throughout the study. Reproduced with permission from Delahay *et al*. (2000).

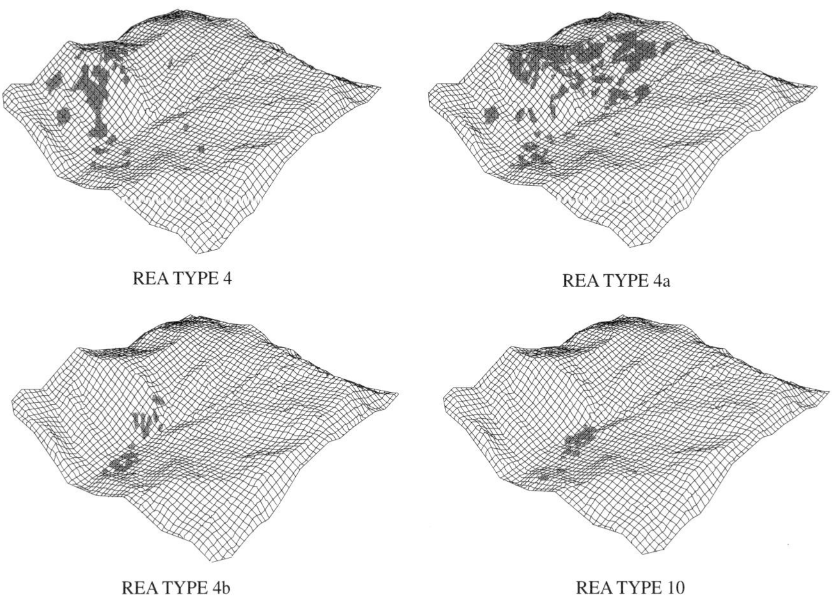

Fig. 10.5. Spatial distribution of restriction endonuclease (REA) types of *Mycobacterium bovis* isolates based on den site locations used by tuberculous possums during a longitudinal study of tuberculosis in possums in the south-east of North Island, New Zealand. Reproduced with permission from Pfeiffer (1994).

epicentre.massey.ac.nz/Information_Theses.htm). The spatial distribution of dens used by brushtail possums infected with *M. bovis* in the first 2 years of the longitudinal study, subdivided on the basis of restriction endonuclease type, is shown in Fig. 10.5. The two major subtypes were focused in different locations within areas of high den density and the two minor subtypes were in areas of low den density. This supports the hypothesis that transmission of *M. bovis* was most likely to occur in areas of high den density.

Some exploratory analytical techniques for spatial data may be used within commercial GIS software; for example, kernel smoothing and kernel extraction methods. However, GIS are generally limited in this area and a broader range of techniques is available in specialized spatial analysis software (see Chapter 5). These packages interface with a GIS, which is used to extract the appropriate data for analysis and to display the results of the analysis. Viewing descriptive maps of fine-scale disease patterns and the results of exploratory analysis can help in the development of hypotheses about possible mechanisms of transmission and risk factors associated with the observed wildlife disease patterns.

10.7 Spatial behaviour of animals

An important component of the study of diseases in wildlife populations is the identification of the spatial behaviour of individuals. This may include identifying home ranges, denning ranges or social activity ranges of individual animals within a population, defining territorial boundaries of individuals or social groups of animals, or identifying dispersal patterns. Displaying the ranges of interest in a GIS facilitates identification of the temporal and spatial overlap of animals within the same species or with those of other species, which may provide insights into routes of disease transmission (Loveridge and MacDonald, 2001). Comparing the spatial behaviour of diseased and non-diseased animals can provide insights into the effect of the disease on individuals and potential opportunities for transmission (Greenwood *et al.*, 1997). Overlaying the spatial extent of an animal's location on other environmental data within a GIS facilitates the building of habitat models for predicting the location of populations over wider geographical areas. Understanding the spatial behaviour of animals is also an important part of developing simulation models of disease in wildlife populations.

There are many methods employed to gather data on locations of animals, including radio-tracking animals fitted with radio collars (Paterson *et al.*, 1995) or injectable passive integrative transponders (Mills and Childs, 1998), satellite tracking, trapping (D.U. Pfeiffer (1994) The role of a wildlife reservoir in the epidemiology of bovine tuberculosis. Unpublished PhD thesis, Massey University, Palmerston North, New Zealand), viewing large animals from vehicles or aeroplanes (Khaemba and Stein, 2000) and the use of coloured pellets administered in feed for badgers – these are visible in the latrines and mark the extremities of the territory of a social group (Delahay *et al.*, 2000). Various techniques can be used to georeference the locations of interest, including GPS, radiotelemetry, which requires at least two reference points with known geographical coordinates (Paterson *et al.*, 1995), and manual digitization of points.

Many analytical methods have been developed to transform the observed set of point locations into an area representing the activity range of interest, the most common being estimation by the minimum convex polygon, harmonic mean and kernel density methods. However, each of these produces a different result with the same data (Staubach *et al.*, 2000). As an example, Fig. 10.6 shows the varying home range estimates for hedgehogs (*Erinaceus europaeus*) on farmland in New Zealand using minimum convex polygons and kernel density estimators (R.J. Gorton (1998) A study of tuberculosis in hedgehogs so as to predict the location of tuberculous possums. Unpublished MSc thesis, Massey University, Palmerston North, New Zealand, http://epicentre.massey.ac.nz/Information_Theses.htm). Furthermore, many factors influence the

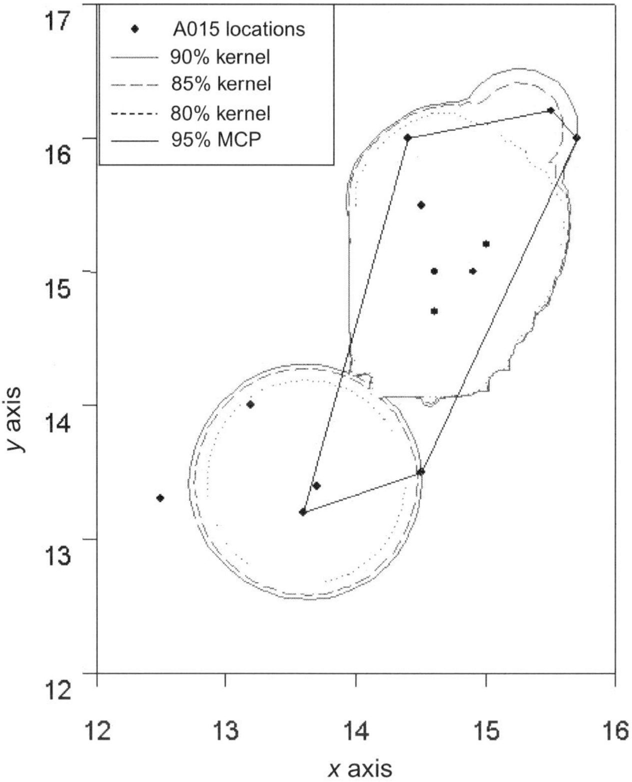

Fig. 10.6. Recorded locations and home range estimates for a female hedgehog (A015) on farmland in the south-east of North Island, New Zealand, showing the variation in areas that arise from different home range estimation methods. The 95% minimum convex polygon (MCP) and kernel density estimates show the 80, 85 and 90% probability isopleths. Units on the *x* and *y* axes are 100-m intervals. Reproduced with permission from Gorton (1998).

calculated area of home ranges, including the number of fixes recorded for an animal, the age of the animal, gender, season and time of day (Staubach *et al.*, 2000). As a result of these many influences, care must be exercised when comparing home range estimates between animals within a study and between different studies.

In some cases, ranges can be estimated in the absence of individual animal movement data. Having identified the location of major badger setts, Hazel and French (2000) estimated the extent of a social group's territory without data on individual badger movements, using Thiessen distance polygons. Thiessen polygons are generated from a set of observed points by dividing the region so that the polygon surrounding each point is closer to the sample point than any other sampled location (Bailey and

Gatrell, 1995). Estimated home range areas may be generated in a GIS by buffering an individual animal's capture location with an area representing the mean home range size for that species. Such areas are most commonly overlaid on environmental data in a GIS to identify habitat factors associated with the location of animals.

10.8 Habitat modelling of wildlife populations and of infected subpopulations

The logistical difficulties of locating wildlife species throughout large geographical areas make predicting their distribution using GIS-based habitat modelling a very useful tool. Guisan and Zimmermann (2000) provide an in-depth review of this area, covering the various steps of predictive modelling from the formulation of the conceptual model to prediction and application. Gough and Rushton (2000) reviewed the different GIS modelling approaches that have been used to investigate the influence of landscape on distributions of Mustelidae, dividing the approaches into two broad categories: associative and process-based modelling. Associative models attempt to determine relationships between the distribution of a species and environmental features without explicitly modelling the population processes of birth, death and dispersal, while process-based models attempt to simulate these key processes within the landscape with the hope that the distribution of the animals will arise as an emergent property. This chapter discusses applications of GIS-based associative modelling, while process-based models are discussed in the chapter on simulation modelling (Chapter 7).

Associative modelling is based on the identification of relationships between the incidence of the species and measured landscape characteristics, usually land-use or vegetation characteristics but also other habitat characteristics considered to have an influence on the distribution of the animals, such as water availability, temperature, elevation and human disturbance. These relationships can potentially be used to predict the distribution of the species in other areas, given information about the landscape. There are many examples of associative habitat modelling in the literature, ranging from simple rule-based models (Ji and Jeske, 2000) to more complex models with mathematical linkages between the distribution of a species and environmental data, such as discriminant analysis (Boone *et al.*, 2000; Guerra *et al.*, 2002), regression techniques (Pereira and Itami, 1991; Lindenmayer *et al.*, 1995; Khaemba and Stein, 2000) and Bayesian modelling (Aspinall, 1992). Habitat models are developed from smaller, focused studies in which it is feasible to obtain detailed data on the distribution of the species and on associated habitat factors (Breininger *et al.*, 1998; McAlpine *et al.*, 1998; Kurki *et al.*, 2000; Staubach *et al.*, 2001), and the results are generalized to predict the distribution of the species over a wider geographical area (Austin *et al.*, 1996; Roseberry and Sudkamp, 1998; Roseberry and Woolf, 1998). Some studies have used GIS in the development of models while others have not. In all cases, GIS-based modelling is the most efficient means of predicting the distribution of a species over large geographical areas. The accuracy of the predicted distribution is dependent on the accuracy with which the digital geographical data used in a GIS represent key habitat factors that influence the distribution of the species of interest.

Habitat may be represented in different ways, the most common being classification into vegetation types or land-cover categories, with the classes represented as the absolute or proportional area of each class. Satellite imagery is a cost-effective source of data from which to derive habitat variables. Images may be classified into land-cover classes or used to produce vegetation indices, the most common being the normalized difference vegetation index (NDVI), which reflects proportional vegetation cover (Haines-Young and Chopping, 1996; Goetz *et al.*, 2000). Landscape pattern analysis provides more detail on the spatial configuration as well as the composition of habitat. Specialized landscape pattern analysis software that interfaces with GIS generates a wide range of landscape variables, including area metrics, patch density, patch size and variability metrics, edge metrics, shape metrics, core area metrics, nearest-neighbour metrics, diversity metrics and contagion and interspersion metrics. Examples of landscape analysis software include: (i) FRAGSTATS (McGarigal and Marks, 1994; McGarigal *et al.*, 2002); (ii) PATCH ANALYST (http://flash.lakehead.ca/~rrempel/patch), which is an extension of ARCVIEW (ESRI, Redlands, CA, USA) that facilitates the spatial analysis of landscape patches and includes a user interface to FRAGSTATS; and (iii) APACK (http://landscape.forest.wisc.edu/projects/APACK/apack.html). Colour Plate 21 shows an example of two levels of homogeneity of habitat on farms, as measured by the contagion metric in FRAGSTATS, in a study to identify farm-level habitat patterns associated with the risk of cattle being exposed to tuberculous brushtail possums (McKenzie *et al.*, 2002).

There are many factors that influence the ability of a study to identify linkages between habitat factors and species distribution (Wilson, 1998). It is important that the scale at which the study is undertaken relates to the scale at which the species of interest interacts with the environment. A study of habitat factors associated with the distribution of elephants will be based on much larger spatial units and a larger geographical area (Khaemba and Stein, 2000) than a study of mice (Boone *et al.*, 2000). There are many issues associated with sampling the population to estimate species distribution accurately, such as the spatial scale used to capture variations in population density and the temporal scale used to capture fluctuations in population density. Both Khaemba and Stein (2000) and Parmenter *et al.* (2000) discuss methods to sample a dynamic population, such as trapping webs, distance sampling and adaptive sampling, which may improve data on species distribution.

A frequent problem encountered in testing the association between disease frequency and geographical risk factors is that the results of a study conducted in one geographical location may not be applicable to another location with different climatic and topographic conditions. Where possible, it is useful to identify the underlying mechanism that is driving the disease process and which is represented by a particular habitat factor. The results can then be generalized to different geographical locations by identifying the local habitat factors associated with the underlying driving factor. For example, analysis of habitat factors in different environments has shown that individual clusters of TB-infected brushtail possums are associated with localized clusters of favourable brushtail possum den sites, which in turn leads to localized crowding of brushtail possums and an increased contact rate, which maintains the disease in such locations (McKenzie and Meenken, 2001). Different habitat is associated with favourable den sites in different geographical locations, and this association can be used to identify habitat with a higher risk of containing clusters of TB-infected brushtail possums in different areas.

Landscape epidemiology involves the application of a landscape ecology approach to understand landscape risk factors associated with diseases (Kitron, 1998). The success of landscape epidemiology in identifying habitat risk factors for disease depends on the disease dynamics and distributions for the population of interest being closely related to measurable habitat variables at a scale that reflects these relationships (Li *et al.*, 2000). Habitat has been successfully used to predict the distribution of diseases with invertebrate vectors, as these species have relatively narrow habitat tolerances. There are fewer examples of the use of habitat to predict the distribution of diseases in wild vertebrate vector species. Boone *et al.* (2000) analysed habitat patterns associated with Sin Nombre virus infection in deermice using eight broad vegetation classes within map units of 100 hectares. McKenzie *et al.* (2002) used a GIS and landscape pattern analysis software to generate habitat and topographic variables that were included in regression analyses to identify farm-level environmental factors that were significantly associated with the risk of cattle being infected with TB by contact with infected possums. Staubach *et al.* (2001) evaluated topographic and habitat factors associated with the distribution of foxes infected with *E. multilocularis* in Germany.

The density of host populations is often considered a common risk factor for infection, and predictors of localized areas of high-density population may be used as a de facto for predicting areas where there is a higher risk of diseased animals being present (McKenzie and Meenken, 2001). However, density effects are scale-dependent and it is important to be looking at the appropriate scale to find any positive association. In the case of Sin Nombre virus in deermice, no simple relationships between host density and antibody prevalence were found, but more complex non-linear relationships appeared to exist (Boone *et al.*, 2000). In the case of TB in brushtail possums there is no association between prevalence of TB and density of population at a large scale, but there is at a very localized scale of less than 1 hectare (Hickling, 1995). The association with disease may be a function not just of density but of connectivity of localized populations. For example, Boone *et al.* (2000) hypothesized that the prevalence of Sin Nombre virus in deermice was lower in salt desert scrub, despite some local dense patches of mice, as there were fewer mice overall and a lower probability of contact between neighbouring populations.

Having identified habitat associations with the distribution of a species or of infected subpopulations, GIS provide tools for building models that combine the data from layers of significant environmental factors and produce a map of distribution using Boolean logic, weighted combinations or probabilistic relationships (Pfeiffer and Hugh-Jones, 2002). Models of the interface between wild animal and livestock populations and the probability of disease transmission between the two have been developed, using habitat as the basis for predicting animal distribution. Howe and Dalrymple (2000) used a spatially integrated disease risk assessment model (SIDRAM) to estimate the risk of brucellosis spreading on the basis of the probability that cattle will come in contact with aborted elk fetuses. The model consists of two parts: (i) spatial modelling of elk feeding grounds and natural habitat where forage availability modelling indicates that there is sufficient forage to support elk should they be dispersed from the feeding ground, and (ii) an integrated disease model to estimate the likelihood of an elk abortion occurring within a defined time step. In a second paper, Howe *et al.* (2000) combined SIDRAM and a spatial ecology model, SAVANNA, which generated population density maps and migration patterns for wildebeest plus the pastoral movement patterns of Maasai cattle. Population density maps for wildebeest were determined through the literature and wildlife models for forage availability during the wet and dry seasons. The SIDRAM model was used to intersect the cattle and wildebeest maps within pixels of 25 km^2 at weekly intervals, and to identify periods when the populations of both species were large enough to support the transmission of infection between the two species.

10.9 Applications of GIS in surveillance and management of wildlife disease

GIS are a powerful tool for surveillance and the management of wildlife diseases, particularly to target disease surveillance and disease control efforts and to record the application of surveillance and control measures on a spatial basis.

10.9.1 Surveillance

Habitat maps are a useful tool to stratify surveillance in wildlife species where links have been made between the distribution of the species of interest and measurable habitat factors (see previous section). The use of such maps can lead to more efficient use of resources by focusing effort on the areas where the species is most likely to be found. Likewise, links between disease distribution and habitat can be used to further stratify surveillance to areas where both the species and the disease are more likely to be found. *Uncertainty maps* can be used to target surveillance in areas where there are gaps in information on the disease status of wildlife populations. There are often multiple sources of information that can contribute to surveillance of diseases in wildlife. By combining maps of data from each source, a spatial orientation of past surveillance activities can be obtained, from which gaps in information can be identified. Uncertainty is defined in this surveillance context as the confidence that one has in the available information on the disease status of a population within an area of interest. For example, different sources of information that contribute to an understanding of the spatial distribution of TB in brushtail possums in New Zealand include on-farm TB testing of cattle and deer, slaughterhouse surveillance for TB lesions in cattle and deer, brushtail possum surveys, surveys of other wildlife species, including ferrets, pigs and deer, individual farmer submissions for the post-mortem examination of sick or dead brushtail possums or ferrets found on their farm, and research projects into TB in wildlife species. Several of the research projects and wildlife surveys are conducted by different organizations, including the regional councils responsible for TB-associated brushtail possum control, AgriQuality NZ (responsible for TB control in livestock) and the Department of Conservation (responsible for the conservation of native flora and fauna). Thus, information is held by different organizations.

Obtaining and overlaying maps of the data from each of these sources can enable a certainty index to be generated for each spatial area of interest. For example, Colour Plate 22 shows a map combining three sources of information on TB status of the underlying brushtail possum population: farms on which cattle have been TB-tested, a survey of ferrets, and a hunter-based survey of deer. These have been overlaid on a vegetation map to provide contextual information on possum habitat. The areas where the TB status of brushtail possums is uncertain, i.e. where there is either no information or very patchy information, have been identified and outlined in red. Surveillance activities can be planned to ensure that these areas are given priority, either by ensuring that livestock have been tested or by conducting additional wildlife surveys. These data can be used in either a qualitative or a quantitative way. Certainty could be quantified by allocating to each source of information a value that represents the certainty one has in regarding disease status as a result of the information. Combining this value across multiple layers would be most easily achieved by converting the data for each layer to raster format and using GIS tools to sum the certainty value across layers, producing a summary certainty value, which could be mapped as a new layer representing the certainty of information of disease status across an area.

Use of a spatial filter within a GIS has been recommended as a technique to identify 'holes' in data as a means of improving surveillance systems that are dependent on notifications of disease cases, such as rabies in raccoons (Curtis, 1999). The method compares the number of cases reported for an area of interest, in this case a county, with that in surrounding counties, using the county as the spatial filter. Repeated randomization of all reported cases across the counties is used to test if the observed number of reported cases in any one county is significantly different from the expected number. The detection of a reporting rate that is significantly lower than expected can provide the basis for investigation of the reasons for the lower reporting rates; possible reasons include a lower detection rate because of a lower human–animal interaction rate due to sparse human and/or animal populations, errors in reporting procedures, and a lower rate of disease. Methods to improve the surveillance system can then be implemented where appropriate.

Using a GIS to generate spatially random points can assist the implementation of wildlife surveys. Several scripts have been prepared to implement this, including Cameron's Survey Toolbox (http://www.ausvet.com.au) and others on the ESRI website (http://arcscripts.esri.com). The generation of points can be restricted to selected polygons within vector coverages of areas of interest. For example, maps of preferred brushtail possum habitat are used to stratify placement of random points for monitoring brushtail possum culling operations carried out in New Zealand as a part of the TB management programme (Fig. 10.7).

10.9.2 Management of wildlife disease

Risk maps can be used to identify areas where there is evidence of a higher risk of disease, as a means of targeting control measures more intensively in such areas. Mapping the incidence of Lyme disease in humans at the zip-code level was found to provide more detailed information than mapping the incidence at the county level, revealing some areas with high incidence that were not obvious in county-level measures because of dilution with neighbouring low-incidence zip-code areas (Frank *et al.*, 2002). This information enables public health efforts to be focused to reduce tick exposure in humans and to increase the

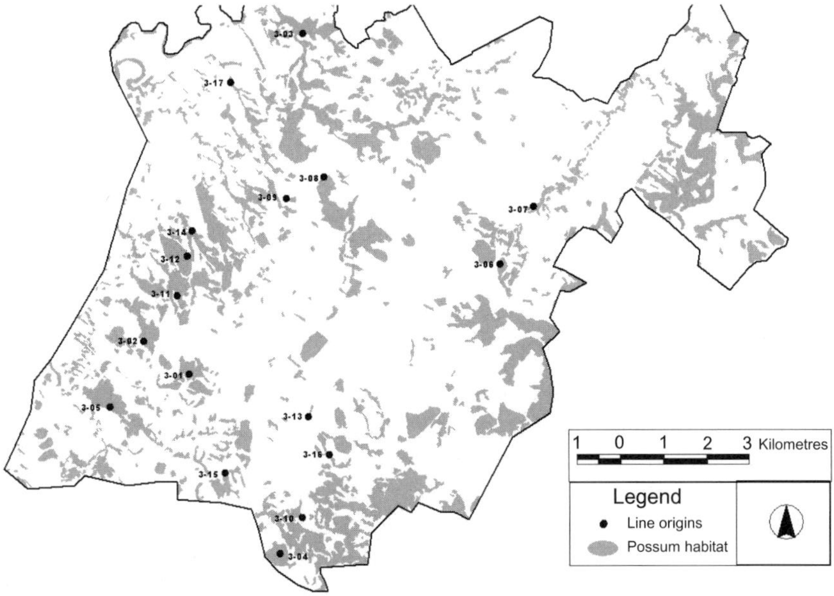

Fig. 10.7. Location of randomly generated start points for trap lines used to monitor the residual density of possums following a cull operation carried out in New Zealand as a part of the TB management programme. Points have been generated within the layer of possum habitat shown in the map. Source of data: J. Lambie, Wellington Regional Council, Masterton, New Zealand.

motivation to use appropriate preventive measures when tick exposure is unavoidable. Farm-level maps of the cumulative incidence of TB in cattle are used as an indication of areas where infected brushtail possum populations are most likely to be located, and the intensity of brushtail possum control is stratified on this information. At a smaller geographical scale, maps of the risk of TB in the brushtail possum associated with habitat can be used to target control efforts within farms (McKenzie *et al.*, 2002).

GPS technology can improve the precision with which control is applied, which can both reduce costs and reduce the risk of environmental contamination if poisons are involved. GPS can also provide an accurate georeferenced record of the geographical area over which control has been applied, by either aerial or ground-based application methods. Attribute data, such as the date of application, operator and control methods, can be stored with the geographical data, providing a historical record of the area over which control was applied. The areas of control can be mapped in a GIS and used to identify gaps in application. Boundaries of control areas may be overlaid on maps of disease incidence, such as maps of farm-level TB incidence in cattle, which represent the incidence of TB in brushtail possums, to evaluate the effectiveness of control and to develop future control strategies.

A further use of GIS in wildlife disease control is the generation of three-dimensional terrain images. In areas where digital terrain data are available to ortho-rectify aerial photographs or satellite images, very realistic images of the area in which control will be applied can be produced in a GIS, enabling operators to evaluate the logistics of working in targeted areas, particularly with respect to issues such as access and terrain. Three-dimensional imaging can be conducted in most of the sophisticated GIS software packages and a three-dimensional analyst add-on is available for ArcView.

Decision-support systems are emerging as useful tools in the management of a number of animal health problems, and a few of these are designed to incorporate spatial data and geographical analyses (Morris *et al.*, 1993). The advantage of such systems is that they can combine complex analytical tools, simulation models and expert systems within one piece of software with a customized interface that makes these tools accessible to decision makers without them having to understand the analytical methods. The advantage of such a system is that it provides field managers with access to spatial information without having to understand how to run a GIS.

An example of a decision-support system that is being developed to manage a wildlife disease is EpiMAN-TB, which is principally designed to assist with the development of effective strategies for the control of TB in brushtail possums in New Zealand (http://epicentre.massey.ac.nz). EpiMAN-TB has four main functions that support possum control decisions:

- Classification of patches of habitat by their risk of supporting tuberculous possums.
- Evaluation of the effectiveness of TB control programmes in possum populations at the farm level using simulation modelling.
- Evaluation of the effectiveness of TB control programmes in possum populations at the regional level using simulation modelling.
- Classification of farms according to the risk of TB possums being present on the farm.

These functions are implemented by combining tools such as a relational database, map display and spatial analysis tools, simulation models of TB in possums at the farm level and at the regional level, and expert systems as illustrated in Fig. 10.8. A key geographical function of the software is a model that combines rasterized vegetation and slope layers to produce a brushtail possum TB risk map, referred to as the 'hotspot predictor'. The resulting risk map can be displayed with vector data, such as a farm boundary, to identify patches of habitat with the highest risk of brushtail possum TB hotspots. Figure 10.9 shows a map

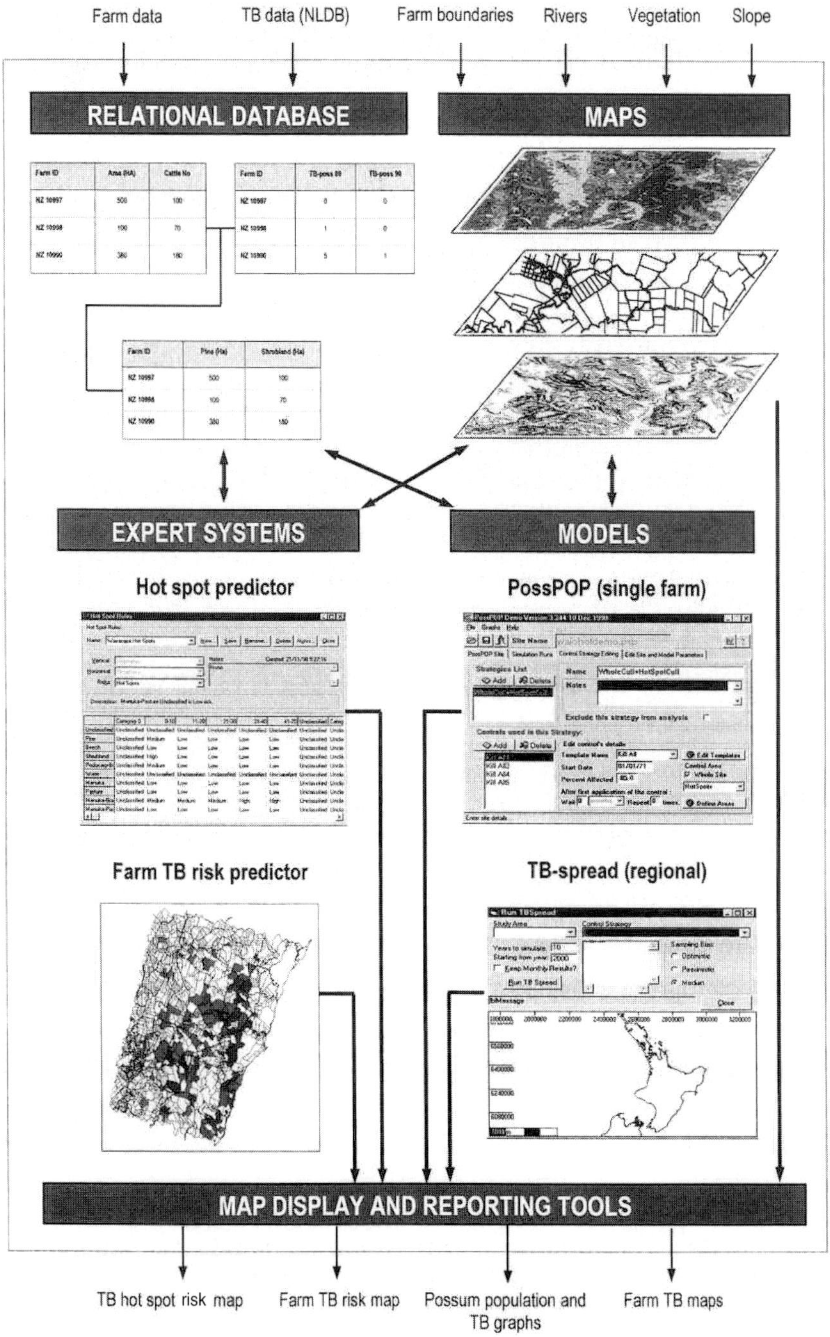

Fig. 10.8. An overview of the structure of EpiMAN-TB (http://epicentre.massey.ac.nz).

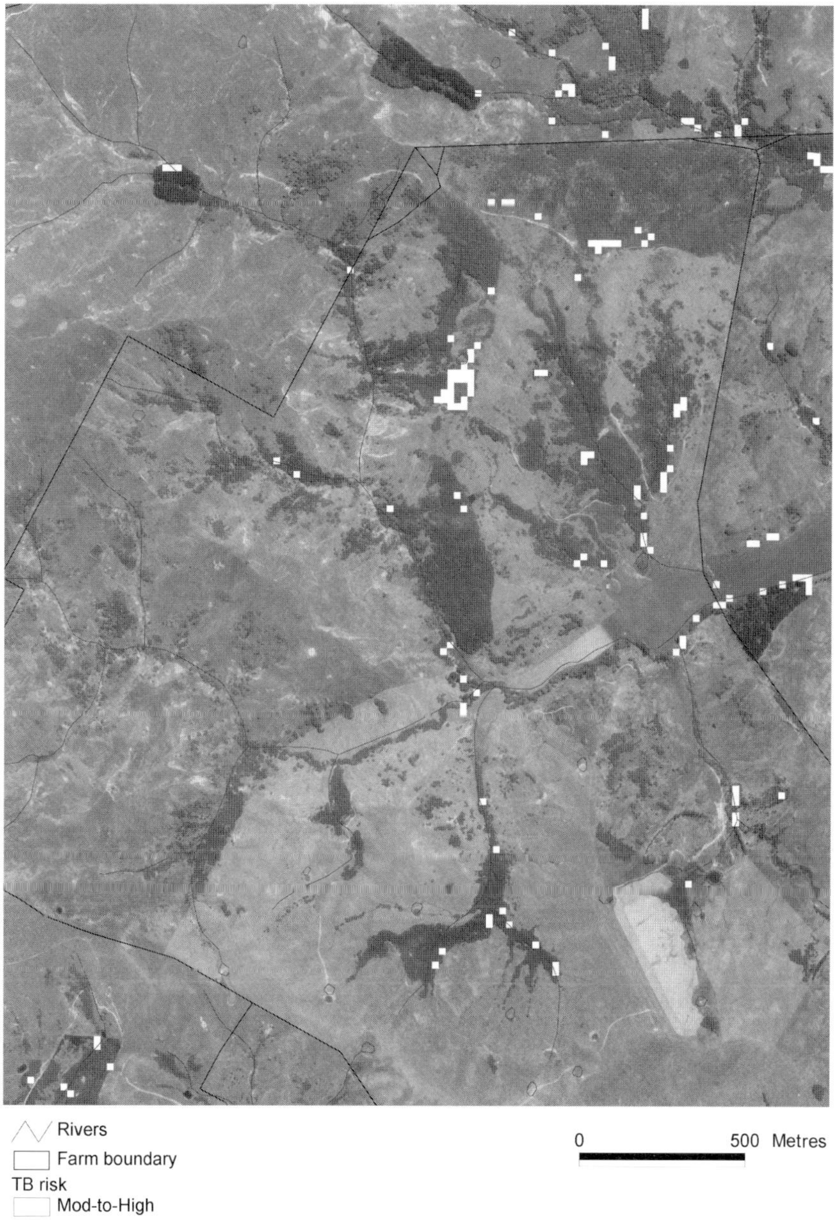

Fig. 10.9. Map of moderate-to-high risk possum hotspots for tuberculosis overlaid on an aerial photograph of a farm to assist with planning an on-farm tuberculosis management programme.

of areas predicted to have a moderate to high risk for TB in brushtail possums. The risk data have been overlaid on an aerial photograph of a farm to provide contextual data, which would assist in planning a TB control programme for the farm.

EpiMAN-TB also incorporates the possum TB simulation model PossPOP, a geographical model representing the ecology and infection dynamics of wild brushtail possum populations (D.U. Pfeiffer (1994) The role of a wildlife reservoir in the epidemiology of bovine tuberculosis. Unpublished PhD thesis, Massey University, Palmerston North, New Zealand). The model uses a real vegetation map in raster format to populate the model with both possums and den sites for the area of interest in the simulation. This gives users the flexibility to model different habitat patterns and to examine the effects of varying control strategies in these. The model can also use the hotspot risk map to adjust the probability of TB transmission between possums, such that it is higher within hotspot areas than outside them. The principal purpose of the model is to evaluate alternative TB control strategies in brushtail possum populations. Strategies can be applied to the whole area being modelled or may be specified for subareas, which can be digitized on-screen. Incorporating the model in the EpiMAN-TB decision-support system provides a user-friendly interface to the model, in particular an interface to select vegetation and possum TB risk maps to run the model for user-defined areas such as specific farms.

10.10 Incorporating GIS into wildlife disease information systems

GIS technology has developed to support the management of spatial data within a standard database management system using tools such as ArcSDE (ESRI, Redlands, CA, USA). This provides a seamless link between spatial and attribute data, maintained within a standard database management system. It is particularly useful for large dynamic databases in which the data are constantly being updated. An information system is being developed in New Zealand to manage the wildlife vector control programme for TB management (personal communication, T. Ryan). This is a NZ$50,000,000 programme involving a large number of culling operations, predominantly of brushtail possum and ferret populations, which are conducted in different areas of the country, and which involve various control methods, delivery systems, frequency, geographical coverage, etc. This national information system will provide a centralized database of the operations based on an 'operational area' as the geographical unit of interest. An operational area is the area covered by a particular culling operation. The system will include geographical coordinates for the boundary of each operational area plus attribute details such as date of control, control methods, contractor and postoperational residual possum numbers (referred to as 'residual trap catch'). The system will be web-based, using ArcIMS (ESRI) as the web-mapping engine. This will allow the uploading of boundaries of operational areas, which have been digitized by regional operators, to the central database via the web, together with attribute data. Such a centralized system enables data from individual areas to be maintained in a standardized format, which will facilitate the use of operational data for research and the evaluation, for example, of the cost-effectiveness of the various control strategies with respect to TB eradication.

Web mapping provides a means of distributing geographical information to a wider audience without the need for each user to have access to a GIS. Clients of web systems require a PC with a web browser but do not need to use GIS software. This can lead to improved efficiencies by maintaining geographical data plus GIS technology and associated expertise at a centralized location where geographical data are processed and maps are produced for distribution via the web. The spatial functionality that can be hosted by the web is considerably more limited than that offered by a GIS, most applications allowing read-only access to the data. Thus the main function is to display maps. The viewer can select the features to be mapped by turning layers on and off, and can scale the view in or out to obtain the required level of detail for their particular purpose. The capabilities to update spatial information via the web are still limited. Some packages will support the insertion of new point locations via the web. However, digitizing and editing of line features is not yet routinely supported. Current developments will allow greater data-editing capability via the web.

An example of this technology can be seen in the web mapping system that has been developed to support surveillance for varroa mite (*Varroa destructor*) infection in honey bees (*Apis mellifera*) in New Zealand (personal communication, R. Sanson). All hives have been georeferenced using a GPS or by reading coordinates off a topographic map, and the data are maintained in a central database. Field officers are able to use the web to produce maps of the hives in their area, which they can then use to develop a programme for visiting hives as a part of the varroa surveillance programme (see Chapter 9). Cases of infection may also be mapped, as can the boundaries of infected areas and buffer zones, which can be used as a guide to appropriate surveillance measures. Web mapping is also used to support the TB management programme in New Zealand (based on the JShape Java applet: http://www.jshape.com) (personal communication, R. Sanson). This system includes data on infected herds by year, represented either as point locations or farm boundaries depending on the scale at which the map is drawn. Other data include multiple layers of topographic data and boundaries of disease control areas. The system allows users to capture new point features, such as the location of a farm homestead or dairy shed. This facility could equally be used to enter point locations of wild animal captures or sightings into a centralized database.

10.11 Conclusions

There have been significant developments in the remote sensing industry that have made it more feasible to collect location data on wild animals, notably GPS and satellite tracking, which enable researchers and managers of wildlife disease to make greater use of GIS. Although it is getting easier to collect more accurate spatial data on wild animals, the major limitation in the application of GIS in the wildlife disease area still lies in the quality of data available for use in the system, because of the logistical challenges of sampling wild animal populations. It is extremely important to understand the biases inherent in data sets being used, and to present maps reflecting spatial patterns of data quality alongside maps of disease measures and disease distribution. When analysing spatial data to identify disease patterns, it is important to be aware of the spatial quality of the data; aspects of data quality include the thoroughness with which the geographical units of interest have been sampled, and whether the gaps in the data are randomly distributed or clustered, the latter being more likely to lead to erroneous conclusions being drawn from spatial pattern analysis.

There is increasing interest in the area of landscape epidemiology to identify environmental risk factors for disease in wild animals and to predict the distribution of populations. The increasing availability of more detailed satellite imagery and more accurate image classification methods, such as the removal of the topographic effect in images, is providing improved data for this application. However, the success of these methods depends on the specificity of habitat use by the species of interest and is more challenging when applied to vertebrate species, which tend to have more generalized habitat requirements compared with invertebrate species. A creative approach is needed to make links between the distribution of species or infected animals and measurable habitat variables, using factors such as the availability of food sources, nest sites and protection from predators for species distribution, and factors that influence the contact rate of animals and, where appropriate, the survival of infective agents in the environment for the distribution of infected animals.

The application of GIS technology to wildlife disease has been predominantly confined to the research domain. However, the improved access to spatial data and the development of veterinarians' skills in using GIS through training programmes is resulting in greater application of the technology in the operational domain. As efforts to include wild animal populations in surveillance and exotic disease response plans increase, greater use needs to be made of GIS to communicate the results of surveillance activity using maps, and to use environmental data plus maps of past surveillance activities to stratify future efforts so that resources are used in the most cost-effective way. There is a need for veterinarians who understand the potential applications of GIS to work with GIS specialists who can provide support by managing spatial data sets, accessing data, customizing GIS software, developing web systems etc., in order to promote the effective use of the technology in surveillance and the management of wildlife disease.

In conclusion, the increase in available spatial data associated with the increase in veterinarians' understanding of how these data may be used, plus the development of web technology and decision support systems, which bring the technology to a wider audience, will all enhance the application of GIS as a valuable tool in the research and management of wildlife disease.

References

Aspinall, R. (1992) An inductive modelling procedure based on Bayes' theorem for analysis of pattern in spatial data. *International Journal of Geographical Information Systems* 6, 105–121.

Austin, G.E., Thomas, C.J., Houston, D.C. and Thompson, D.B.A. (1996) Predicting the spatial distribution of buzzard *Buteo buteo* nesting areas using a geographical information system and remote sensing. *Journal of Applied Ecology* 33, 1541–1550.

Bailey, T.C. and Gatrell, A.C. (1995) *Interactive Spatial Data Analysis*. Longman, Harlow, UK.

Barling, K.S., Sherman, M., Peterson, M.J., Thompson, J.A., McNeill, J.W., Craig, T.M. and Adams, L.G. (2000) Spatial associations among density of cattle, abundance of wild canids, and seroprevalence to *Neospora caninum* in a population of beef calves. *Journal of the American Veterinary Medical Association* 217, 1361–1365.

Bengis, R.G. (Coordinator) (2002) *Infectious Diseases in Wildlife: Detection, Diagnosis and Management.* Office International des Épizooties, Paris.

Bengis, R.G., Kock, R.A. and Fischer, J. (2002) Infectious animal diseases: the wildlife/livestock interface. *Revue Scientifique et Technique Office International des Epizooties* 21, 53–65.

Bengston, S.D. and Rogers, F.R. (2000) Prevalence of sparganosis by county of origin in Florida feral swine. In: Salmon, M.D., Morley, P.S. and Ruch-Gallie, R. (eds) *Proceedings of the 9th Symposium of the International Society for Veterinary Epidemiology and Economics, Breckenridge, Colorado, August 6–11, 2000*, pp. 1321–1323.

Boone, J.D., McGwire, K.C., Otterson, E.W., DeBaca, R.S., Kuhn, E.A., Villard, P., Brussard, P.F. and St Jeor, S.C. (2000) Remote sensing and geographical information systems charting Sin Nombre virus infections in deer mice. *Emerging Infectious Diseases* 6, 248–258.

Breininger, D.R., Larson, V.L., Duncan, B.W. and Smith, R.B. (1998) Linking habitat suitability to demographic success in Florida scrub-jays. *Wildlife Society Bulletin* 26, 118–128.

Caley, P., Hone, L.J. and Cowan, P.E. (2001) The relationship between prevalence of *Mycobacterium bovis* infection in feral ferrets and possum abundance. *New Zealand Veterinary Journal* 49, 195–200.

Cheeseman, C.L., Jones, G.W., Gallagher, J. and Mallinson, P.J. (1981) The population structure, density and prevalence of tuberculosis (*Mycobacterium bovis*) in badgers (*Meles meles*) from four areas in south-west England. *Journal of Applied Ecology* 18, 795–804.

Cheeseman, C.L., Wilesmith, J.W., Stuart, F.A. and Mallinson, P.J. (1988) Dynamics of tuberculosis in a naturally infected badger population. *Mammalian Review* 18, 61–72.

Cleaveland, S., Appel, M.G.J., Chalmers, W.S.K., Chillingworth, C., Kaare, M. and Dye, C. (2000) Serological and demographic evidence for domestic dogs as a source of canine distemper virus infection for Serengeti wildlife. *Veterinary Microbiology* 72, 217–227.

Curtis, A. (1999) Using a spatial filter and a geographic information system to improve rabies surveillance data. *Emerging Infectious Diseases* 5, 603–606.

Deem, S.L., Karesh, W.B. and Weisman, W. (2001) Putting theory into practice: wildlife health in conservation. *Conservation Biology* 15, 1224–1233.

Delahay, R.J., Langton, S., Smith, G.C., Clifton-Hadley, R.S. and Cheeseman, C.L. (2000) The spatio-temporal distribution of *Mycobacterium bovis* (bovine tuberculosis) infection in a high-density badger population. *Journal of Animal Ecology* 69, 428–441.

Frank, C., Fix, A.D., Pena, C.A. and Strickland, G.T. (2002) Mapping Lyme disease incidence for diagnostic and preventive decisions, Maryland. *Emerging Infectious Diseases* 8, 427–429.

Goetz, S.J., Prince, S.D. and Small, J. (2000) Advances in satellite remote sensing of environmental variables for epidemiological applications. In: Hay, S.I., Randolph, S.E. and Rogers, D.J. (eds) *Remote Sensing and Geographical Information Systems in Epidemiology*. Academic Press, London, pp. 289–307.

Gough, M.C. and Rushton, S.P. (2000) The application of GIS-modelling to mustelid landscape ecology. *Mammalian Review* 30, 197–216.

Greenwood, R.J., Newton, W.E., Pearson, G.L. and Schamber, G.J. (1997) Population and movement characteristics of radio-collared striped skunks in North Dakota during an epizootic of rabies. *Journal of Wildlife Diseases* 233, 226–241.

Guerra, M.A., Walker, E.D., Jones, C., Paskewitz, S., Cortinas, M.R., Stancil, A., Beck, L., Bobo, M. and Kitron, U. (2002) Predicting the suitability of Lyme disease: habitat suitability for *Ixodes scapularis* in the north central United States. *Emerging Infectious Diseases* 8, 289–297.

Guisan, A. and Zimmermann, N.E. (2000) Predictive habitat distribution models in ecology. *Ecological Modelling* 135, 147–186.

Haines-Young, R. and Chopping, M. (1996) Quantifying landscape structure: a review of landscape indices and their application to forested landscapes. *Progress in Physical Geography* 20, 418–445.

Halpin, K., Young, P.L., Field, H. and Mackenzie, J.S. (1999) Newly discovered viruses of flying foxes. *Veterinary Microbiology* 68, 83–87.

Hazel, S.M. and French, N.P. (2000) The effect of habitat on the spatial ecology of badgers and the implications for the epidemiology of bovine tuberculosis. In: Salmon, M.D., Morley, P.S. and Ruch-Gallie, R. (eds) *Proceedings of the 9th Symposium of the International Society for Veterinary Epidemiology and Economics, Breckenridge, Colorado, August 6–11, 2000*, pp. 626–628.

Hazel, S.M., Bennett, M., Chantrey, J., Bown, K., Cavanagh, R., Jones, T.R., Baxby, D. and Begon, M. (2000) A longitudinal study of an endemic disease in its wildlife reservoir: cowpox and wild rodents. *Epidemiology and Infection* 124, 551–562.

Hickling, G. (2000) Clustering of tuberculosis infection in brushtail possum populations: implications for epidemiological simulation models. In: Griffin, F. and de Lisle, G. (eds) *Tuberculosis in Wildlife and Domestic Animals. Proceedings of the Second International Conference on Mycobacterium Bovis, University of Otago, 28 August–1 September, 1995.* University of Otago Press, Dunedin, New Zealand, pp. 174–177.

Howe, R. and Dalrymple, M. (2000) A spatially integrated brucellosis model for elk/livestock interactions in the Greater Yellowstone Area. In: Salmon, M.D., Morley, P.S. and Ruch-Gallie, R. (eds) *Proceedings of the 9th Symposium of the International Society for Veterinary Epidemiology and Economics, Breckenridge, Colorado, August 6–11, 2000*, pp. 629–631.

Howe, R., Boone, R., DeMartini, J., McCabe, T. and Coughenour, M. (2000) A spatially integrated disease risk assessment model for wildlife/livestock interactions in the Ngorongoro conservation area of Tanzania. In: Salmon, M.D., Morley, P.S. and Ruch-Gallie, R. (eds) *Proceedings of the 9th Symposium of the International Society for Veterinary Epidemiology and Economics, Breckenridge, Colorado, August 6–11, 2000*, pp. 629–631.

Ji, W. and Jeske, C. (2000) Spatial modeling of the geographic distribution of wildlife populations: a case study in the lower Mississippi River region. *Ecological Modelling* 132, 95–104.

Kaneene, J.B., Fitzgerald, S.D., Schmitt, S., Miller, R.A., Bruning-Fann, C., O'Brien, D. and Judge, L. (2000) Epidemiological studies of *Mycobacterium bovis* in wildlife and domestic livestock, Michigan, USA. In: Salmon, M.D., Morley, P.S. and Ruch-Gallie, R. (eds) *Proceedings of the 9th Symposium of the International Society for Veterinary Epidemiology and Economics, Breckenridge, Colorado, August 6–11, 2000*, pp. 1217–1219.

Khaemba, W.M. and Stein, A. (2000) Use of GIS for a spatial and temporal analysis of Kenyan wildlife with generalised linear modelling. *International Journal of Geographical Information Science* 14, 833–853.

Kitron, U. (1998) Landscape ecology and epidemiology of vector-borne diseases: tools for spatial analysis. *Journal of Medical Entomology* 35, 435–445.

Kramer, M., Fiedler, J., Teuffert, J., Selhorst, T. and Schlüter, H. (2000) Classical swine fever among wild boar – experiences of large-scale surveillance in Germany. In: Salmon, M.D., Morley, P.S. and Ruch-Gallie, R. (eds) *Proceedings of the 9th Symposium of the International Society for Veterinary Epidemiology and Economics, Breckenridge, Colorado, August 6–11, 2000*, pp. 1324–1326.

Kurki, S., Nikula, A., Helle, P. and Linden, H. (2000) Landscape fragmentation and forest composition effects on grouse breeding success in boreal forests. *Ecology* 81, 1985–1997.

Li, H.B., Gartner, D.I., Mou, P. and Trettin, C.C. (2000) A landscape model (Leemath) to evaluate effects of management impacts on timber and wildlife habitat. *Computers and Electronics in Agriculture* 27, 263–292.

Lindenmayer, D.B., Ritman, K., Cunningham, R.B., Smith, J.D.B. and Horvath, D. (1995) A method for predicting the spatial distribution of arboreal marsupials. *Wildlife Research* 22, 445–456.

Loveridge, A.J. and MacDonald, D.W. (2001) Seasonality in spatial organization and dispersal of sympatric jackals (*Canis mesomelas* and *C. adustus*): implications for rabies management. *Journal of the Zoological Society of London* 253, 101–111.

Lugton, I.W., Wilson, P.R., Morris, R.S. and Nugent, G. (1998) Epidemiology and pathogenesis of *Mycobacterium bovis* infection of red deer (*Cervus elaphus*) in New Zealand. *New Zealand Veterinary Journal* 46, 147–156.

Mbassa, G.K., Pereka, A.E., Matovelo, J.A., Mgasa, M.N., Kaita, M. and Mwangalimi, M.O. (2000) Risks and causes of mortalities in wild ungulates of Tanzania. In: Salmon, M.D., Morley, P.S. and Ruch-Gallie, R. (eds) *Proceedings of the 9th Symposium of the International Society for Veterinary Epidemiology and Economics, Breckenridge, Colorado, August 6–11, 2000*, pp. 1201–1204.

McAlpine, C.A., Mott, J.J. and Sharma, P. (1998) Mapping the kangaroo habitat mosaic in a semi-arid rangeland using vegetation survey and thematic mapper data. *Geocarto International* 13, 5–18.

McGarigal, K. and Marks, B.J. (1994) FRAGSTATS: spatial pattern analysis program for quantifying landscape structure. Version 2.0. USDA Forest Service General Technical Report PNW-351. http://www.umass.edu/landeco/pubs/pubs

McGarigal, K., Cushman, S.A., Neel, M.C. and Ene, E. (2002) FRAGSTATS: spatial pattern analysis program for categorical maps. Version 3.0. Computer software program produced by the authors at the University of Massachussetts, Amherst. www.umass.edu/landeco/research/fragstats/fragstats.html

McKenzie, J.S. and Meenken, D. (2001) *Spatial Clustering of Low-density Possum Populations and Association with Habitat.* Animal Health Board Report, EpiCentre, Massey University, Palmerston North, New Zealand.

McKenzie, J.S., Morris, R.S., Pfeiffer, D.U. and Dymond, J.R. (2002) Application of remote sensing to enhance the control of wildlife-associated *Mycobacterium bovis* infection. *Photogrammetric Engineering and Remote Sensing* 68, 153–159.

Michel, A.L. and Maré, L. (2000) The molecular epidemiology of *Mycobacterium bovis* infection in the Kruger National Park, South Africa. In: Salmon, M.D., Morley, P.S. and Ruch-Gallie, R. (eds) *Proceedings of the 9th Symposium of the International Society for Veterinary Epidemiology and Economics, Breckenridge, Colorado, August 6–11, 2000*, pp. 1205–1207.

Mills, J.N. and Childs, J.E. (1998) Ecological studies of rodent reservoirs: their relevance for human health. *Emerging Infectious Diseases* 4, 529–538.

Morris, R.S., Sanson, R.L., McKenzie, J.S. and Marsh, W.E. (1993) Decision support systems in animal health. In: Thrusfield, M.V. (ed.) *Proceedings of the Society for Veterinary Epidemiology and Preventive Medicine, University of Exeter, 31st March – 2nd April, 1993*, pp. 188–199.

Parmenter, C.A., Yates, T.L., Parmenter, R.R. and Dunnum, J.L. (2000) Statistical sensitivity for detection of spatial and temporal patterns in rodent population densities. *Emerging Infectious Diseases* 5, 118–125.

Paterson, B.M., Morris, R.S., Weston, J. and Cowan, P.F. (1995) Foraging and denning patterns of brushtail possums, and their possible relationship to contact with cattle and the transmission of bovine tuberculosis. *New Zealand Veterinary Journal* 43, 281–288.

Pereira, J.M.C. and Itami, R.M. (1991) GIS-based habitat modelling using logistic multiple regression: a study of the Mt. Graham red squirrel. *Photogrammetric Engineering and Remote Sensing* 57, 1475–1486.

Pfeiffer, D.U. and Hugh-Jones, M. (2002) Geographical information systems as a tool in epidemiological assessment and wildlife disease management. *Revue Scientifique et Technique Office International des Epizooties* 21, 91–102.

Roehrig, J.T., Layton, M., Smith, P., Campbell, G.L., Nasci, R. and Lancotti, R.S. (2002) The emergence of West Nile Virus in North America: ecology, epidemiology and surveillance. *Current Topics in Microbiology* 267, 195–221.

Roseberry, J.L. and Sudkamp, S.D. (1998) Assessing the suitability of landscapes for northern bobwhite. *Journal of Wildlife Management* 62, 895–902.

Roseberry, J.L. and Woolf, A. (1998) Habitat–population density relationships for white-tailed deer in Illinois. *Wildlife Society Bulletin* 26, 252–258.

Sanson, R. and Pearson, A. (1997) Agribase – a national spatial farm database. In: *Proceedings of the VIII International Symposium on Veterinary Epidemiology and Economics, Paris, 8–11 July, 1997*, pp. 12.16.1–12.16.3.

Staubach, C., Stiebling, U., Ziller, M., Tackmann, K., Thulke, H.H. and Schlüter, H. (2000) The consequences of using different analysis techniques on wildlife study data to model disease transmission. In: Salmon, M.D., Morley, P.S. and Ruch-Gallie, R. (eds) *Proceedings of the 9th Symposium of the International Society for Veterinary Epidemiology and Economics, Breckenridge, Colorado, August 6–11, 2000*, pp. 885–887.

Staubach, C., Thulke, H.H., Tackmann, K., Hugh-Jones, M. and Conraths, F.J. (2001) Geographic information system-aided analysis of factors associated with the spatial distribution of *Echinococcus multilocularis* infections of foxes. *American Journal of Tropical Medicine and Hygiene* 65, 943–948.

Tackmann, K., Löschner, U., Mix, H., Staubach, C., Thulke, H.-H. and Conraths, F.J. (1998) Spatial distribution patterns of *Echinococus multilocularis* (Leuckart 1863) (Cestoda: Cyclophyllidea: Taeniidae) among red foxes in an endemic focus in Brandenburg (Germany). *Epidemiology and Infection* 120, 101–109.

Wacker, K., Rodriguez, E., Garate, T., Geue, L., Tackmann, K., Selhorst, T., Staubach, C. and Conraths, F.J. (1999) Epidemiological analysis of *Trichinella spiralis* infections of foxes in Brandenburg, Germany. *Epidemiology and Infection* 123, 139–147.

Wilson, M.L. (1998) Distribution and abundance of *Ixodes scapularis* (Acari: Ixodidae) in North America: ecological processes and spatial analysis. *Journal of Medical Entomology* 35, 446–457.

Resources Guide: Software, Data and GisVet Web

11

Peter A. Durr, Nigel Tait and Christoph Staubach

11.1 Introduction

Spatial epidemiology involves obtaining data and using software as well as understanding fundamental geographical concepts and learning how to think spatially about disease (see Chapter 2). The first two of these tasks can both be challenging, even allowing for the comparative user-friendliness of modern desktop GIS and the accessibility of a range of spatial data sets via the World Wide Web. A key constraint is that a considerable investment is needed to obtain a GIS package and spatial data, and thus for those on a limited research budget, getting things right the first time can make or break the project.

In this section we provide some advice on these matters. This guidance reflects our experience, and all the comments must be taken as informed opinions rather than definitive judgements. We also introduce an initiative, the GisVet Web site (http://www.gisvet.org) to provide an information gateway to those wishing to commit to the use of GIS in animal health for the long term.

11.2 Which GIS software package?

The first commercial GIS software (ArcInfo) was released only in 1982, but due to the enormous increase in the use of GIS in retailing, government and the utilities, there are now a large number of packages on the market. As these are all mature products, generally using sophisticated graphical user interfaces (GUIs), they resemble each other superficially.

However, this belies differences in how the geographical data are stored and handled, and especially how they interact with other essential software, such as databases, spreadsheets, statistical analysis software and drawing packages. One way of classifying GIS software is via its provenance; it may have been originally designed for desktop cartography, querying and manipulation of vector objects (points, lines and polygons) or for processing remotely sensed images. Although many packages now have the capacity to do all three tasks, they either require the purchase of extensions or do not perform all these functions equally well. ArcView, MapInfo and idrisi are the predominant GIS currently used in animal health research and disease control, and here we provide a brief introduction, focusing particularly on their strengths and limitations.

ArcInfo, from ESRI (http://www.esri.com), has managed to retain its strong position, the last major release (8.0) being in 2000. This release represented a significant revision, with major changes including the introduction of a GUI, the replacement of the proprietary macro language (AML) with Visual Basic for Applications (VBA), and more sophisticated data storage, essentially replacing the 'Info' component with a single unified object-oriented database structure. There has also been convergence with its sister package, ArcView, which, although originally introduced as a desktop GIS package in 1991 to compete with MapInfo (see below), quickly became the preferred software in many universities and research institutes. This arose particularly from the ease with which it allowed users to develop their own tailor-made extensions and modules through a sophisticated scripting language (Avenue), furthered by the support ESRI gave to developers via their website. The recent release of ArcView 8.0 saw the replacement of Avenue by VBA; this new version has an improved GUI and superior string manipulation, mathematical functionality and memory management. Nevertheless, the object model is much harder to learn and program. Furthermore, the introduction of VBA to replace Avenue has made hundreds of Avenue extensions unusable, and no doubt has been an important reason why the migration of users from ArcView 3.2 to ArcView 8.0 has been slower than anticipated. ESRI seems to have taken note and continues to develop the 'old' ArcView, a new version of which (3.3) was issued in April 2003.

MapInfo Professional 1.0, released by MapInfo (http://www.mapinfo.com) in 1985, was designed to run on personal computers (PCs) rather than Unix workstations, the platform then used by most GIS software. Designed for small to medium-sized businesses, its philosophy was that '20% of GIS functionality would satisfy 80% of users'. From the outset it was menu-driven and had an intuitive task-based interface, so that activities such as geocoding, basic spatial queries and the production of maps could be performed quickly and simply with a minimum of training. Although MapInfo has lost its distinctive advantage as other GIS vendors have largely adopted many of these features, it is still a more user-friendly package than most of its rivals. The most recent version of MapInfo Professional (7.0) was released in 2002, the main change being its improved database connectivity. However, it still lacks many key spatial analytical tools and in particular it cannot do sophisticated raster (grid) manipulations. In addition, it has had more limited involvement from its user community in developing freeware extensions as compared with ESRI's ArcView.

The package idrisi was first released around the same time as MapInfo Professional 1.0, but shares little else in its provenance, having been developed by a team of academics in the Geography Department at Clark University in Worcester, Massachusetts (http://www.clarklabs.org). The impetus for its initial development came largely from the United Nations Environment Programme (UNEP), whose interest was in developing appropriate software for environmental monitoring, particularly through the use of remote sensing. This meant that idrisi initially used a raster (grid) as its fundamental data model, as opposed to the vector model of ArcInfo and MapInfo. However, with the release of idrisi32 in 2000 its capacity to handle vector data was considerably enhanced. Nevertheless, its strength still lies in raster manipulation, which, besides the processing of remotely sensed imagery, now includes sophisticated spatial modelling. This enables, for example, dynamic cell-based ('cellular automata') modelling, Bayesian classification and statistical procedures such as regression.

The total cost of investing in a GIS package can be considerable, if one includes the investment in time that is needed to learn how to master it. Accepting the need to provide a recommendation as to which package to buy, and at some risk of offending partisans of each package, we offer the following suggestions:

- For generalist epidemiologists essentially wanting to produce simple maps of where animal disease occurs and/or to explore such data infrequently with the minimum of learning effort, MapInfo Professional is probably the best choice.
- For regular users of spatial data, the ESRI products are undoubtedly the best choice, as there is more sophisticated data manipulation capacity and associated tools to support them. The more difficult question currently is which product to choose (ArcInfo 8.3, ArcView 8.3 or ArcView 3.3). There is currently no easy answer to this question, but hopefully a consensus will arise soon and be accessible on many of the web GIS discussion forums, such as those at the ESRI Support Center (http://support.esri.com).
- idrisi is the preferred solution for anyone wishing to undertake intermediate-level analysis of remote sensing data, particularly if the

interest is in investigating (and modelling) change over time. IDRISI also comes with two excellent training manuals, which serve as one of the better introductions to the processing of remotely sensed imagery. It is also the cheapest package and includes novel analytical methods.

As a final note, analysis of spatial data does not always require a GIS. Database management systems, as general-purpose software products, can store and also analyse large amounts of geographical data sets without visualization. Spatial extensions to relational database systems, such as IBM DB2, Informix, Microsoft SQL Server and Oracle, provide the software to store, manage, edit and query large spatial data sets in a multi-user environment. These extensions support spatially indexed data in vector, image and raster format that can be accessed and queried by different GIS clients.

11.3 Obtaining spatial data

One of the surprises for those purchasing a commercial GIS for the first time is how little effective work can be done with the data that are supplied. This tends to comprise some sample data sets to permit the completion of introductory exercises, and it is then up to the new user to obtain their own spatial data. This is a task which generally proves more costly (in time as well as money) than the initial software purchase. This is recognized by the vendors, who nowadays provide listings of data suppliers on their websites; an example being ESRI's Geography Network (http://www. geographynetwork.com).

The *critical data set* is a vector base-map of the country of interest, providing as a minimum the coastline and/or national borders, and preferably subnational boundaries, roads, rivers and major towns (Table 11.1). In countries with long-established national mapping agencies, such data sets are readily available, but they can be expensive and prices tend to rise rapidly with increasing detail and spatial resolution. For example, in the UK the Ordnance Survey (http://www.ordsvy.gov.uk) produces a number of vector data sets, the cheapest that covers all of Great Britain (Strategi) costing 'only' £2000. By contrast, the most complete (MasterMap) costs almost £100,000 for a 30 × 30 km area.

As many countries either do not have national mapping agencies or have not commercialized their spatial data, a third-party industry has grown up to supply it. This is a specialized area in which companies or institutes concentrate on different themes and/or areas of the world. For example, the EROS data centre (http://edc.usgs.gov) is the central data repository for free and commercial data of the US Geological Survey. Similarly, ACASIAN (http://www.asian.gu.edu.au), a university-based research institute in Queensland, Australia, has become a clearing house for a large amount of digital data for China and south Asia. Reflecting to some extent their monopoly position for these data, prices are high: the non-academic cost of a digital map of China's administrative boundaries at 1:1,000,000 costs US$2500 and yearly updates cost US$250.

Many of the third-party suppliers of both vector data and gazetteers (see below) derived their data initially from the pioneering Digital Chart of the World, which was released in 1992 and provided the first readily available digital data set with global coverage. This can be bought from a number of vendors (e.g. ESRI), but a good site from which individual countries and layers can be downloaded is that of the Pennsylvania State University Libraries (http://www.libraries.psu.edu/maps).

Inevitably, anyone wishing to go beyond simple mapping of disease cases requires other data sets, particularly a spatially referenced denominator, be it of farms or of animal populations. In many situations data may need to be collected for the specific study. Even when the data are available – for example, from a pre-existing national animal health information system or trade association, such as a milk recording scheme – they may need to be 'ground-truthed' to establish the extent of error. Three tools are important georeferencing resources to assist in these tasks:

1. A *global positioning system* (GPS), for direct on-site recording of location. Quality hand-held sets are now available for less than US$200, all with a spatial resolution of less than 20 metres. There are now a number of manufacturers who are market leaders in low-cost products, including Garmin (http://www.garmin.com) and Magellan (http://www.magellangps.com/en). These all have similar features such that the decision as to which brand or model to buy may best be decided upon after examining the available range of accessories.

2. A *georeferenced postal code database* to operate within an appropriate GIS. Many GIS software companies are developing these databases as extensions (e.g. ESRI's STREETMAP for the USA). However, before investing in a proprietary solution, it is worthwhile investigating whether there is alternative third-party geocoding software. For example, in the UK there is a package, MATCHCODE (http://www.capscan.co.uk), which enables batch-processing of large lists of postal codes and provides frequent updates, as part of the licence. This is ideal if geocoding is an ongoing need, but possibly inappropriate for a small, one-off project. A pragmatic alternative is to use online location finders that give latitude and longitude (e.g. in the UK, http://www.streetmap.co.uk). However, some sites restrict the number of permissible queries per day, and not all (e.g. http://www.mapquest.com in the USA) offer or are able to provide latitude and longitude as output.

3. An alternative where postal code data are lacking or unreliable is the use of an *electronic gazetteer*, which provides listings of latitudes and

Table 11.1. Some guidelines on the main agro-ecological spatial data sets required for studies relating animal disease to environmental covariates. This table is mainly based on the experience in Great Britain and the recommendations, particularly as regards spatial resolution, may not necessarily apply for less densely settled countries. In addition, this list largely excludes remotely sensed data sets, which may act as effective surrogates for some of the variables, particularly climatic ones (Hay and Lennon, 1999). From Durr *et al.* (2000); reproduced by permission of the Society for Veterinary Epidemiology and Preventive Medicine.

Variable group	Minimum variables	Other variables	Spatial resolution	Temporal resolution	Cost and availability
(a) Ecological variables					
Physical geography	Rivers Altitude	Streams Slope Aspect	1:10,000–1:50,000 (vector data)	Dependent upon rate of landscape change. Updates generally necessary every 5–10 years	Good, except for altitude, which requires a digital terrain model and is relatively expensive
Climate	Temperature Rainfall	Relative humidity Evapotranspiration Solar radiation Wind speed and direction	10–100 km^2	Long-term (30-year) averages vs. annual summaries, depending on requirement	Good availability at coarse resolution; generally poorer availability at fine resolution
Geology and soils	Rock stratum Soil classification Soil geochemistry	Soil texture Soil pH Available water capacity	Due to considerable spatial heterogeneity, 1 km^2 is preferable	For some elements with significant industrial pollution (e.g. S), may need updates every 10 years	Generally good for geology and soil as most countries have specific mapping agencies; however, resolution is often coarser than optimum. Generally poor for geochemistry
Vegetation	Land cover	Vegetation classes	If vegetation maps remotely sensed, may be as high as 25 m^2	At a minimum, mapping needs to be updated every 10 years	Currently few countries have complete vegetation maps at high resolution, but these will become increasingly available

Wildlife populations	Distribution (presence/absence) of disease vectors or reservoir hosts	Abundance (density) estimates	Dependent upon wildlife. 10–25 km^2 reasonable for larger mammals	At a minimum, estimates should be available for 10-year periods	Generally poor, unless specific surveys have been undertaken
(b) Agricultural variables					
Human geography	Roads Cities and towns Administrative boundaries	Country lanes Livestock markets Slaughterhouses Import and export ports	1:10,000–1:50,000 (vector data)	Depends on rate of landscape change. Updates every 5–10 years generally necessary	In GB the relevant administrative boundary is the civil parish
Farm details	Farm location Farm area	Farm boundaries	For farms of size 100 ha, maps needed at 1:10,000 scale	Depends on rate of landscape change. Updates every 5–10 years generally necessary	Farm boundary information not available in GB
Pastures	Grassland area	Area of leys, permanent pasture, etc. Species	If vegetation maps remotely sensed, may be as high as 25 m^2	At a minimum, mapping needs to be updated every 10 years	May be available through census collection, but variable quality and may be restrictions on disclosure
Livestock	Stock numbers Predominant breed	Stratification of livestock by breed Management (housing, culling, etc.)	Depends on enterprise and confidentiality requirements	Many countries with agricultural support policies have annual census	May be available through census collection, but variable quality and may be restrictions on disclosure

longitudes of cities, towns and sometimes even villages. There are a large number of country-specific products available, e.g. Bartholomew's Great Britain Place Name Gazetteer (http://www.bartholomewmaps.com) and in Germany the Bundesamt für Kartographie und Geodäsie (http://www.geodatenzentrum.de) GN250 digital gazetteer. The GEOnet Names Server (GNS) of the National Imagery and Mapping Agency (http://www.nima.mil/gns/html) is a worldwide database of geographical feature names. The GNS contains approximately 3.84 million features with 5.28 million names in the WGS84 coordinate system. Two other products which provide worldwide coverage are by Europa Technologies (http://www.europa-tech.com) and ADCi (http://www.adci.com). These are similar datasets that currently provide locational and boundary data for approximately 500,000 locations worldwide.

As spatial epidemiology is so much about relating disease to its environment, many users will need to obtain covariate data sets, particularly for climate, vegetation and soils (Table 11.1). This frequently is the most difficult data to obtain, as these will rarely be obtainable at both low cost and appropriate spatial resolution (Durr *et al.*, 2000). In addition, all these data sets (except the underlying geology) have a temporal aspect, most obviously for climate and vegetation, but even soil values change with time. For example, as a result of acid rain, topsoil sulphur levels may be raised over a wide area within a time frame of a few decades. Thus the metadata recording details, such as by whom, when and how the data were collected, are of critical importance, and without it such data sets are of dubious value. A further problem associated with data sets without accompanying metadata is an unknown projection and coordinate system, although websites for identifying projections (http://www.geocities.com/capecanaveral/1224/prj/prj.html) and coordinate systems (http://www.geocities.com/capecanaveral/1224/mapref.html) may help overcome this. The absence of metadata is particularly a problem with data sets that are available freely to download from the web, and sometimes the difference between such a download and the purchase of the data offline on a CD (for several hundred dollars) is that the CD comes with a booklet of metadata.

There are a number of websites that act as referencing points for environmental data. A good starting point for global data sets is the GEO Data Portal collated by the United Nations' various programmes, e.g. UNEP (http://geodata.grid.unep.ch). Similarly, the FAO has collated a large number of data sets during their many projects, particularly in developing countries. Finding these can be difficult, as each project tends to have its own website, but a recent initiative to collate them into a central 'GeoNetwork' indexing site (http://www.fao.org/geonetwork) is a promising development. A downloadable global land cover data set derived from AVHRR (Advanced Very High Resolution Radiometer) imagery is available at 1-km resolution (http://edcdaac.usgs.gov), but is now largely out of date, having been compiled in 1992. Key sites for finding the large number of climate data sets available include the World Meteorological Organization (http://www.wmo.ch), which includes links to a catalogue of data sets held by national meteorological agencies. Also, the Intergovernmental Panel on Climate Change (IPCC) (http://ipcc-ddc.cru.uea.ac.uk) data distribution centre provides a consistent set of up-to-date scenarios of changes in climate and related environmental and socioeconomic factors for use in climate impact assessments.

At a national and subnational level, one can find a number of websites with a more regional and national focus, often maintained by national mapping agencies. For example, a good portal for environmental data in Australia is the Environmental Resources Information Network (http://www.ea.gov.au/erin) and in the USA there is the EROS Data Center (http://edc.usgs.gov). This is an instance where spending a couple of hours on the web will generally show whether a data set of interest is available.

Satellite imagery is readily available over the web, though that from the USA is made somewhat confusing by a number of websites supplying imagery from different programmes. Key sites for obtaining AVHRR data (the predominant imagery used in epidemiology to date) are the Goddard Space Flight Center's Distributed Active Archive Center (http://daac.gsfc.nasa.gov) for the Pathfinder AVHRR 64-km^2 resolution image set; the Land Processes Distributed Active Archive Center (http://edcdaac.usgs.gov) for the Global Land 1-km AVHRR Project; and NOAA's Satellite Active Archive (http://www.saa.noaa.gov) for downloads of current imagery. MODIS (Moderate Resolution Imaging Spectroradiometer) imagery is likely to be of increasing importance in epidemiological studies because of its reasonably high spatial resolution, and selected data sets are now starting to become available (http://modis.gsfc.nasa.gov).

11.4 Statistical analysis of spatial data

When commercial GIS software became readily available 10–15 years ago, a frequent complaint was of the lack of accompanying statistical routines in spatial analytical software (Anselin and Getis, 1992). Although the situation has improved somewhat, the major GIS packages still do not provide for the types of statistical spatial analysis shown within the present book. A note of caution is needed here, as 'spatial analysis' has come to have a somewhat different meaning in the GIS literature than might be expected. For example, ESRI sells a Spatial Analyst extension, but this is simply a set of routines mainly for grid-based data manipulation. However, the Geostatistical Analyst extension provides tools for inverse distance weighting and spline interpolation as well as semivariogram modelling and kriging (ordinary, simple, universal, probability, indicator and disjunctive), including cokriging and cross-validation. As mentioned above, IDRISI32 has a number of interesting statistical routines, but these are confined to grid-based data, with no functions to analyse points, lines or polygon data.

An acceptable alternative may be to treat the GIS simply as a means to store, manipulate and map spatial data, which is then exported (or coupled) to a standard statistical package. This appeared to be the chosen route when S-Plus (http://www.insightful.com) introduced the S+ Spatial Stats module in 1996; this contains routines for spatial regression, kriging and tests for the spatial randomness of point patterns. This module is still available but, except for the introduction of dialogue boxes to lead users through each procedure, has not been developed further. GENSTAT for Windows 6ed (http://www.nag.co.uk) also contains some basic geostatistical routines, but as for S + Spatial Stats, there does not appear to be active development under way. Of the other main statistical packages, SAS offers variogram and kriging procedures, while SPSS, Minitab and Statistica, do not currently offer any spatial statistical functions. This is somewhat surprising in view of the volume of potential users from disciplines such as geography, geology, ecology and economics.

As a result of the lack of support from the commercial statistical software industry, spatial statistical software retains a somewhat cottage industry approach, with a number of stand-alone packages and freeware extensions available. Some important ones that have been used in epidemiology include:

- STAT! This was one of the first commercialized products (released 1994), offering a range of tests for space and space–time clustering, such as Cuzick and Edwards' test and Knox's method. This package has now been replaced by CLUSTERSEER (http://www.biomedware.com), which has a Windows front end and enhanced functionality and display.
- A freeware alternative, developed to analyse crime incident location data but applicable to other point pattern analysis, is CRIMESTAT 2.0 (http://www.icpsr.umich.edu/NACJD/crimestat.html). Although chiefly for hotspot detection, it has some good additional functions, such as adaptive kernel density estimation.
- Another freeware package for analysing point pattern data is SATSCAN 3.0 (http://srab.cancer.gov/satscan), developed by Martin Kulldorf while at the National Cancer Institute (Kulldorff, 1997). This uses a circular window which moves systematically over all the centroids in an area, and enables clusters to be ranked with an indication of whether they are 'significant'.

- SPLANCS (http://www.maths.lancs.ac.uk/~rowlings/Splancs) is a set of library routines developed by Peter Diggle and Barry Rowlingson at the University of Lancaster for advanced spatial point pattern analysis, such as space–time *K*-functions (Rowlingson and Diggle, 1993). Although it is downloadable freeware, it requires S-Plus or its freeware alternative 'R' (http://www.r-project.org) to run.
- SPACESTAT differs from the above software in being designed mainly for the analysis of area data. Developed by an econometrician, Luc Anselin, it also allows local analysis through a set of specific statistics, the G_i and G_i^* statistics (Anselin, 1995). Although essentially a stand-alone DOS package, it now has an interface with ARCVIEW to allow visualization of output. SPACESTAT is a commercial product and is currently available from Biomedware (http://www.biomedware.com).
- GEOBUGS 1.1 (http://www.mrc-bsu.cam.ac.uk/bugs) is an add-on module to WINBUGS, a package used for Bayesian analyses of complex statistical models using Markov chain Monte Carlo (MCMC) methods. GEOBUGS provides an interface that creates the matrices needed for spatial smoothing and in addition can produce maps from other packages, including S-Plus. GEOBUGS and WINBUGS are both freeware.

A more complete listing and description of spatial statistical software can be found at http://www.ai-geostats.org/software as well as GisVet Web (see Section 11.5).

All of the listed packages, except SPLANCS, operate through menus and are relatively easy to master, although each tends to have individual quirks and limitations. For example, SATSCAN does not have any edge correction for its cluster detection routines, and although CRIMESTAT can allow for edges in its kernel density function, this is restricted to a square bounding box. Because of these limitations, for anyone wishing to undertake serious spatial statistical analysis or to develop their own routines, the preferred package remains either S-Plus or R. However, these require users to master a difficult command-line language, and although much of the code is freely available through Statlib (http://lib.stat.cmu.edu/S), an advanced understanding of statistical principles is necessary in order to avoid errors in procedures or interpretation.

11.5 GisVet Web

The above comments on software and data were written in April 2003 and checked for accuracy through searches on the Web several weeks later. However, the information will date rapidly (for example, IDRISI shortly after released a replacement for IDRISI32 (Idrisi Kilimanjaro)), and it is likely that by the time this book is being read other information will be inaccurate, particularly the web addresses. This simply reflects the current state of the GIS industry, in which change and innovation are dominating characteristics. Accordingly, a number of resources have arisen to keep the GIS community in touch and up to date, including regular magazines and newsletters, such as *GeoWorld* (http://www.geoplace.com) and *GeoSpatial Solutions* (http://www.geospatial-online.com). In addition, there are several excellent portals/directories, such as GeoCommunity (http://www.geocom.com) and GISmonitor (http://www.gismonitor.com), that point to a wealth of online resources, such as data providers and software reviews. The problem then becomes not one of insufficient information but of too much, and keeping up to date with developments can become an end in itself, to the inevitable detriment of research or teaching activities.

For the first GisVet conference held at Lancaster University in September 2001, we set up a website to inform delegates about the conference and permit online booking. Arising out of interest expressed by delegates at the conference, we developed this site as an information source, with a number of pages providing links to software, data, upcoming training courses and so on. This was an ambitious undertaking, as the GisVet community (*senso stricto*) is very small. We did, however, hope that the site would be of interest to a much wider community of users interested in biomedical applications of GIS and spatial analysis, who essentially have the same resource and information requirements. However, this raised the problem that the site would only be of much use if it was kept up to date, which might entail an enormous drain on our resources.

To overcome this, we have reformulated the site and renamed it GisVet Web (http://www.gisvet.org) to reflect a more international outlook, as well as a fundamental change in the technology behind it (Fig. 11.1). The concept is that instead of static HTML pages, which need to be rewritten and uploaded to the web server every time there are changes in the information content, the site uses active HTML pages, which are rebuilt afresh from a database each time the page is downloaded. Consequently, we only need to make a change in the database and not rewrite the page, for example, to add a new reference or update a link. Better still, this also means that we can potentially provide an upload facility for anyone visiting the site to similarly make changes, although such changes need to be first approved by a site editor before the database is updated. This effectively means that the users of the site become responsible for its content, and ideally it will become self-maintaining. Whether this happens remains to be seen, but in committing ourselves to this project we are simply stating our confidence that GIS and spatial analysis have an assured future in animal health and disease investigation and control.

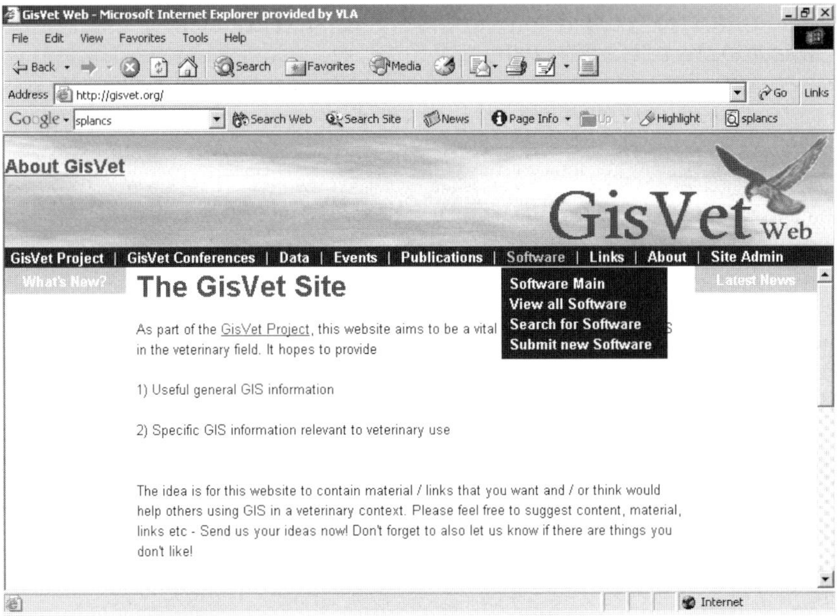

Fig. 11.1. Screen shot of the home page of GisVet Web (www.gisvet.org).

Acknowledgements

Thanks to Alice Froggatt, who initially developed GisVet Web, and Vincent Adcock and Stuart Eastland, who undertook the major rewrite to enable its current interactivity. Thanks also to Megan Powers and Dirk Pfeiffer for their helpful comments on earlier drafts of this chapter.

References

Anselin, L. (1995) Local indicators of spatial association – LISA. *Geographical Analysis* 27, 93–115.

Anselin, L. and Getis, A. (1992) Spatial statistical analysis and geographical information systems. *Annals of Regional Science* 26, 19–33.

Durr, P.A., Argyraki, A., Ramsey, M. and Clifton-Hadley, R.S. (2000) Agro-ecological databases for spatial correlation studies: methodological issues. In: Thrusfield, M.V. and Goodall, E.A. (eds) *Proceedings of the Society for Veterinary Epidemiology and Preventive Medicine, University of Edinburgh, 29th–31st March, 2000*, pp. 225–235.

Hay, S.I. and Lennon, J.J. (1999) Deriving meteorological variables across Africa for the study and control of vector-borne disease: a comparison of remote sensing and spatial interpolation of climate. *Tropical Medicine and International Health* 4, 58–71.

Kulldorff, M. (1997) A spatial scan statistic. *Communications in Statistics: Theory and Methods* 26, 1481–1496.

Rowlingson, B.S. and Diggle, P.J. (1993) SPLANCS: spatial point pattern analysis code in S-Plus. *Computers and Geosciences* 19, 627–655.

Index